AF667262

BDJ Clinician's Guides

This series enables clinicians at all stages of their careers to remain well informed and up to date on key topics across all fields of clinical dentistry. Each volume is superbly illustrated and provides concise, highly practical guidance and solutions. The authors are recognised experts in the subjects that they address. The *BDJ Clinician's Guides* are trusted companions, designed to meet the needs of a wide readership. Like the *British Dental Journal* itself, they offer support for undergraduates and newly qualified, while serving as refreshers for more experienced clinicians. In addition they are valued as excellent learning aids for postgraduate students.

The BDJ Clinicians' Guides are produced in collaboration with the British Dental Association, the UK's trade union and professional association for dentists.

Ewen McColl • Aws Alani
Editors

Practical Tips in Clinical Dentistry

Achieving Optimal Outcomes

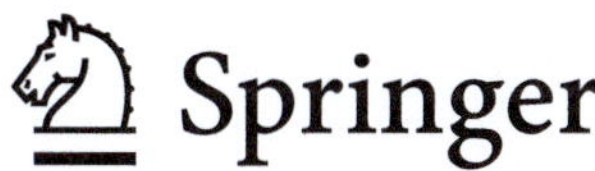

Editors
Ewen McColl
Peninsula Dental School
Plymouth, UK

Aws Alani
Peninsula Dental School
Plymouth, UK

ISSN 2523-3327 ISSN 2523-3335 (electronic)
BDJ Clinician's Guides
ISBN 978-3-031-90354-0 ISBN 978-3-031-90355-7 (eBook)
https://doi.org/10.1007/978-3-031-90355-7

This Springer imprint is published by the registered company Springer Nature Switzerland AG
The registered company address is: Gewerbestrasse 11, 6330 Cham, Switzerland

Foreword

What are the things you wish someone had told you in dental school, but never did? *Practical Tips in Clinical Dentistry* is a treasure chest of authoritative insights and advise—nuggets of experience-tempered information to complement your education and training, enhance your clinical practice and enable you to better meet the needs and expectations of your patients in primary care.

Practical Tips in Clinical Dentistry is based on a series of short, accessible articles published in the *British Dental Journal*—a brainchild of the journal's readership panel. The first 'top tips' article was published in November 2021. The series now runs to some 60 articles, authored by approximately 80 accomplished practitioners, academics and other experts. The topics covered range from top tips in, for example, improving crown preparations, the immediate management of dental trauma and complete denture prosthetics to top tips in incorporating research, utilising dental therapists, leading a team and optimising clinical governance in primary care. Certain themes emerge from reading the series, including get to know and understand your patients, establish a diagnosis before embarking on treatment, in the event of untoward events, don't panic, keep calm and follow established protocols, work as a team, and, for materials and devices, if all else fails, read the instructions. Such guidance may seem to be blindingly obvious to some, but it is always worth reinforcing, as it can be forgotten or inadvertently overlooked in the 'cut and thrust' of 'frontline' clinical practice.

Delving into the top tips articles, there are countless 'gems', many of which I wish someone had shared with me during my time in clinical practice. No one knows all there is to know about dentistry; there are always new things to be learned and applied in the care of patients. Even to this day, 51+ years after graduating, it is a sad day if I don't learn something new about dentistry. *Practical Tips in Clinical Dentistry* highlights the need, as frequently stated in the top tips articles, to read journals and contemporary textbooks presenting state-of-the-art information; too often colleagues limit their continuing professional development to joining webinars and attending the occasional lecture, which, good as they may be, are at best an overview, rather than an in-depth, detailed, referenced consideration of a topic. Huge time and effort go into preparing and producing high-quality, peer-reviewed articles and books, which it is hoped *Practical Tips in Clinical Dentistry* will encourage readers to access and read—no greater privilege than to be a student for life (*sic.* GV Black) when it comes to be a committed oral healthcare professional.

In the meantime, I congratulate the *British Dental Journal* for running the top tips series, all of the authors who have collectively produced a unique source of invaluable guidance and advice, specifically Professor Ewen McColl, who in addition to having authored, or at least co-authored many of the articles, has been the driving force behind the initiative and the team which published the articles and this book—a great team effort to be applauded.

Now time for you to use *Practical Tips in Clinical Dentistry* for its intended purpose. If you do, you will be able to say, I was told many things at dental school, but I have subsequently come to know them, thanks to the timely top tips series, and have become a better practitioner in the process. Your team and your patients will be grateful that you have read and applied all that this book offers.

President Emeritus College of General Dentistry Prof. Sir Nairn Wilson
Emeritus Professor of Dentistry
2025

Preface

The precursor to this compendium textbook stemmed from a long running series in the *British Dental Journal*. The series was originally commissioned by the *British Dental Journal* readers panel, who recognised the need for bite-sized practical tips for the busy practitioner. The series became very popular and has remained over the years one of the most accessed group of articles in the journal, which highlights the value and relevance the readership placed in this work.

The idea grew to include a very wide range of authors who the editors had worked with over many years and at times had learned from their clinical expertise. As both editors of *Practical Tips* have a very broad clinical background, we wanted readers to be able to pick up gems of knowledge and micro-solutions gained through years of experience. Often these micro-solutions had taken years of practising dentistry to gain, and the hope was to provide a shortcut for busy clinicians. In imparting this knowledge in written form, the aspiration was that this would directly impact on patient care whilst supporting colleagues to deliver treatment efficiently and effectively. Given the volume of online accesses, the series became a readily available resource in a wide range of dental disciplines. The textbook takes these articles in a structured, logical manner so that the dental team can learn from and adapt to their individual circumstances to further develop as clinicians. All contributors are experts in their field and have contributed in the spirit of advancing knowledge and improving patient care.

The textbook is organised in subject-related sections, each containing chapters that cover various key topics. The chapters themselves outline key learning points before detailing contemporary approaches to every day clinical challenges. We thank all the authors for sharing so generously their expertise and hope this textbook will be a ready resource for busy clinicians across the dental team.

> Pure logical thinking cannot yield us any knowledge of the empirical world; all knowledge of reality starts from experience and ends in it
>
> —Albert Einstein

Plymouth, UK — Ewen McColl
Plymouth, UK — Aws Alani

Contents

Part I

Restorative Dentistry

1 Practical Tips on Occlusion

Andrew Harris, Christopher Tredwin, and Ewen McColl

Learning Points

- Understand the key role that occlusal analysis plays in the provision of all aspects of restorative dentistry.
- Recognise the various ways in which the occlusion can be examined.
- Recall the various ways in which the occlusion can be recorded through the utilisation of equipment such as facebows and articulators.
- Appreciate aspects of denture construction that require an appreciation of the occlusion.
- Understand the interrelationship between occlusion and the periodontal apparatus.

1.1 Introduction

On a daily basis, primary care clinicians may impact on occlusion whether placing a single restoration or more complex multiples in fixed prosthodontics. Whilst it is crucial to consider the dynamic nature of occlusion, this area is often overlooked. Neglecting to analyse the occlusion and the effect our interventions may have on it can significantly affect successful outcomes and accelerate failure if not managed carefully.

A. Harris
Peninsula Dental School (University of Plymouth), Derriford Dental Education Facility, Plymouth Science Park, Plymouth, UK

C. Tredwin
Institute of Dentistry, Queen Mary, University of London, The Royal London Dental Hospital, London, UK

E. McColl (✉)
Peninsula Dental School, Plymouth, UK
e-mail: ewen.mccoll@plymouth.ac.uk

E. McColl, A. Alani (eds.), *Practical Tips in Clinical Dentistry*, BDJ Clinician's Guides, https://doi.org/10.1007/978-3-031-90355-7_1

In this short paper, we discuss practical tips for occlusion, highlighting that occlusion should be at the forefront of our thinking in order to improve patient outcomes.

1.2 Simple Occlusal Analysis

Terminology alone can be confusing in occlusion with a plethora of different terminologies for the same positional/occlusal concepts.

You need to think separately about those with teeth and without teeth. For the dentate, there are three key occlusal positions that are relevant to the clinician:

(a) The intercuspal position (ICP)—also known as maximal intercuspation position (MIP): this is the complete intercuspation of the opposing teeth independent of condylar position, sometimes referred to as the best fit of the teeth regardless of the condylar position [1].This is the most closed the mandible can be.
(b) Retruded axis position (RAP)—also known as centric relation (CR): This is a non-tooth determined position and dictated by anatomical structures (hard and soft tissues/muscles/ligaments). It is when the condyles articulate in the anterior-superior position against the posterior slopes of the articular eminences [1].
(c) Retruded contact position (RCP)—This is the first tooth contact on closure of the mandible when in RAP and may or may not be coincident with ICP. The presence of an RCP–ICP discrepancy has to be considered the norm for the majority of the population, with between 56 and 100% of patients in multiple studies reporting a discrepancy between the two [2–5].

There is a great capacity for adaptation and compensation, and as long as you remain within aesthetic parameters, freeway space is not a pivotal consideration in the dentate.

Most of the time in general practice, you will accept the current occlusal scheme and conform to it (conformative approach). If this is not possible, e.g. a severe tooth surface loss case where there is lack of occlusal space, then you will need to reorganise the occlusion at an increased vertical dimension (OVD) (Reorganised approach). When reorganising, there is only one reference point that can be used to restore from, and that is RAP.

1.3 Occlusion and Restorations

If conforming, a simple tip is to check that the occlusal contacts (ICP) on other teeth are the same before and after the restoration is placed.

It is important that any restoration has contact in the intercuspal position, as teeth may move if not in contact [6, 7]. Shearing forces are damaging for posterior restorations, and in order to prevent fracture, dynamic tooth guided movement should not involve posterior restorations where possible, i.e. the occlusion discludes off the restoration in any excursions.

It is important to identify where the slide from RCP to ICP is located prior to restoration. If the tooth to be restored is involved in producing that slide, you may unknowingly alter the slide between RCP and ICP. This unplanned occlusal adjustment may result in the created space for the restoration being lost.

If the slide from RCP to ICP involves your planned restoration, then articulated study casts should be made before tooth preparation and mounted in RAP. A planned occlusal adjustment can then be made on the casts prior to being duplicated in the mouth and the slide removed from the tooth.

1.4 Facebows (Earbows)

The most commonly used facebows are average value ones, and if occlusal analysis/changes are planned, a facebow needs to be utilised in order to accurately set the models up on a semi-adjustable articulator. These approximate the position of the hinge axis (axis of opening of the mandible) of the condyle to the maxilla.

Additional patient information is obtained through a horizontal reference plane and allows an aesthetic perspective (often by paralleling to the interpupillary line) to be transferred to the articulator and then to the laboratory. Due to the aesthetic utility offered by a facebow, it is wise to make use of one if performing multiple anterior restorations.

1.5 Articulators

If conforming to ICP, an articulator may not be required (as in most cases in primary care), and often hand-holding the casts or a simple plain line articulator will suffice. As cases get more complex and multiple units are involved, then using an articulator may be more helpful.

If changes are required in the occlusal scheme, then a semi-adjustable articulator should be used and the casts mounted on the articulator in RAP. An example of this is the management of a patient with severe tooth surface loss, whereby you intend on increasing their vertical dimension.

The main parameter that determines how much to increase the OVD by will be the aesthetics of the upper anterior teeth. As a rule of thumb, the upper incisors and canines should follow the contour of the lower lip line during smiling.

A diagnostic wax up can then be transferred from the models to the mouth utilising putty or a suck down splint, containing an acrylic based temporary crown material. The proposed occlusal scheme and aesthetics can then be assessed prior to definitive restoration preparation.

1.6 Occlusion and Dentures

For partially dentate patients, if there are sufficient tooth-to-tooth contacts to ensure a stable ICP, adequate inter-arch space for the denture, and few aesthetic concerns, generally, they conform.

For partial dentures, the occlusal plane and prosthetic tooth forms are usually dictated by the patient's established occlusal pattern in order to function harmoniously. Whilst the abutment teeth on either side of a saddle can impart a degree of denture stability, partial denture teeth should not interfere with natural tooth contact in ICP or be involved in lateral excursions. Where possible, denture tooth contact should be limited to bilateral and simultaneous contact of prosthetic teeth in ICP (Fig. 1.1).

Historically, the adopted occlusal scheme for complete dentures has been based around the concept of providing a balanced bilateral occlusion (BBO)/articulation; denture stability is provided by simultaneous posterior occlusal contact of prosthetic teeth in ICP and eccentric positions. The conceptual importance of BBO has been challenged recently; BBO is difficult to technically achieve, and a systematic review indicated little difference in masticatory performance or quality of life/satisfaction between BBO and other occlusal schemes [8].

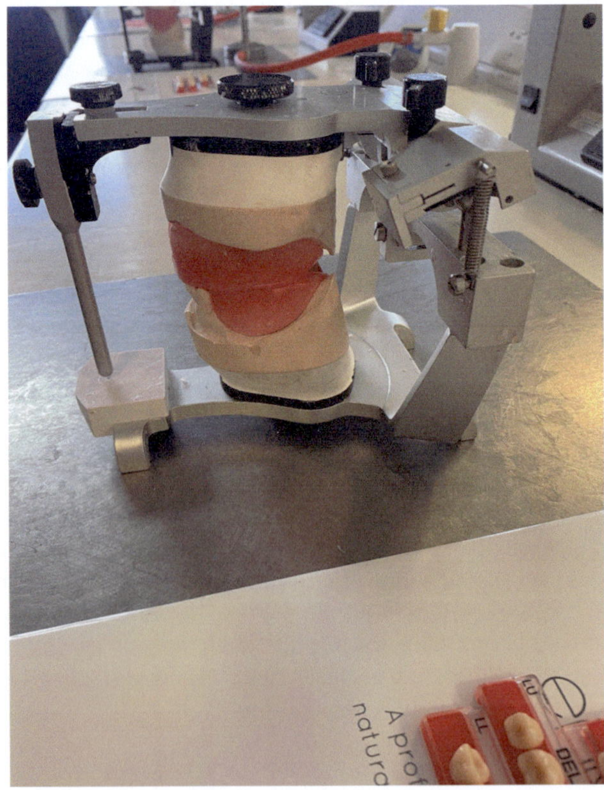

Fig. 1.1 Occlusal considerations in denture construction

More importantly, setting the occlusion in RAP is pivotal to the success of complete dentures. With the loss of periodontal mechanoreceptors and subsequent depletion of tactile sensory input to the central nervous system [9], RAP is the only reproducible reference position that patients possess. Freeway space also becomes important as the ability for adaptation and compensation as with teeth is lost. When a patient closes in RAP, the mandible should rotate into ICP, and patients can simply reseat prostheses loosened by function by closing gently together. If not coincident, patients have to guess where their ICP is located, upper and lower teeth clash and move, border seals break, and dentures loosen. If you are having difficulties obtaining an accurate RAP record, remove the patient's existing lower denture or place a cotton wool roll between the dentures to allow some deprogramming to occur [10].

Even for those complete dentures set up correctly in RAP, instability can result from prosthetic tooth position. Avoid setting molar teeth posteriorly on the upward sweep of the mandible because dislodging forces can be created in function. It is quite acceptable for the occlusal scheme to finish at the first molars. For those with poor neuromuscular control, there should be some freedom of movement in ICP to avoid occlusal locking and subsequent movement—consider occlusal adjustment or utilising cuspless teeth [11].

1.7 Occlusion and Periodontology

Studies by Ericson and Lindhe [12]suggested that, in the presence of uncontrolled periodontitis, greater attachment loss could occur in the presence of occlusal trauma. This suggested that occlusal trauma may exacerbate periodontitis. However, this effect has only been shown in some animal studies, and the evidence for this so-called co-destructive effect is weak. Such effects have not been shown in human studies, and there is a lack of evidence from such human studies to implicate occlusal trauma in the progression of attachment loss in periodontitis.

Whereas some clinicians advocate occlusal intervention to reduce occlusal trauma in periodontitis patients, a relatively recent Cochrane systematic review showed that there was insufficient evidence to justify such treatment in periodontitis cases [13]. The World Workshop on the Classification of Periodontal and Peri-implant Diseases and Conditions (2018) [14] has stated that there is no evidence that traumatic occlusal forces cause periodontal attachment loss in humans.

1.8 Conclusion

Understanding occlusion and the effect our clinical interventions have on occlusion is an essential element of daily clinical practice affecting all disciplines in dentistry. In this chapter, we have presented tips and observations that we have found to help in managing occlusion to avoid occlusal disharmony and the complications this may bring. We hope these tips will be useful in allowing clinicians to think about occlusion and dispel some of the confusion that often exists around discussions in this area.

References

1. The Glossary of Prosthodontic Terms: Ninth Edition. J Prosthet Dent 2017; doi: https://doi.org/10.1016/j.prosdent.2016.12.001.
2. Kattadiyil MT, Alzaid AA, Campbell SD. The relationship between centric occlusion and the maximal intercuspal position and their use as treatment positions for complete mouth rehabilitation: best evidence consensus statement. J Prosthodont. 2021;30:26–33.
3. Posselt U. Studies in the mobility of the human mandible. Copenhagen: Acta Odontologica Scandinavica; 1952.
4. Hodge LC Jr, Mahan PE. A study of mandibular movement from centric occlusion to maximum intercuspation. J Prosthet Dent. 1967;18:19–30.
5. Rieder CE. The prevalence and magnitude of mandibular displacement in a survey population. J Prosthet Dent. 1978;39:324–9.
6. Love W, Adams R. Tooth movement into edentulous areas. J Prosthet Dent. 1971;25:271–8.
7. Craddock HL, Youngson CC. A study of the incidence of overeruption and occlusal interferences in unopposed posterior teeth. Br Dent J. 2004;196:341–248.
8. Lemos CAA, Verri FR, Gomes JML, Santiago Júnior JF, Moraes SLD, Pellizzer EP. Bilateral balanced occlusion compared to other occlusal schemes in complete dentures: a systematic review. J Oral Rehabil. 2018;45:344–54.
9. Klineberg I, Murray G. Osseoperception: sensory function and proprioception. Adv Dent Res. 1999;13:120–9.
10. Blakely L, Beare WAV, Harris A, McColl E. Top tips for complete denture prosthetics in primary care. Br Dent J. 2022;232:498–500.
11. McCord JF, Grant AA. Identification of complete denture problems: a summary. Br Dent J. 2000;189:128–34.
12. Lindhe J, Ericsson I. The effect of elimination of jiggling forces on periodontally exposed teeth in the dog. J Periodontol. 1982;53:562–7.
13. Weston P, Yaziz YA, Moles DR, Needleman I. Occlusal interventions for periodontitis in adults. Cochrane Database Syst Rev. 2008;3:CD004968.
14. Caton JG, Armitage G, Berglundh T, et al. A new classification scheme for periodontal and peri-implant diseases and conditions—introduction and key changes from the 1999 classification. J Clin Periodontol. 2018 https://doi.org/10.1111/jcpe.12935.

The Application of Restorative Dentistry Materials

2

Steve Bonsor and Ewen McColl

Learning Points

- Appreciate the need to understand how materials work to best apply them to clinical situations.
- Recognise that reading the product instructions is a valuable starting point in applying dental materials optimally.
- Understand that some materials are best applied for one role, whereas others may be applicable to various clinical indications.

2.1 Introduction

Keeping abreast of advances in dental materials is a challenge for even the most enthusiastic of clinicians. However, product development offers the dental team the opportunity to optimise their clinical skills and, hence, outcomes for patients in primary dental care. The present paper discusses some fundamental and some specific points with the intention of helping busy practitioners to make the best use of dental materials in practice, although all the tips offered may be extended to the practice of restorative dentistry in general.

S. Bonsor
GDP, The Dental Practice, Aberdeen, UK

University of Edinburgh, Edinburgh, UK

E. McColl (✉)
Peninsula Dental School, Plymouth, UK
e-mail: ewen.mccoll@plymouth.ac.uk

E. McColl, A. Alani (eds.), *Practical Tips in Clinical Dentistry*, BDJ Clinician's Guides, https://doi.org/10.1007/978-3-031-90355-7_2

2.2 Know How Beats Guess How

It has long been said that know-how surpasses guess-how, and it is of utmost importance in using dental materials in order to get the most out of these often-expensive materials. Clinical dentistry, in particular restorative dentistry, involves a series of problem-solving steps, each demanding an understanding by the clinician of the pathology and how this may be best managed by operative intervention. A critical factor in this treatment is the selection of the most appropriate dental material or materials for the situation. It therefore goes without saying that a thorough understanding of the properties, indications, contraindications, and handling of each dental material or biomaterial is critical to the optimum outcome for the treatment in question [1].

This knowledge and understanding may be gained by personal reading from textbooks or peer-reviewed literature, attendance at quality assured postgraduate lectures and courses, and by interaction with the materials companies themselves. Establishing, building, and continuing a professional relationship with representatives of reputable companies is a very useful way of learning about dental materials and keeping this knowledge contemporary. These colleagues possess a wealth of knowledge and, in many cases, experience, which may be invaluable to the busy practitioner. Furthermore, should the representative not be in a position to answer any specific enquiries, then technical support is readily available from their company.

It is critical and obvious that all members of the dental team are involved in this education and training. Almost universally, the operator will be assisted in surgery by a dental nurse whose responsibility it will be to handle, mix (if necessary), and present the dental material or biomaterial to the treating clinician. The knowledge, understanding, and skills of all members of the dental team must be current and of a high level in order to properly support the clinician in the treatment of the patient. Learning together as a team fosters excellent communication, trust, and teamworking skills, the importance of which can never be underestimated in the clinical environment.

2.3 Utilise the Product Instructions

Like the previous tip, reading the instructions or product directions for use (DFU) seems an obvious statement to ensure its appropriate and correct usage [1]. In the same way it is wise when assembling flat-packed furniture to read the instructions in its entirety before embarking on the construction of the product, the DFU should be consulted by all members of the dental team before clinical use (Fig. 2.1). Following these instructions fastidiously will yield consistent and predictable results every time. The DFU of each new batch of material should be studied as products may change with time due to evolution, which may necessitate different usage or handling demands. It is good practice to retain a copy of the most recent DFU in a file in an area of the clinic accessible to all staff members for reference. This file can be maintained by the team member responsible for stock control.

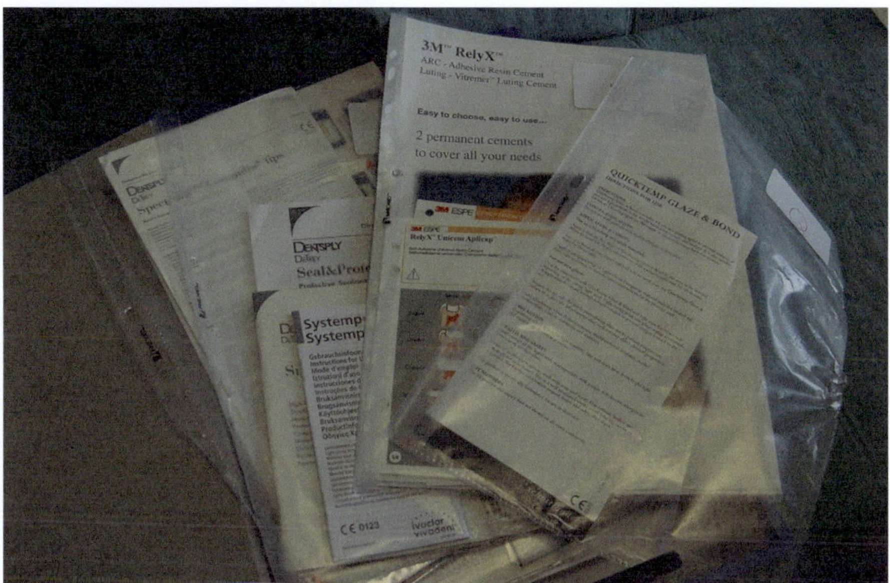

Fig. 2.1 The directions for use file (DFU file)

Contained in the DFU of the material, the manufacturer will impart information that will inform the reader of the indications and contraindications of the product. It is important to stress that all materials should be used only in accordance with these instructions and the operator should never be tempted to 'ski off-piste', so to speak, and use the product for an indication not explicitly stated in the DFU. This dangerous strategy will surely lead to failure and unfortunate medico-legal consequences should a complaint be pursued. Similarly, should there be any issues with treatment failure by the correct prescription and usage of the product, then the dental team will be supported by the manufacturer in whose commercial interests it is to find a solution to the problem. It is worth noting at this point that products such as bonding agents and resin composite materials, which have been designed to be used together, should be consistent in terms of their manufacturer, in other words from the same stable. Choosing products from different companies and attempting to use them together can lead to failure as they may be chemically incompatible. Furthermore, the manufacturer will not be in a position to offer assistance, as discussed earlier, should a problem arise.

Very often products, particularly those which demand a more involved clinical protocol such as requiring many procedural steps, for example, dental bonding, are supplied with step-by-step pictorial guides for use at the chairside (Fig. 2.2). There is nothing to be ashamed of by using these guides to ensure that the clinical protocol is followed exactly, and in fact, it could be argued that this good practice should be encouraged to yield best clinical outcomes. It is wise to explain to the patient why this is being done, and they will be reassured and grateful that the team is providing them with the best of care.

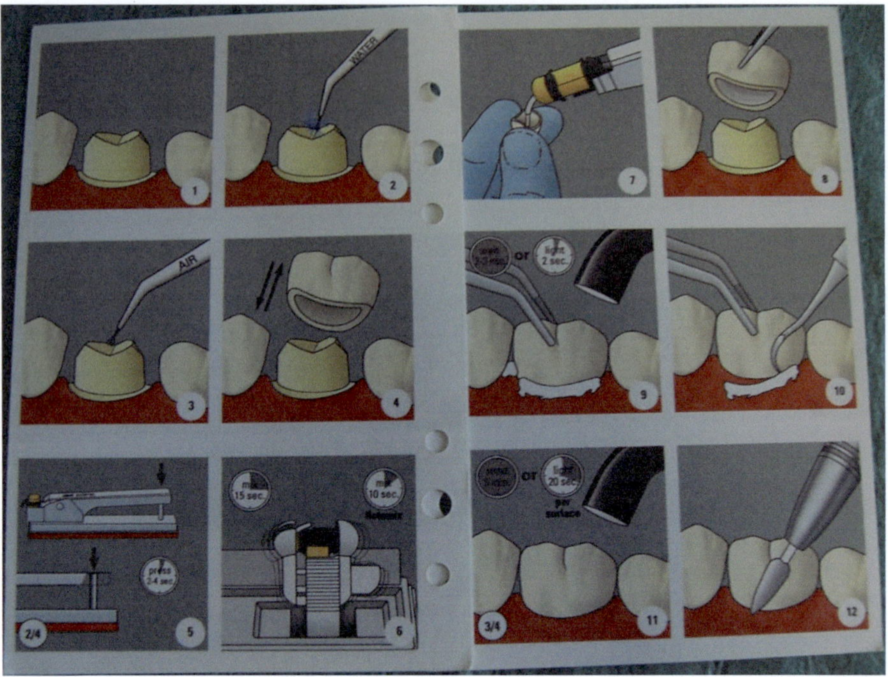

Fig. 2.2 Useful step-by-step pictorial guide

2.4 Spend to Save: Choose Bona Fide Materials From Reputable Companies

Dental material and biomaterial manufacturing companies invest huge sums of money in research and development to ensure the consistent and predictable performance of their products. This may not always be said for all materials that are available on the market, in particular 'own-label' products [2, 3]. The clinical performance of these latter materials may not be supported by any robust scientific evidence with behaviour even varying between batches [4–7]. Premature failure of inferior products will invariably lead to loss of reputational damage to the dentist [3] and their practice with an associated financial cost to remediate the treatment for the potentially unhappy patient. It is wise, therefore, to select products manufactured by reputable companies whose quality control and assurance procedures are of a high standard. Very often, these products may be more expensive, but with this investment comes a reassurance that the product being used to treat the patient is of the highest quality, with research data to support its use and clinical performance.

2.5 Using Materials to Their Full Extent

An example of a resin composite adhesive cementation system is Panavia V5 (Kuraray Noritake, Osaka, Japan), which is widely used for the cementation of resin-bonded bridges (RBB) [8] and, indeed, for other restorations that require bonding to dental hard tissue, such as lithium disilicate ceramics. Prior to its use clinically, it is essential to lay out the product and follow the instruction card, explaining to the patient that this is a highly technical cementation process. It can be useful for the dental nurse to read out the instructions as this acts as a valuable checklist with good communication being the key throughout. This particular material is often not used to its full utility, and it is important to remember five distinct shades, which are available, namely, white, brown, universal, clear, and opaque. In the aesthetic zone, although an opaque resin cement is frequently selected, it is advisable to utilise the try-in pastes, which are included in the kit, to assess the effect of metal 'shine-through' before final bonding. This stage is one that can pay dividends as the aesthetics of the definitive restoration can often be enhanced. Prior to cementation, the surface of the tooth should be prepared by ultrasonic scaling followed by the application of a pumice slurry on a bristle brush. If the tooth surface has previously supported an RBB retainer or has been restored with resin composite, then the surface should be particle air abraded with 50-μm alumina under rubber dam isolation before undertaking the bonding stages. In order to facilitate excess cement removal post-bonding, it is wise to place polytetrafluoroethylene (PTFE) tape interproximally between the abutment tooth and its adjacent.

2.6 Using Materials for Many Indications

Glass ionomer cements (GICs), or to use their proper chemical name the glass polyalkenoate cements, are a versatile group of materials. While physically weaker than resin composites, they can be utilised to provide aesthetic outcomes and have a wide range of uses. These include definitive restorations in class III and V restorations, temporary restorations including inter-appointment visits in endodontics, deep margin elevation, and definitive restorations in paediatric dentistry. They are also available to lute cast restorations such as crowns although the powder to liquid ratio differs from those restorative products listed above.

GICs chemically attach to dental hard tissue via calcium chelation and subsidiary collagen bonding, which makes them particularly useful in the management of class V cavities associated with non-carious tooth surface loss, especially where such lesions are associated with symptoms of dentine (hyper) sensitivity. For many class V cavities, visibility and access to the gingival margin can be assisted by using a retraction cord, which, in addition, controls gingival crevicular fluid ingress into the treatment area, which may compromise moisture control. As with most branches of restorative dentistry, the use of magnification when working clinically is strongly recommended [9, 10].

In endodontics and in the restorative stabilisation phase, Fuji Triage (GC, Leuven. Belgium) is a useful material as the orange colouring allows for ease of removal without risk of concomitant excessive tooth substance while maintaining coronal seal. The concept of colouring materials is not a new one and was used by American military dentists in the Vietnam war where IRM (Dentsply, Konstanz, Germany) was coloured with a dye which indicated whether the tooth required restorative treatment (blue) or endodontics or extraction in which case the cement was coloured red [11].

Further development of glass ionomer cements in recent years has led to the appearance of products such as Equia Forte HT (GC) whose indications include the restoration of class I and II cavities and to build-up cores. This has been made possible by incorporating filler particles of different sizes, a so-called hybrid arrangement, in addition to the utilisation of high-molecular-weight polyacrylic acids and other polyacrylic acids. This product should be used in conjunction with a coating agent, which is supplied in that after the material has cured, the coating is applied to its surface and light cured. It is claimed that this step increases the wear resistance and durability of the restoration.

As has been illustrated by the foregoing, dental materials are constantly developing and evolving to improve outcomes for patients and ease of use at the chairside for clinicians. It is hoped that these tips will provide food for thought for busy clinicians on how best to optimise the use of dental materials across a range of disciplines. Given the broad topic area, further reading is essential to grasp more of this fascinating and critically important area of dentistry [1].

2.7 Conclusions

A good grasp of basic science and the relatively optimal working protocols for dental materials is imperative for the provision of restorative dentistry. In this chapter, we have outlined tips to improving clinician's approach to utilising materials to their full potential through pragmatism and awareness of material properties and their applicability to clinical situations.

References

1. Bonsor SJ, Pearson GJ. A clinical guide to applied dental materials. 1st ed. Edinburgh: Churchill Livingstone Elsevier; 2013.
2. Burke FJT. Own label materials: scientific evidence. Dent Update. 2017;44:273.
3. Burke FJT. Enhancing adhesive restoration effectiveness. Dent Update. 2020;47:545–7.
4. Burke FJ. The evidence base for 'own label' resin-based dental restoratives. Dent Update. 2013;40:5–6.
5. Johnsen GF, Thieu MK, Hussain B, et al. Own brand label restorative materials—a false bargain? J Dent. 2017;56:84–98.
6. Mickenautsch S. How well are GIC product labels related to current systematic review evidence? Dent Update. 2011;38:634–8. 641–642, 644

7. Shaw K, Martins R, Hadis MA, Burke T, Palin W. 'Own-label' versus branded commercial dental resin composite materials: mechanical and physical property comparisons. Eur J Prosthodont Restor Dent. 2016;24:122–9.
8. Gulati JS, Tabiat-Pour S, Watkins S, Banerjee A. Resin-bonded bridges—the problem or the solution? Part 2: practical techniques. Dent Update. 2016;43:608–16.
9. Bonsor SJ. The use of the operating microscope in general dental practice. Part 1: magnification in general. Dent Update. 2014;41:912–9.
10. Bonsor SJ. The use of the operating microscope in general dental practice. Part 2: if you can see it, you can treat it! Dent Update. 2015;42:60–6.
11. Sirona D. Over a century of storied history and innovative leadership. https://www.dentsply-sirona.com/en-us/company/our-company/history.html (Accessed 2 April 2022).

Practical Tips for Restorative Prognosis

3

Prashanti Eachempati, Guy Lambourn, Andrew Harris,
and Ewen McColl

Learning Points

- Recognise the importance of assessing restorative prognosis during treatment planning.
- Understand the multiple prognostic factors that need to be taken into consideration for restorability and longevity.
- Appreciate the various biomechanical factors and their interrelationship that play a role in the prognostic process.

3.1 Introduction

Assessing the likelihood of a tooth's long-term stability within a patient's oral cavity, thereby determining its suitability for inclusion in comprehensive rehabilitation, poses a formidable challenge in the field of dentistry [1]. As treatment complexity increases, designing a well-structured and achievable treatment plan becomes increasingly important. Whilst the treatment plan often needs adaptation as treatment progresses, it serves as a useful road map for the stages of treatment. The foundation of robust treatment planning hinges upon accurate diagnosis and prognosis evaluations, particularly when exploring various treatment options [1].

P. Eachempati
Peninsula Dental School (University of Plymouth), Derriford Dental Education Facility, Plymouth Science Park, Plymouth, UK

Prosthodontics, Manipal University College Malaysia, Melaka, Malaysia

G. Lambourn · A. Harris
Peninsula Dental School (University of Plymouth), Derriford Dental Education Facility, Plymouth Science Park, Plymouth, UK

E. McColl (✉)
Peninsula Dental School, Plymouth, UK
e-mail: ewen.mccoll@plymouth.ac.uk

E. McColl, A. Alani (eds.), *Practical Tips in Clinical Dentistry*, BDJ Clinician's Guides, https://doi.org/10.1007/978-3-031-90355-7_3

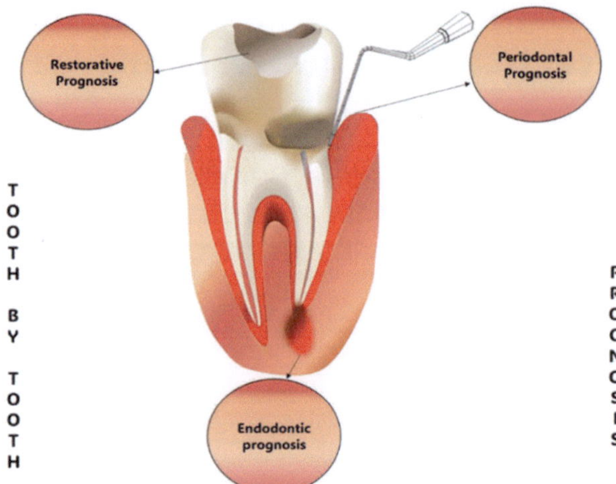

Fig. 3.1 Diagram representing the three critical areas for tooth-by-tooth prognosis

Prognosis, in this context, refers to the predictive estimation of the probable course and outcome of a dental condition, as well as the likelihood of recovery [2]. This prognostic assessment operates on two distinct levels: the patient level and the individual tooth level [1].

In the evaluation of patient-level prognosis, factors such as biologic risks, environmental influences, financial, behavioural, and personal considerations must be taken into account. Once relevant clinical information has been gathered along with necessary investigations (e.g. radiographs), the phase prior to developing the treatment plan involves considering individual tooth-by-tooth prognosis. This is a key stage and allows an open discussion in the consent process as to what teeth can and cannot be saved so that the patient enters the treatment pathway with sufficient information to provide informed consent [3, 4].

Tooth-specific prognosis examines three critical areas: restorative, periodontic, and endodontic assessments for each tooth (Fig. 3.1). In this chapter, we focus on the restorative prognostic factors.

3.2 Classification System for Assessing Prognosis

Various classifications have been suggested in the literature [5] for tooth-by-tooth prognosis, encompassing terminology such as 'favourable' and 'questionable' [6], or employing prognostic categories of 'good', 'questionable', and 'hopeless' [7]. Some systems utilise descriptors like 'good', 'fair', 'poor', 'questionable', and 'hopeless' [8]. In order to enhance accessibility and reader comprehension, the present article adopts a simplified approach, utilising the terms 'good', 'questionable', and 'poor' to characterise prognosis.

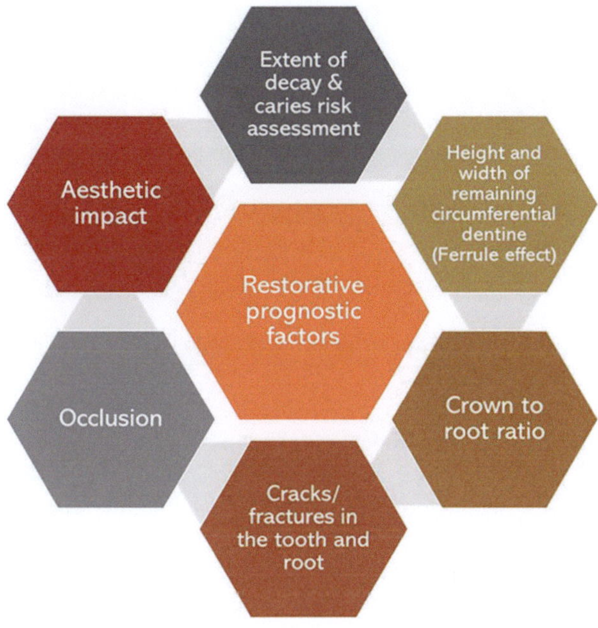

Fig. 3.2 Restorative factors to be considered for tooth-by-tooth prognosis

3.3 Restorative Factors

The figure presented below provides a comprehensive overview of the factors essential for tooth-by-tooth prognosis, with a specific focus on the restorative aspects (Fig. 3.2).

3.3.1 Assessing the Extent of Decay or Caries

One of the primary considerations in determining restorative individual tooth prognosis is the thorough assessment of decay or caries present in a tooth. This evaluation involves a comprehensive examination to identify the extent of the decayed areas within the tooth structure. Clinical examination, visual inspection, and radiographs help to precisely gauge the depth and spread of the decay (Fig. 3.3). This assessment guides the clinician in making informed decisions about the prognosis of the tooth and aids in selecting the most suitable restorative or endodontic interventions based on the severity of the carious lesions. As part of the dental examination for caries, it is essential to conduct a caries risk assessment [9]. This evaluation is pivotal in determining whether a tooth's prognosis can be classified as good, questionable, or poor.

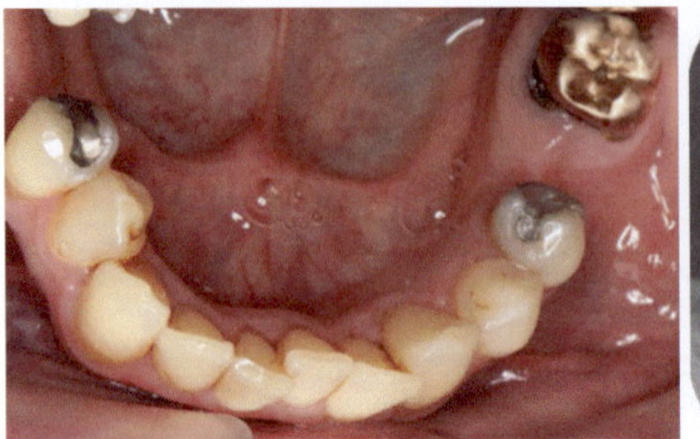
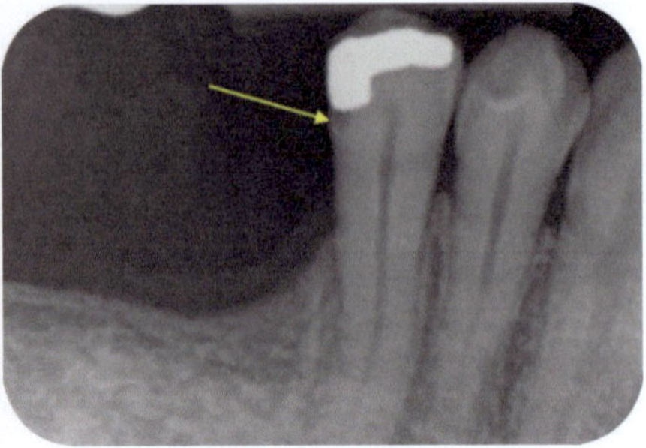

Fig. 3.3 Clinical and radiographic evaluation to determine the extent of caries

3.3.1.1 Caries Risk Assessment

A thorough caries assessment demands a comprehensive evaluation that encompasses various critical factors. These include an examination of the patient's historical and current experiences with dental caries, dietary habits, exposure to fluoride, the presence of cariogenic bacteria, salivary conditions, and overall medical history. Additionally, the assessment should extend to encompass behavioural and physical factors, as well as broader medical and demographic characteristics that may contribute to or influence the development of dental caries. While there exist various methods to categorise caries risk, Fontana and Zero 2006 [10] propose an initial decision-making process that revolves around three primary categories: high risk, moderate risk, and low risk. Illustrated in the accompanying figure, their classification model commences with an assessment of caries experience (Fig. 3.4).

A comprehensive caries risk assessment must not overlook factors that could potentially impede the patient's ability to maintain optimal oral hygiene. These obstacles may include challenges such as crowded dentition, the presence of deep fissures, wide-open restorative margins, or the use of oral appliances.

3.3.1.2 Considering the Size and Location of Cavities

The size and location of cavities are critical factors influencing the prognosis of individual teeth. The size of a cavity directly correlates with the amount of healthy tooth structure that remains after decay removal. Larger cavities may compromise the structural integrity of the tooth, impacting its long-term stability. Additionally, the location of cavities, whether they are on occlusal surfaces, proximal surfaces, or extend onto the root surface, can influence the complexity of restorative procedures and their success. Restorative treatments for root caries lesions exhibit a poor prognosis, primarily attributable to the close proximity of the gingival margin, challenges in isolation, and difficulties associated with bonding to dentine [11] (Fig. 3.5).

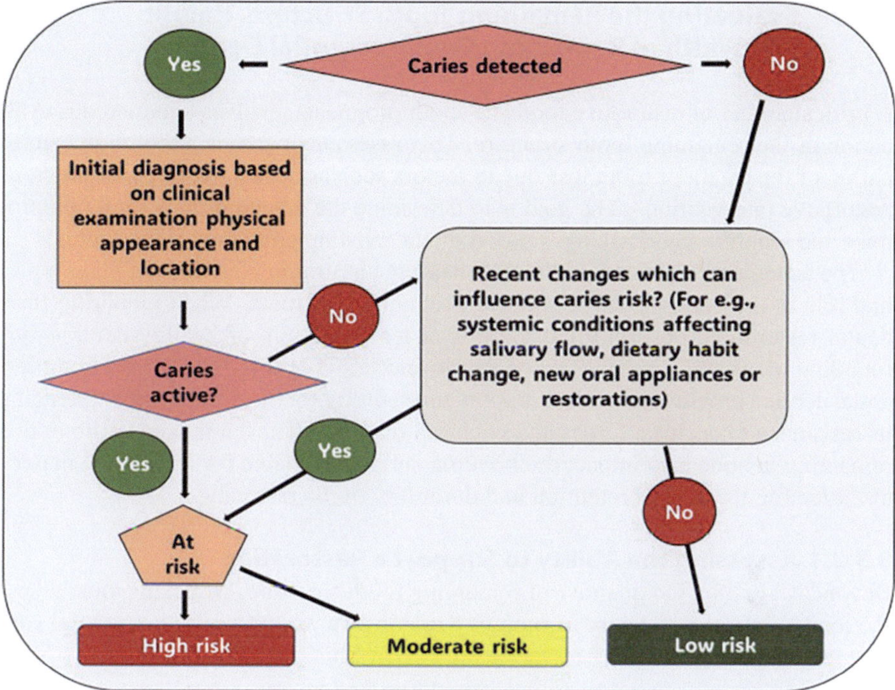

Fig. 3.4 Caries risk assessment decision chart: adopted from Fontana and Zero 2006 [10]

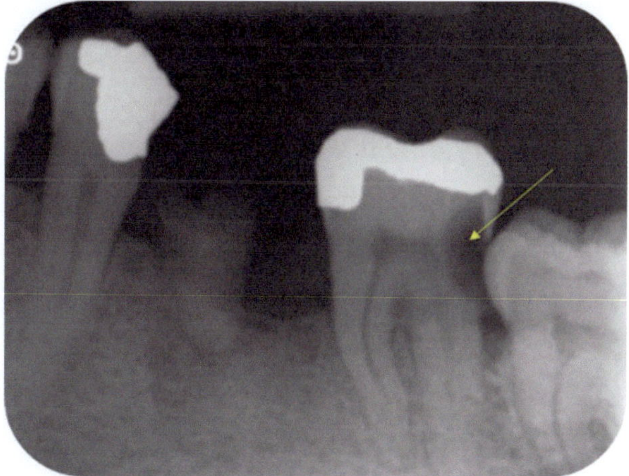

Fig. 3.5 Location of caries—extending on to root surface influences prognosis

3.3.2 Evaluating the Remaining Tooth Structure: Height and Width of Remaining Circumferential Dentine

A critical aspect of restorative tooth-by-tooth prognosis involves a meticulous evaluation of the remaining tooth structure. This assessment entails a thorough examination of the extent of tooth loss due to factors such as decay, fractures, or previous restorative interventions. The goal is to determine the degree of structural compromise and identify any challenges posed by the existing condition of the tooth.

The adequate height and width of remaining circumferential dentine plays a pivotal role in determining the restorative prognosis of a tooth. When preparing for a dental restoration, ensuring that there is at least 2–3 mm of healthy dentine surrounding the tooth is crucial for long-term success [12] (Fig. 3.6). This circumferential dentine provides structural support and stability for the restoration, influencing its resistance to occlusal forces and potential fractures. The height and width of this remaining dentine also impact the bonding surface available for restorative materials, affecting the overall retention and durability of the restoration.

3.3.2.1 Assessing the Ability to Support a Restoration

Beyond evaluating the quantity of remaining tooth structure, clinicians must assess the tooth's inherent capacity to support a restoration. Compromised structural support influence the feasibility of various restorative options [13] (Fig. 3.7).

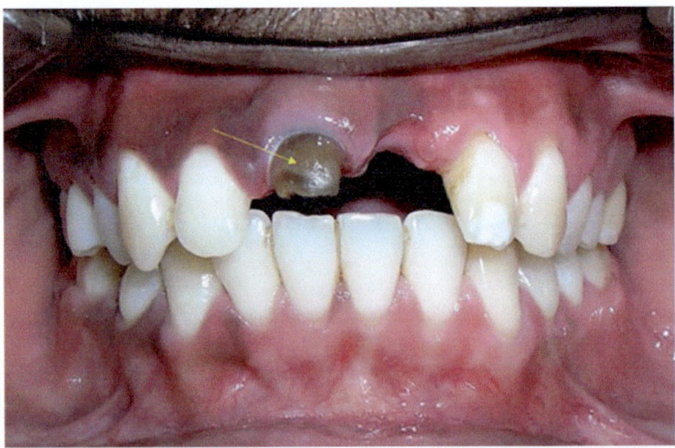

Fig. 3.6 Evaluating the amount of healthy dentine surrounding the tooth influences prognosis

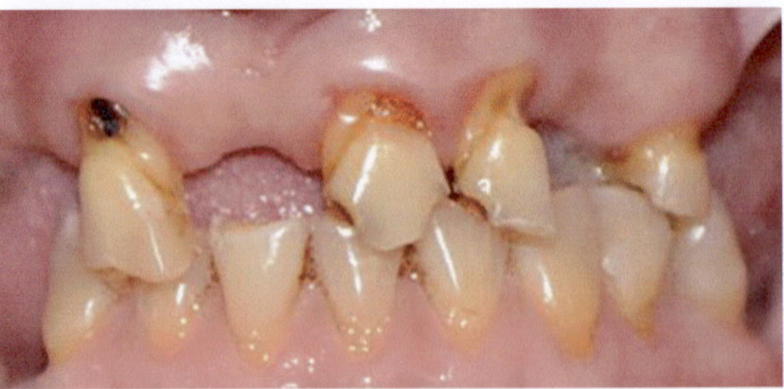

Fig. 3.7 Compromised structural support influences restorability of the teeth

3.3.2.2 Ferrule Effect

The ferrule effect refers to the presence of a continuous band of sound tooth structure encircling the crown of a tooth above the level of the preparation margin. This circular rim of tooth structure plays a crucial role in providing stability and support for the final restoration. It contributes significantly to the overall success of restorative treatments, particularly in cases where a tooth requires a crown. The ferrule effect helps distribute occlusal forces more evenly, enhances resistance against fractures, and promotes the long-term durability of the restoration. A favourable prognosis for a crown restoration is typically associated with a minimum ferrule height of 2 mm or greater [14, 15].

3.3.3 Crown-to-Root Ratio

The crown-to-root ratio is a critical factor in predicting the prognosis of individual teeth especially when the tooth is a potential abutment for a fixed or removable prosthesis. It is the ratio of the length of the part of a tooth that appears above the alveolar bone versus what lies below it (Fig. 3.8). Ideally, a minimum ratio of 1:2 is considered favourable, ensuring a balance between the tooth's crown and root dimensions. Additionally, a minimum ratio of 1:1.5 is generally accepted [16]. Clinicians should regard teeth with a reduction of more than one-third of their periodontal support as having questionable suitability as abutments. Notably, a reduced crown-to-root ratio is often associated with a more favourable prognosis compared to an increased ratio. The reduction in crown height results in a shorter lever arm length, leading to a decreased application of lateral force on the attachment apparatus. This, in turn, seems to diminish the horizontal mobility of the abutment.

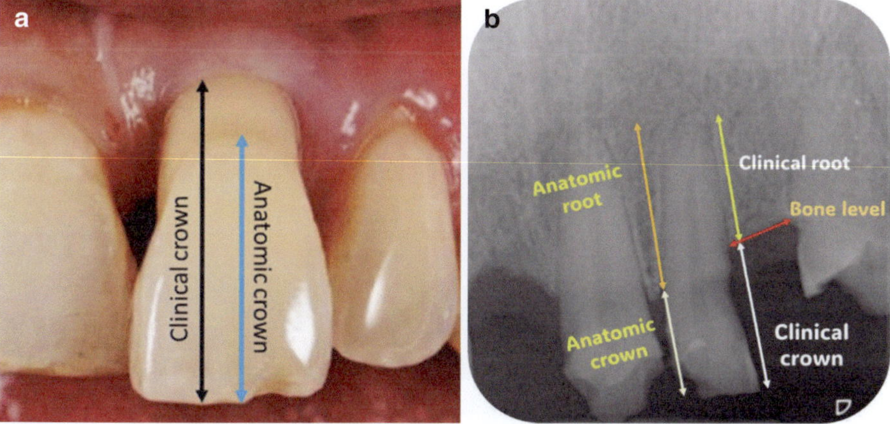

Fig. 3.8 (**a**) The difference between clinical and anatomical crown. (**b**) A radiograph illustrating the difference between clinical and anatomical crown and root dimensions

Table 3.1 gives the requirements to consider when determining the prognosis of a tooth based on remaining tooth structure, ferrule, and crown-to-root ratio [1]. To simplify, we have refined the classification system by consolidating certain categories initially proposed by the author into three overarching classifications: good, questionable, and poor (Table 3.1).

3.3.4 Identifying Cracks or Fractures in the Tooth Structure

Another crucial element in determining restorative prognosis is the identification of cracks or fractures within the tooth structure. Clinicians employ various diagnostic methods, including visual examinations, tactile assessments, and imaging techniques and magnification, to detect any signs of structural compromise. Cracks can manifest in different forms, such as craze lines, fractured cusps, or vertical root fractures (Fig. 3.9). The early identification of these issues is essential for making

Table 3.1 Tooth-by-tooth prognosis based on amount of remaining tooth structure (adapted from Samet N and Jotkowitz A 2009 [1])

Remaining tooth structure	Parameters to consider	Prognosis [colour code]	
80–100%	2 mm ferrule, ideal crown-to-root ratio	Good [green]	Good [green]
50–80%	Adequate ferrule, good crown-to-root ratio	Fair [yellow]	
30–50%	Achieving adequate ferrule would result in compromising the crown-root ratio to some extent	Questionable [cream]	
>30%	Does not enable a good ferrule to be achieved	Compromised [light brown]	Poor [red]
No remaining supragingival sound coronal tooth structure	Loss of tooth structure deep into the root dentine/canals	Non-salvageable [dark brown]	

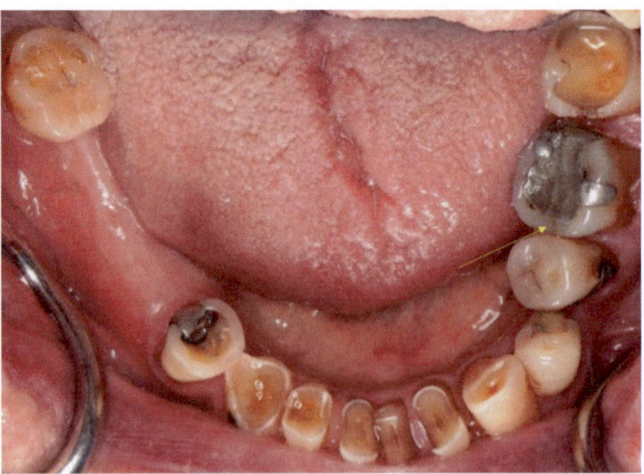

Fig. 3.9 Fracture in the mesial margin of the 36

informed decisions regarding the appropriate restorative or endodontic interventions necessary [17].

3.3.4.1 Assessing If Fractures Extend Into the Root

In addition to identifying cracks or fractures, it is crucial to assess whether these structural compromises extend into the root of the tooth. Vertical root fractures pose a significant challenge to the tooth's prognosis, as they may not always be readily apparent in clinical examinations. Advanced imaging techniques, such as cone-beam computed tomography (CBCT), can be particularly valuable in determining the presence and extent of root fractures. The involvement of the root can influence treatment decisions, and in some cases, extraction may be considered if the fracture compromises the tooth's long-term stability [17].

3.3.5 Considering the Patient's Occlusion and Its Impact on the Restoration

An integral component of tooth-by-tooth prognosis involves a careful consideration of the patient's occlusion, and its potential impact on the longevity of dental restorations. In cases where adverse occlusal conditions, such as a deep overbite or inadequate interocclusal space, are present, the feasibility of tooth restoration may be impeded with a diminished likelihood of successful restoration (Fig. 3.10a, b). Consequently, the prognosis for such cases is inherently deemed unfavourable. Issues such as malocclusion, bruxism (teeth grinding), or temporomandibular joint (TMJ) disorders can significantly affect the success of a restoration and need to be considered when tooth prognosis is being considered. The orientation of the occlusal plane and tooth position constitutes another crucial aspect that can significantly influence prognosis. For instance, severely supra-erupted teeth may create challenges by limiting space for restoration in the opposing arch, thereby impacting the available treatment options [1].

Table 3.2 gives the requirements to consider when determining the prognosis of a tooth based on occlusal plane and tooth position [1].

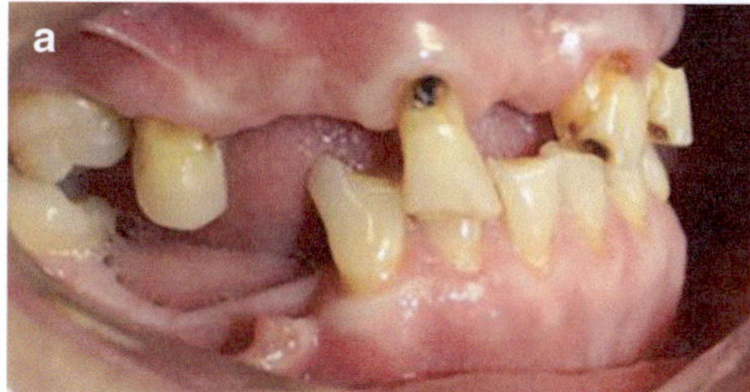

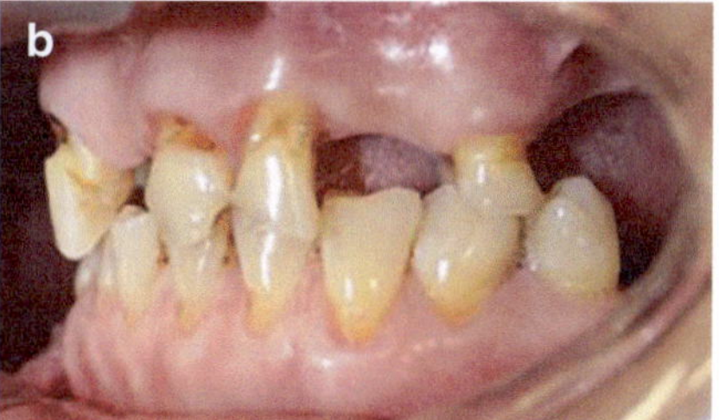

Fig. 3.10 (**a**, **b**) Right and left lateral views of the occlusion illustrating challenging contacts, planes of occlusion, and tooth positioning

Table 3.2 Tooth-by-tooth prognosis based on occlusal plane and tooth position (adapted from Samet N and Jotkowitz A 2009 [1])

	Parameters to consider	Prognosis [colour code]	
Occlusal plane and tooth position	Correct occlusal plane and/or position/needs minimal enameloplasty	Good [green]	Good [green]
	Out of occlusal plane and may require tooth modifications and methods to seal the exposed dentine	Fair [yellow]	
	Out of the occlusal plane and requires multiple procedures to function within the occlusal plane	Questionable [cream]	
	Severely out of occlusal plane and its position impacts the adjacent structures	Compromised [light brown]	Poor [red]
	Super-erupted or tilted out of the occlusal plane that it cannot be restored into correct function and interferes with restoration of opposing arch	Non-salvageable [dark brown]	

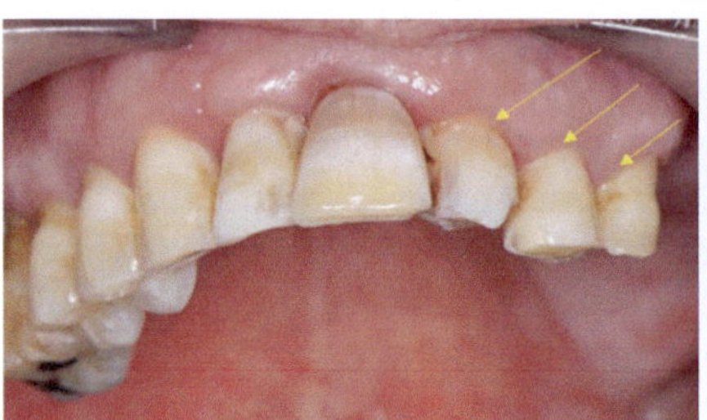
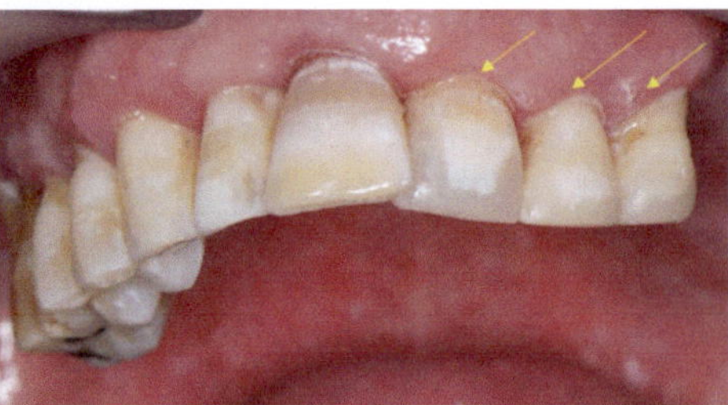

Fig. 3.11 Restoration must integrate with natural appearance of neighbouring teeth

3.3.6 Evaluating the Aesthetic Impact of the Restoration

Aesthetic considerations hold substantial influence in a patient's treatment decision-making process, even though they do not inherently impact the prognosis of the tooth. Beyond functional considerations, the aesthetic implications of a restoration need to be evaluated by the clinician, especially when located in visible areas of the oral cavity. It is crucial to assess whether the intended restoration can seamlessly integrate with the natural appearance of neighbouring teeth, ensuring harmony in terms of colour, shape, and contour. The objective is not only to restore functional aspects but also to elevate the overall aesthetic appeal of the patient's smile (Fig. 3.11). Incorporating this aspect elevates the clinical judgement to a more advanced level [1].

3.4 Conclusion

The consideration of multiple presenting clinical factors and formulating a prognosis from these that the patient can consider for decision-making is a difficult task. Communication is key in instances where the tooth presents in a borderline where a definitive decision on 'favourable' or 'unfavourable' prognosis cannot be utilized. An objective assessment of tooth structure and longevity needs to be balanced against the potential subjective opinion of the patient, who is likely to want to maintain their teeth for as long as possible.

References

1. Samet N, Jotkowitz A. Classification and prognosis evaluation of individual teeth—a comprehensive approach. Quintessence Int. 2009;40:377–87.
2. Mordohai N, Reshad M, Jivraj S, Chee W. Factors that affect individual tooth prognosis and choices in contemporary treatment planning. Br Dent J. 2007;202:63–72.
3. DDU. Guide to consent to dental treatment. 14 September 2022. https://www.theddu.com/guidance-and-advice/guides/quick-guide-to-consent (accessed September 2023).
4. General Dental Council. Standards for the dental team. Principle Three: Obtain valid consent. 2013. https://standards.gdc-uk.org/pages/principle3/principle3.aspx (Accessed September 2023).
5. Halperin-Sternfeld M, Levin L. Do we really know how to evaluate tooth prognosis? A systematic review and suggested approach. Quintessence Int. 2013;44:447–56.
6. Hirschfeld L, Wasserman B. A long-term survey of tooth loss in 600 treated periodontal patients. J Periodontol. 1978;49:225–37.
7. Becker W, Berg L, Becker BE. The long term evaluation of periodontal treatment and maintenance in 95 patients. Int J Periodontics Restorative Dent. 1984;4:54–71.
8. McGuire MK, Nunn ME. Prognosis versus actual outcome. II. The effectiveness of clinical parameters in developing an accurate prognosis. J Periodontol. 1996;67:658–65.
9. Carounanidy U, Sathyanarayanan R. Dental caries: a complete changeover (part II)—changeover in the diagnosis and prognosis. J Conserv Dent. 2009;12:87–100.
10. Fontana M, Zero DT. Assessing patients' caries risk. J Am Dent Assoc. 2006;137:1231–9.
11. Hellyer P. Root caries. Br Dent J. 2021;231:32.
12. Koosha S, Jebelizadeh MS, Mostafavi AS. Effect of ferrule location on fracture resistance of maxillary premolars: an in vitro study. Int J Dent. 2023; https://doi.org/10.1155/2023/9513804.
13. Fichera G, Mazzitelli C, Picciariello V, et al. Structurally compromised teeth. Part I: clinical considerations and novel classification proposal. J Esthet Restor Dent. 2024;36:7–19.
14. Skupien JA, Luz MS, Pereira-Cenci T. Ferrule effect: a meta-analysis. JDR Clin Trans Res. 2016;1:31–9.
15. Ma PS, Nicholls JI, Junge T, Phillips KM. Load fatigue of teeth with different ferrule lengths, restored with fiber posts, composite resin cores, and all-ceramic crowns. J Prosthet Dent. 2009;102:229–34.
16. Grossmann Y, Sadan A. The prosthodontic concept of crown-to-root ratio: a review of the literature. J Prosthet Dent. 2005;93:559–62.
17. Lee TY, Yang SE, Kim HM, Kye MJ. Characteristics, treatment, and prognosis of cracked teeth: a comparison with data from 10 years ago. Eur J Dent. 2021;15:694–701.

Minimally Invasive Dentistry

4

Yen Lin, Ewen McColl, and Henry F. Duncan

Learning Points

- Understand the risk assessment process for dental caries management.
- Appreciate the importance of instilling a preventative regime for the patient and the various methods that this can be achieved.
- Recognise lesions that require restoration and how previous stages require compliance prior to invasive management.
- Understand the atraumatic restorative technique and its application to the clinical setting.
- Recognise situations where the use of resin infiltration can halt demineralisation and halt the caries process.

4.1 Introduction

Minimally invasive dentistry (MID) (or minimal intervention dentistry) is defined as a holistic approach that respects the dental tissues and the patient's comfort and aims to help maintain long-term oral health centred around preventive, patient-focused care plans with the management of patients' needs and expectations [1, 2]. It recognises that caries is a multifactorial, lifestyle-associated condition, which can be modified with behavioural modifications [3]. Caries can also be managed without removing all microorganisms involved, with the focus shifting to arresting the

Y. Lin
Dental Education, Peninsula Dental School (University of Plymouth), Plymouth, UK

E. McColl (✉)
Peninsula Dental School, Plymouth, UK
e-mail: ewen.mccoll@plymouth.ac.uk

H. F. Duncan
Division of Restorative Dentistry and Periodontology, Dublin Dental University Hospital, Trinity College Dublin, Dublin, Ireland

E. McColl, A. Alani (eds.), *Practical Tips in Clinical Dentistry*, BDJ Clinician's Guides, https://doi.org/10.1007/978-3-031-90355-7_4

lesion instead [4]. Management can be divided into four stages: Identify, prevent, restore, and recall.

In this paper, we discuss the top tips for carrying out MID and further explore the four stages involved in the management of caries.

4.2 Identify

This stage allows clinicians to identify the aetiology behind the prevalence of caries for each patient and also assess the extent of damage [1]. A risk assessment-based approach aimed at disease prevention and patient management should be undertaken, considering risk indicators, risk factors, and protective factors, which can lead to the demineralisation of teeth and plan for prevention or restoration of them in the subsequent phases [2, 5]. This also aids in tailoring the individual patient care plan and recall intervals.

Risk indicators include previous caries experience, presence of active cavitated lesions and white spot lesions, as well as the number of restorations in the last 6 months. The site of the lesions may also play a role; for example, patients with defective restorations, exposed root surfaces, and posterior teeth with deep fissures may increase caries risk as these are recognised as difficult-to-clean areas.

Sociodemographic factors should also be considered, and this can include age, educational background, and disabilities, which can impact their ability to access and maintain dental care. The following patient groups are considered high risk based on their sociodemographic background: dependent elderly people, disabled people, people with chronic conditions, people from disadvantaged socioeconomic backgrounds, migrant and prison populations, pregnant women, people with drug-induced xerostomia, as well as people who have had head and neck radiotherapy or who are involved in the food industry [6].

Risk factors can be categorised as local, systemic, and behavioural. Systemic risk factors include an individual's environment, and this can include their living conditions, disorder and medication, age, genetics, and physiological behaviours [6]. Behavioural risk factors relate specifically to the individual and can be modified, which usually encompasses their dietary habits, oral hygiene measures, smoking habits, or emotional stress. Lastly, local risk factors are involved in the disease activity, and these include salivary flow, plaque retention factors, periodontal biotype, and structural dental abnormalities.

Protective factors mainly encompass the frequency of fluoride exposure, and this can stem from toothbrushing habits with fluoride toothpaste as well as living in an area that has fluoridated water.

In children, the recommended age for a dental visit is by the first year of age or eruption of the first deciduous tooth [7]. This will allow the dentist to establish rapport with the patient as well as encourage participation amongst members of the family. The use of distractors and positive reinforcement will aid the clinician in assessing the dentition and surrounding soft tissues. Risk assessment of children is important, too, as it allows all parties involved to identify patients at high risk of early childhood caries and design treatment and preventative protocols to manage this. In addition to the above risk factors, additional risk factors would include assessing whether the child sleeps with a bottle or consumes liquids other than water for an extended period.

In detecting the activity state of a carious lesion, the appearance and position of the lesion should be considered in conjunction with gentle tactile probing and the gingival status of the surrounding tissues [8]. Pre-cleaning the teeth can improve direct visual examination, and this can be carried out with a rotary brush and prophy paste. The teeth are then air-dried, and the use of magnification with good illumination should be considered, which can improve the detection rate of carious lesions. Clinical indicators of lesion activity can include the presence of biofilm on the lesion, gingival condition, as well as lesion texture, hardness, and appearance (Fig. 4.1) [4].

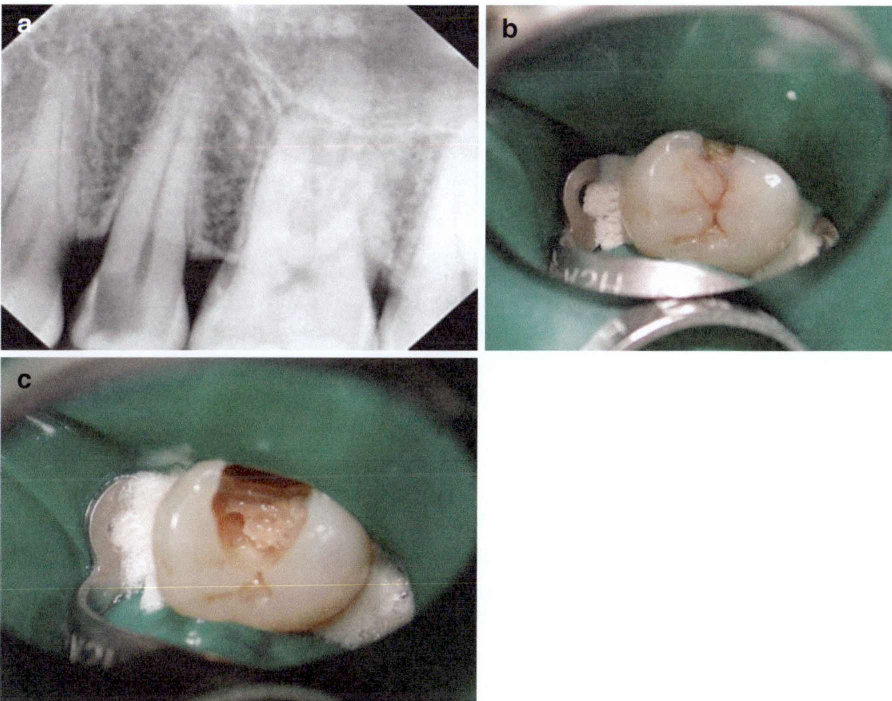

Fig. 4.1 (**a**) Periapical radiograph of the upper left second premolar showing a mesial radiolucency indicative of deep caries (extending into the inner third of dentine radiographically). (**b**) Clinical photograph of the same tooth as 1a with cavitation evident mesially and 'yellow' carious tissue. (**c**) Cavity after unsupported caries removal reveals soft 'yellow' carious dentine indicative of an active lesion. Nonselective (complete) removal of the carious tissue around the margins and periphery of the cavity will facilitate 'carious' dentine to be left over the aspect of the cavity in proximity to the pulp, avoiding pulp exposure

Bitewing radiographs are the gold standard for detecting proximal lesions and should also be used in the detection of carious lesions [8, 9]. Radiographs will also allow at least a cursory division of the depth of caries into shallow, moderate, deep, and extremely deep caries, which will aid in treatment planning. Recently, there has been the development of new diagnostic tools, e.g. dyes, transillumination, infrared lasers, LED cameras, electrical conductance, and fluorescence systems in caries detection, but these should be used with care as they may under- or over-detect the presence of caries.

4.3 Prevent

This stage aims to restore balance between the pathological and protective factors involved as well as eliminate and minimise disease risk factors by modifying lifestyle behaviour [1, 10]. Preventive measures aimed at remineralisation of the tooth surfaces should be initiated and encouraged. This involves an emphasis on promoting oral hygiene and good dietary habits and the cessation of smoking and destructive drinking habits as well as drug use [4]. Patients should be encouraged to undergo plaque removal at least twice a day with a manual toothbrush, a rotating or oscillating toothbrush, and a 'pea-sized' amount of 1350–1500 ppm fluoride toothpaste. Interproximal cleaning should also be encouraged via the use of interdental brushes, floss, or soft toothpicks [6]. One can consider the use of a water jet in patients who lack manual dexterity as well as the use of a disclosing dye to highlight areas that are missed during brushing.

In addition, a diet diary as part of a caries-risk assessment can be considered, which can monitor patients' 'acid attacks' [8]. Once oral hygiene measures are optimal, the prescription of topical fluoride supplements can be considered, e.g. 5000 ppm fluoride toothpaste, 0.05% sodium fluoride mouthwash as well as the placement of fissure sealants (resin, GIC, RMGIC, or compomers), or topical 22,600 ppm fluoride varnish at 3–6-month intervals, depending on the caries risk. Products containing CPP-ACP (casein phosphopeptide-amorphous calcium phosphate) have also been recently introduced, but these should be used with caution as there is a lack of evidence regarding their effectiveness [11].

In children, the correct use of toothbrushing techniques should be demonstrated to the carer via the 'tell-show-do' technique [7]. The amount of toothpaste required should also be reduced, with a smear being sufficient for children under the age of 2 years.

Behaviour management not only applies to children but adults as well, and successful motivation will aid in reducing their modifiable risk factors. This can be undertaken via understanding the patients' views on their oral health, identifying their limitations, improving their self-esteem by paying attention to them, and setting SMART objectives in the long term [6].

4.4 Restore

In this stage, the decision to intervene should take into consideration lesion activity, cavitation, depth, and the cleansability of the lesion [4]. Treatment should be focused on minimally invasive operative intervention, resolution of symptoms if present, and the repair instead of replacement of defective restorations. The former will preserve tooth structure and pulp sensibility, whereas the latter increases the size of the cavity and can weaken the overall structural integrity of the tooth [1, 10, 12]. It should also be noted that the success of this stage is affected by previous stages and can lead to the failure of restorations if aetiological factors are not identified and managed. Restoration of a carious lesion aims to reduce any further loss of dental tissue; remove any plaque retentive factors, which may present in a cavity; as well as restore occlusion, function, and aesthetics of an individual. The use of durable, bioactive, adhesive, restorative materials, e.g. resin-based composite, glass ionomer cement (GIC), and hydraulic calcium silicate cements, is also advocated, as this negates the need to destroy 'sound' tooth structure to achieve mechanical retention [12].

4.5 Atraumatic Restorative Treatment

Atraumatic restorative treatment (ART) can be considered as an initial stabilisation phase prior to a definitive restoration. This can be used as an alternative to selective caries removal in deep caries lesions that are in close proximity to the pulp radiographically, which run the risk of pulpal exposure should nonselective removal of carious dentine be undertaken (Fig. 4.1) [13]. This technique can also be used in children if there is insufficient compliance to employ the use of a fast handpiece under local anaesthesia [7].

This technique is carried out by selective removal of necrotic tissue and leaving a layer of affected carious dentine on the floor of the cavity to reduce the microbial load. Hard-stained and discoloured dentine should be left in situ as this has the potential to remineralise. Any unsupported enamel that is thin and weak should be removed as these are prone to fracture. The use of rotary instrumentation relies on tactile feedback that results in the unnecessary removal of 'sound' tooth tissues as clinicians tend to want to remove all soft, affected dentine. Isolation of the surrounding area with cotton wool rolls is usually sufficient to reduce contamination of the area and aid moisture control.

Following this, the smear layer is removed using a dentine conditioner before a GIC restoration is placed, which reduces the surface area for retention of the plaque biofilm and allows for ion exchange, leading to remineralisation of any demineralised tissues [3]. GIC also provides a long-lasting seal via chemical adhesion that deprives any remaining bacteria of nutrients as well as reduces the risk of inducing inflammation in the pulp. Pits and fissures can also be sealed using the 'finger-press technique', which reduces the risk of bacterial ingress leading to decay [14].

4.6 Resin Infiltration

Resin infiltration is more commonly used in the management of white spot non-carious lesions but can also be used in the management of caries, which halts the demineralisation process and stabilises the carious lesion [15]. It is usually indicated in initial proximal lesions and non-proximal smooth surfaces but should not be used on cavitated lesions as resin infiltration is poor. Fifteen percent hydrochloric acid gel should be applied for 2 min to etch the tooth, followed by dehydration of the tooth with 99% ethanol and air. A low-viscosity TEGDMA-type resin is then applied, which forms a mechanical barrier that removes the source of nutrients for bacteria to feed on. It also impedes further acid diffusion and mineral loss [4].

4.7 Sono-Abrasion

Sono-abrasion works on the principles of vibration, abrasion, thermal, and cavitation, which can be selectively used in the treatment of small lesions and aims to preserve tissue as much as possible and stimulate pulpal repair mechanisms [16]. A variety of abrasive powders can be used, which allows for conservative cavity preparations and produces rounded cavity line angles, which reduces stress during polymerisation shrinkage [12]. This reduces the risk of chipping, loss of residual enamel, and damage to adjacent tooth surfaces and optimises marginal adaptation of restorations. It is also used in the operative management of primary and secondary lesions and the improvement of the quality of occlusal, approximal, and cervical margins. This technique also has its uses in aesthetic dentistry, as it can be used for the preparation, recontouring, and finishing of margins of ceramic or indirect resin-based composite restorations.

4.8 Other Techniques

Other minimally invasive techniques for caries removal include chemo-mechanical caries removal using a hypochlorite/amino acid-based gel system, which allows for selective removal of infected and affected dentine [17]. This technique however is technique-sensitive and requires sufficient clinician training to ensure its proper use.

4.9 Recall

Lastly, this stage focuses on establishing an appropriate recall period depending on the individual's caries risk to allow for monitoring of the disease and maintenance of the dentition [1]. This also allows for reinforcement of the patient's education, monitoring the effectiveness of preventative and control measures implemented by the clinician, as well as checking the integrity of any restorations provided in the previous stage [7]. Any potential failures can be identified and a new caries risk and recall interval assigned to the patient. Any suspicious lesions should be monitored with preventative strategies before invasive intervention if there are any doubts about the disease activity, as this will reduce the potential of over-treatment [11].

4.10 Conclusions

A good grasp of basic science and the relatively optimal working protocols for dental materials is imperative for the provision of restorative dentistry. In this chapter, we have outlined an approach to improving clinicians' approach to utilising materials to their full potential through pragmatism and awareness of material properties and their applicability to clinical situations.

References

1. Featherstone JDB, Doméjean S. Minimal intervention dentistry: part 1. From 'compulsive' restorative dentistry to rational therapeutic strategies. Br Dent J. 2012;213:441–5.
2. Banerjee A. 'Minimum intervention'—MI inspiring future oral healthcare? Br Dent J. 2017;223:133–5.
3. Ngo H, Opsahl-Vital S. Minimal intervention dentistry II: part 7. Minimal intervention in cariology: the role of glass-ionomer cements in the preservation of tooth structures against caries. Br Dent J. 2014;216:561–5.
4. Banerjee A, Splieth C, Breschi L, et al. When to intervene in the caries process? A Delphi consensus statement. Br Dent J. 2020;229:474–82.
5. Doméjean S, Banerjee A, Featherstone JDB. Caries risk/susceptibility assessment: its value in minimum intervention oral healthcare. Br Dent J. 2017;223:191–7.
6. Lallam C, Decup F. Minimal intervention dentistry II: part 2. Management of caries and periodontal risks in general dental practice. Br Dent J. 2014;216:179–85.
7. Ramos-Gomez FJ, Crystal YO, Domejean S, Featherstone JDB. Minimal intervention dentistry: part 3. Paediatric dental care—prevention and management protocols using caries risk assessment for infants and young children. Br Dent J. 2012;213:501–8.
8. Guerrieri A, Gaucher C, Bonte E, Lasfargues JJ. Minimal intervention dentistry: part 4. Detection and diagnosis of initial caries lesions. Br Dent J. 2012;213:551–7.
9. Fontana M, Gonzalez-Cabezas C. Minimal intervention dentistry: part 2. Caries risk assessment in adults. Br Dent J. 2012;213:447–51.
10. Dawett B, Atkins B, Banerjee A. A guide to building 'MI' oral healthcare practice. Br Dent J. 2017;223:223–7.
11. Holmgren C, Gaucher C, Decerle N, Doméjean S. Minimal intervention dentistry II: part 3. Management of non-cavitated (initial) occlusal caries lesions—non-invasive approaches through remineralisation and therapeutic sealants. Br Dent J. 2014;216:237–43.
12. Mackenzie L, Banerjee A. Minimally invasive direct restorations: a practical guide. Br Dent J. 2017;223:163–71.
13. Duncan HF, Galler KM, Tomson PL, et al. European Society of Endodontology position statement: management of deep caries and the exposed pulp. Int Endod J. 2019;52:923–34.
14. Holmgren CJ, Roux D, Doméjean S. Minimal intervention dentistry: part 5. Atraumatic restorative treatment (ART)—a minimum intervention and minimally invasive approach for the management of dental caries. Br Dent J. 2013;214:11–8.

15. Lasfargues JJ, Bonte E, Guerrieri A, Fezzani L. Minimal intervention dentistry: part 6. Caries inhibition by resin infiltration. Br Dent J. 2013;214:53–9.
16. Decup F, Lasfargues JJ. Minimal intervention dentistry II: part 4. Minimal intervention techniques of preparation and adhesive restorations. The contribution of the sono-abrasive techniques. Br Dent J. 2014;216:393–400.
17. Banerjee A. Minimal intervention dentistry: part 7. Minimally invasive operative caries management: rationale and techniques. Br Dent J. 2013;214:107–11.

The Provision of Direct Posterior Restorations

5

R. J. R. Smith, G. E. Bryce, and Ewen McColl

Learning Points

- Appreciate the need to decide which restorative material suits the cavity needs prior to treatment.
- Understand the handling properties of composite and how to prepare the residual tooth tissue to accept the material.
- Recall the challenges with restoring cavities that are subgingival.
- Recognise the need for appropriate isolation and moisture control.
- Appreciate the different failure modes and how best to manage them.

5.1 Introduction

The British Society of Restorative Dentistry (BSRD) defines restorative dentistry as the study, examination, and treatment of diseases of the oral cavity, the teeth, and their supporting structures. Restorative dentistry includes the dental monospecialties of endodontics, periodontics, and prosthodontics (including implantology), and its foundation is based upon how these interact in the management of cases requiring multifaceted care [1].

It is impossible to cover the extensive scope of all the domains that encompass restorative dentistry within the limits of this series of articles. Subsequently, the challenges that we discuss are those that we have experienced from our own clinical trial and error, questions that have been frequently posed, or observations of failing

R. J. R. Smith
Defence Centre for Rehabilitative Dentistry, Aldershot, UK

G. E. Bryce
Restorative Dentistry, Defence Centre for Rehabilitative Dentistry, Aldershot, UK

E. McColl (✉)
Peninsula Dental School, Plymouth, UK
e-mail: ewen.mccoll@plymouth.ac.uk

E. McColl, A. Alani (eds.), *Practical Tips in Clinical Dentistry*, BDJ Clinician's Guides, https://doi.org/10.1007/978-3-031-90355-7_5

treatments. These tips are experiential in many respects, and whilst we are fully cognisant of the time pressures and fiscal demands dental teams face, we hope that the advice given can not only improve outcomes for patients but also help hard-pressed clinicians to manage the clinical challenges they face daily.

5.2 Choosing a Posterior Restorative Material

(a) Amalgam restorations can be selected for use in posterior teeth where isolation is suboptimal and can be especially useful in the following situations: (a) the restoration of partially erupted third molars and (b) the restoration of distal cervical caries lesions in mandibular second molars, where impacted third molars have been extracted and in conjunction with a deep circumferential matrix band.
(b) Glass-ionomer cement (GIC), with its inherent ability to bond to tooth tissue, makes it particularly useful for the management of class V cavities associated with non-carious tooth surface loss, especially where such lesions are associated with symptoms of dentine (hyper)sensitivity.
(c) Composite can be used for all other definitive restorations.

5.3 Working with Composite

(a) Compared to total etch techniques, a selective etching technique can increase bond strengths to dentine [2] whilst reducing the risk of post-operative sensitivity and other pulp-related complications. In practice, this could be achieved via the following protocol: (a) selective placement of etch on the enamel of the cavity margin (a periodontal probe can be used to place the etch); (b) rinsing off the etch after 20 s and drying (not desiccating); (c) Application of a self-etch adhesive (e.g. Scotchbond Universal Adhesive, 3 M ESPE, St. Paul, USA), to both the dentine and enamel with microbrush; iv. rubbing the adhesive into the dentine for up to 20 s, as rubbing has been shown to increase the bond strength; [3] v. incremental placement and curing of composite prior to finishing procedures.
(b) Warming composite increases flowability and aids adaptability of the material [4]. A variety of appliances have been specifically manufactured for composite warming, but alternate approaches include the use of coffee-cup warmers or placing the composite capsules in a sealed bag within a bowl filled with hot water. Non-stick contouring instruments (e.g. OptraSculpt, Ivoclar Vivadent, Amherst, USA) and brushes are ideal for layering and shaping.

5.4 Placement of Composite Within the Subgingival Cavity Zone

(a) Moisture control. Gingival bleeding control can be assisted with intra-papillary infiltrations of a local anaesthetic (LA) solution containing a vasoconstrictor. Subgingival placement of a retraction cord soaked in a vasoconstrictor containing LA can be used as an adjunct in cases where gingival bleeding is particularly troublesome. A rubber dam should be placed to control the saliva. A suitable matrix should then be placed and wedged, ensuring that the matrix closely approximates the cavity margins.
(b) Following the etching and application of a dental adhesive, an increment of composite should first be placed, adapted, and cured in the deep submarginal aspect of the cavity; this will tend to further stabilise the matrix prior to the addition of further layers.
(c) Plastic matrices may often be too flexible to displace the gingival tissue from deep class III cavity margins on anterior teeth, and metal matrices can often help in these situations, as long as either labial or lingual access for light curing is maintained to the proximal surface. Further light curing should be undertaken following the removal of the metal band to ensure a complete curing.
(d) In deep cavities, where there is an absence of enamel to bond to, marginal elevation of the cavity floor with RMGIC should be considered [5].

5.5 Placement of the Matrix alongside the Rubber Dam

(a) When placing a circumferential matrix system on a posterior tooth, the tooth under treatment and those adjacent to it (where present) should be isolated with a rubber dam, the clamps being placed on the teeth adjacent to that being treated. The matrix can then be placed and wedged as required without interference from the clamps.
(b) When restoring a class II cavity, the tooth undergoing the procedure and (where present) the tooth adjacent to the cavity should be isolated. The more posterior of the teeth will need a clamp to resist the tension in the dam. The dam can be secured on the more anterior tooth by either another clamp, floss ligature, or elastic stabilising cord (e.g. Wedjets, Coltene/Whaledent, Cuyahoga Falls, USA).
(c) Placement of unbonded composite onto the outside surface of the matrix can also help stop the rubber dam from slipping whilst also improving moisture control.

5.6 Polishing Composites: Reducing the Risk of Staining?

(a) The oxygen-inhibited layer on the external surface of newly placed composite resin restoration contains unpolymerised monomer, which is liable to adsorb stain [6]. Polishing to remove this layer can be challenging in hard-to-reach areas, such as fissures and interproximal areas.
(b) Coating the final layer of composite, prior to curing, with glycerol delivered with a microbrush reduces this problem. Most polishing systems on the market are effective if the entirety of the recommended polishing protocol is followed.

5.7 Repairing/Replacing Fractured Composite

(a) Firstly, carry out an assessment to determine the type of the composite fracture (e.g. adhesive vs cohesive failure), and identify and manage any contributing factors, such as the following: caries, an occlusal interference, or parafunctional habits.
(b) If the failure is due to loss of adhesion, then the composite will need to be replaced. The composite bulk can be removed using a high-speed handpiece and then a slow-speed handpiece and a composite-removing bur used to carefully remove the tooth-surface adhered layer. Resin tags from the tooth surface can be removed using a sandblaster, with the oral cavity shielded from the tooth using a rubber dam.

In the event that the cohesive fracture and the remainder of the restoration are assessed to be satisfactory with no secondary caries or voids, then the restoration may be repaired. The surface layer of composite should be removed with a bur and the surface further roughened via sandblasting under a rubber dam, prior to etching, bonding, and re-restoring with composite.

5.8 Conclusions

A good grasp of basic science and the relatively optimal working protocols for dental materials is imperative for the provision of restorative dentistry. In this chapter, we have outlined an approach to improving clinicians' approach to utilising materials to their full potential through pragmatism and awareness of material properties and their applicability to clinical situations.

References

1. The British Society of Restorative Dentistry. https://www.bsrd.org.uk/Index.aspx (accessed 17 January 2022).
2. Goracci C, Rengo C, Eusepi L, Juloski J, Vichi A, Ferrari M. Influence of selective enamel etching on the bonding effectiveness of a new all-in-one adhesive. Am J Dent. 2013;26:99–104.
3. Dal-Bianco K, Pellizzaro A, Patzlaft R, de Oliveira BJR, Loguercio AD, Reis A. Effects of moisture degree and rubbing action on the immediate resin-dentin bond strength. Dent Mater. 2006;22:1150–6.
4. Deb S, Di Silvio L, Mackler HE, Millar BJ. Pre-warming of dental composites. Dent Mater. 2011;27:51–9.
5. Van Dijken JW, Kieri C, Carlen M. Longevity of extensive class II open-sandwich restorations with a resin-modified glass-ionomer cement. J Dent Res. 1999;78:1319–25.
6. Park SH, Noh BD, Ahn HJ, Kim HK. Celluloid strip-finished versus polished composite surface: difference in surface discoloration in microhybrid composites. J Oral Rehabil. 2004;31:62–6.

Crown Provision

6

James Baker, Ewen McColl, and Christopher Tredwin

Learning Points

- Appreciate the need to balance risk vs benefit when deciding to crown a tooth and how this may impact the patient and their future oral health.
- Understand the process of comprehensively assessing the residual tooth tissue and how this influences crown provision.
- Recognise techniques in optimising the process of tooth preparation in terms of protecting adjacent units and the dental pulp.
- Recall techniques in improving impression accuracy to minimise errors in subsequent working models.
- Understand the various stages of the crown fit process and how to navigate when issues arise.

6.1 Introduction

Mastering crown preparations can be one of the most rewarding areas of dentistry but comes with a range of challenges requiring a broad skill set to overcome them. Although technical excellence and manual dexterity are essential skills, close consideration needs to be given to the biological system we are working with, and pulpal anatomy and preservation of residual tooth substance should never be far from the forefront of a clinician's thoughts. As with all areas of dentistry, prior

J. Baker
James Baker Dental Practice, London, UK

E. McColl (✉)
Peninsula Dental School, Plymouth, UK
e-mail: ewen.mccoll@plymouth.ac.uk

C. Tredwin
Institute of Dentistry, Queen Mary, University of London, The Royal London Dental Hospital, London, UK

E. McColl, A. Alani (eds.), *Practical Tips in Clinical Dentistry*, BDJ Clinician's Guides, https://doi.org/10.1007/978-3-031-90355-7_6

preparation and planning prevent poor performance. This prior preparation will involve careful prognostication of teeth, consideration of occlusion, and close coordination with nursing colleagues and laboratory technicians to facilitate success. Whilst obtaining the ideal crown preparation can be time-consuming, the tips below should allow realistic improvements for clinicians whilst improving outcomes for patients.

6.2 Pre-Operative Considerations

- To crown or not—even the most conservative of clinicians needs to closely consider the biological risks when embarking on crowning a tooth. The necessary tooth removal and use of an air turbine rotating at 350,000 RPM means there is always a risk of devitalisation [1] and patients need to be aware of this risk during the consent process. As is always the case, consider a range of available options and opt for the most conservative. Do your most destructive option last, never first, which will delay further progress down the restorative cycle. There are many clinical scenarios where traditionally a crown might have been prescribed that could now be treated in a much more conservative manner. With a combination of bleaching, orthodontics, additive resin composite, and sympathetic enameloplasty, crowns on anterior teeth now occupy a very small treatment niche. Posteriorly, where cuspal protection may be indicated, a partial coverage restoration, whether direct or indirect, is generally a more conservative approach.
- Take photographs—under normal and polarised conditions, with shade tabs adjacent to the teeth before tooth preparation to give the technician a reference shade.
- Consider the occlusion of the preparation—before putting bur to tooth, it is essential to decide if the final restoration will be a guiding contact during lateral movements of the mandible or not and to remove suitable amounts of tissue from the occlusal aspect of the preparation. If the tooth is to disclude, make sure there is space between the preparation and opposing tooth not only when the patient is in ICP [intercuspal position] but also when they make mandibular excursions. If the tooth is to provide a guiding contact, then it may contact the opposing tooth in excursion even after being prepared. When recording the jaw relationship, ensure the recording material is only placed between the preparations and opposing teeth, not between intact occluding teeth, as this will give an inaccurate recording.

6.3 Assess Restorability

- Strip everything back—in the process of deciding if a crown is truly indicated, removal of all existing restorations is essential to eliminate the possibility of caries, diagnose structural cracks, ensure good retention of the core and therefore the crown, and assess the remaining structural dentine for retention of the crown.

Once stripped of all restorations, photographs and sectional impressions serve as a useful record of the remaining dentine if the tooth is not being prepared for the crown at the same visit. A pre-operative radiograph is essential to eliminate periodontal or endodontic pathology.

- Start with the end in mind—it is rarely the case that the desired form of the final crown will be the same as the starting situation. When placing the structural core, it is useful to create the desired final form so that when the tooth is prepared for the crown, it is easy to visualise the correct amount of tooth reduction. If this is not possible or practical, then a putty reduction guide made on a lab-made diagnostic wax up can serve the same purpose. Make a second putty to be used to construct the provisional crown.

6.4 Optimising the Preparation

- Use rubber dam—it will retract gingiva and other soft tissues, improving visibility and access. It will make the procedure more comfortable for the patient by containing the coolant spray, and it will save you time by making the process more streamlined.
- *Wetter, the better*—use copious irrigation as it takes only a five-degree increase in temperature to cause pulpal necrosis [2, 3].
- Protect the adjacent teeth—break the proximal contacts with a narrow flamed-shaped diamond bur and leave a slither of tooth protecting the contact point to avoid inadvertently damaging the adjacent teeth with the bur. This works better than proximal strips, which limit visibility and are easily perforated with a bur.
- Handpiece control is key—use a two-handed finger rest to ensure complete control of the handpiece and bur. This will also prevent the inherent over-tapering created by the rotation of the wrist joint.
- Use the right handpiece and burs—in the authors' experience, the use of a 1:5 speed-increasing handpiece rather than an air turbine improves preparations because the bur will run with less wobble and higher torque, thus giving more control of the preparation process. Select burs with round rather than flat ends to prevent creating sharp internal line angles that can produce stress concentrations, risking fracture of the abutment.

6.5 Improve Impression Accuracy

- Double cord—place one narrow retraction cord before refining the margin preparation, followed by a second larger cord 5 min before taking the working impression (Fig. 6.1). Record the bite whilst you're waiting to save time. Wet the area before removing the larger cord, and then wash thoroughly and dry. Scrutinise the margins and tuck in the smaller cord if it has been dislodged anywhere. Apply a haemostatic agent if there is any bleeding, no matter how minor, as this will spoil the impression.

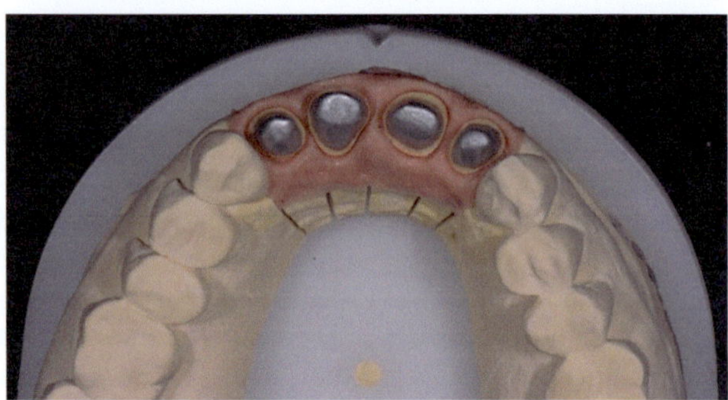

Fig. 6.1 Crown preparations on anterior teeth

- Use rigid trays—to prevent flexure and distortion of the impression. Ensure the tray is completely free of teeth or bony anatomy. Apply suitable tray adhesive and allow time for it to become tacky. Use a heavy body in the tray and light body wash on the teeth. Apply the light body just before inserting the tray as it will set faster in the mouth than the material in the tray. Insert the tray with a rolling action and a slight jiggle to prevent air entrapment. Hold completely still with both hands for the entire setting time.
- Use a face bow—when providing crowns for teeth that will guide mandibular movement, when providing multiple crowns in the aesthetic zone to prevent introducing a cant, and when restoring the last tooth in the arch to prevent the tipping of hand-held models.

6.6 Optimising Temporaries

- Make good temporaries—well-made temporary crowns can provide lots of valuable information about occlusal function, aesthetics, and phonetics that can be transferred to the lab. When making temporaries, apply a thin layer of Vaseline to prevent bonding to any freshly placed composite cores. Re-marginate using flowable composite to ensure excellent marginal closure. When trimming the excess from margins, always orientate the cutting instrument to the long axis of the crown to prevent damaging the margin. After checking and adjusting the occlusion, clean off the oxygen-inhibited layer with an alcohol wipe, and apply and cure a layer of glaze coat to the surface to provide a smooth surface that is comfortable and resists stain. Before cementing, sandblast the fit surface; this ensures a neater clean-up later when removing the crown as the temporary cement preferentially adheres to the temporary crown rather than the tooth. Always use non-eugenol temporary cement since eugenol may mask pulpitic symptoms that simply return when the definitive crown is cemented.

6.7 Crown Fit

- In the authors' experience using local anaesthetic when fitting crowns improves success—it's tempting not to, especially when the crown is on a non-vital tooth, but the surrounding tissue is still very much alive and sensitive, and not anaesthetising these will inhibit proper removal of cement residue (Fig. 6.2a, b, c).
- Removing the temporary crown—try to avoid levering a metal instrument between the preparation margin and the temporary crown as this can damage the tooth and affect the fit of the final crown. Instead, invest in some crown removing forceps. Once removed, clean the preparation thoroughly with a slurry of water and pumice in a prophy cup. You can also use a mild acid as a pre-GIC conditioner to ensure a very clean preparation.
- Have a system for crown fitting—the order in which you check various aspects of the final crown is important. First, is the shade correct? You can check this before even removing the temporary crown. If it's wildly out, this may require a remake, so waste no more time. Next, will it seat? Check and adjust the proximal contacts first, and then if it still doesn't fit, examine the margins for any obvious overextension. Finally, look at the fit surface and any damage to the die. Once the crown is fully seated with firm but flossable contact points, check there are light holding contacts in ICP using a suitable marking medium—not a thick paper or ribbon but a thin mylar-based product. Last, check contacts in mandibular

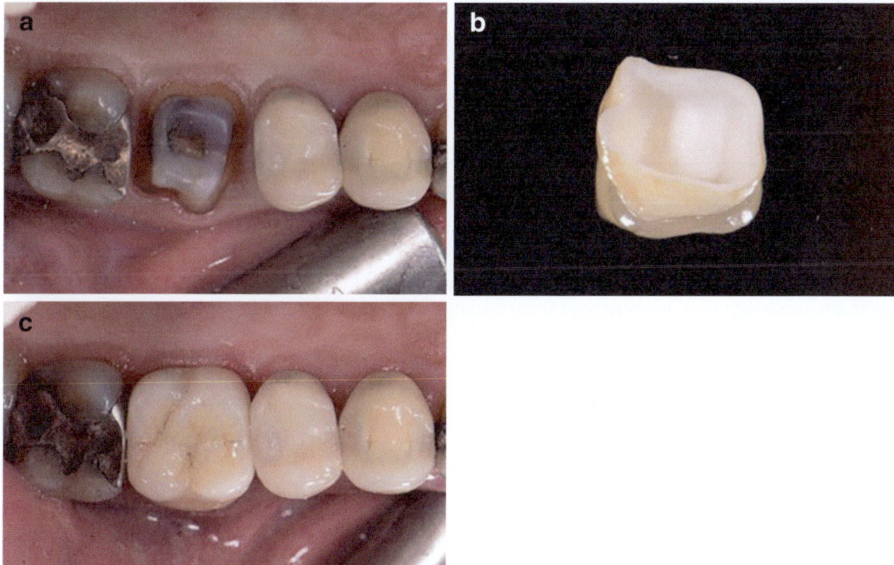

Fig. 6.2 (**a**) Crown preparation of a heavily restored molar demonstrating precise handpiece control to define margins. (**b**) The fit surface of the constructed crown. (**c**) The restoration cemented

excursions. Again, you need to know in advance if you want contact on the crowns in the excursion or not and adjust the crown accordingly.
- Following the IFUs—instructions for use from the manufacturers of crown luting cements and resins are there for a reason. Ignore them at your peril!

6.8 Post-Operative Care and Maintenance Are Key

- Take a post-op radiograph—to check for cement residue and to act as a baseline to compare the marginal appearance at subsequent review appointment [4].
- Look after the new crown—provide the patient with detailed oral hygiene instructions on how to maintain their new crown and impress on them the importance of regular follow-up to pick up any complications at an early stage. If the patient is prone to clenching or grinding, then a rigid maxillary occlusal splint is a very sensible investment to protect your work and their teeth.

6.9 Conclusions

While crown preparations are less commonly carried out due to advances in adhesive techniques, they are an important skill set in the clinician's armamentarium. The above tips will hopefully assist hard-pressed clinicians to plan and deliver well-designed and constructed crowns in close conjunction with technician colleagues. As always, control of active disease prior to commencing treatment, meticulous planning, and informed consent are key elements in optimising outcomes for our patients.

References

1. Saunders W, Saunders E. Prevalence of periradicular periodontitis associated with crowned teeth in an adult Scottish subpopulation. Br Dent J. 1998;185:137–40.
2. Zach L, Cohen G. Pulp response to externally applied heat. Oral Surg Oral Med Oral Pathol. 1965;19:515–30.
3. Kwon SJ, Park YJ, Jun SH, et al. Thermal irritation of teeth during dental treatment procedures. Restor Dent Endod. 2013;38:105–12.
4. Horner K, Eaton KA. Selection criteria for dental radiography. 3rd ed. FGDP(UK); 2018.

Practical Tips for the Immediate Replacement of Teeth

7

Prashanti Eachempati and Ewen McColl

Learning Points

- Understand that immediate restoration provision is more difficult than standard tooth replacement in a healed site as the stages in the construction of the prosthesis rely on predicting the final edentate site post-extraction.
- Recall the different methods in the provision of immediate tooth replacement.

7.1 Introduction

Loss of teeth can be an extremely upsetting event for patients, and concerns around immediate replacement of teeth for aesthetic and functional reasons can weigh heavily on patients' minds [1, 2]. Replacing missing teeth immediately after extraction, without restrictions for future solutions, is clearly attractive for both patients and dentists [3]. There are a wide range of options available for immediate placement of teeth (Fig. 7.1), and in this short article, we discuss the options available with relevant advantages and disadvantages and tips on how to optimise outcomes in support of our patients.

P. Eachempati
Peninsula Dental School (University of Plymouth), Derriford Dental Education Facility, Plymouth Science Park, Plymouth, UK

Prosthodontics, Manipal University College Malaysia, Melaka, Malaysia

E. McColl (✉)
Peninsula Dental School, Plymouth, UK
e-mail: ewen.mccoll@plymouth.ac.uk

E. McColl, A. Alani (eds.), *Practical Tips in Clinical Dentistry*, BDJ Clinician's Guides, https://doi.org/10.1007/978-3-031-90355-7_7

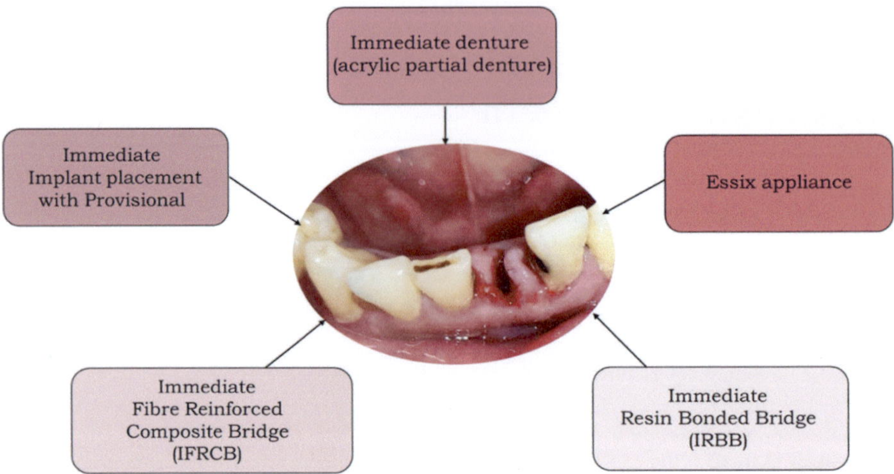

Fig. 7.1 Different options for immediate replacement of teeth

7.2 Immediate Dentures

Immediate dentures, whether complete or partial, are dentures that are inserted on the same day as the removal of natural teeth [4]. This means that patients do not have to endure a waiting period of several weeks for their tissues to heal before receiving their dentures (Fig. 7.2). By offering immediate dentures to patients, we can swiftly reinstate both their aesthetic appearance and functional capabilities, thereby mitigating the potentially distressing experience of adjusting to tooth loss.

One of the significant advantages of immediate dentures is their ability to closely mimic the patient's natural dentition, including tooth shape, colour, position, arch form, and inter-occlusal relationship. This imitation helps maintain the existing occlusal vertical dimension when done optimally [4]. Research studies have also shown that wearing immediate dentures, whether for partial or complete tooth loss, can reduce the rate of alveolar resorption around extraction sites, preserving bone structure [5–7].

Furthermore, immediate dentures act as a kind of protective 'plastic bandage'. They help minimise disturbances, trauma, or insults caused by factors like opposing teeth, oral fluids, and food debris, as they are inserted immediately after tooth extraction [8]. This approach can enhance the overall patient experience and facilitate a smoother transition to a denture-supported lifestyle.

While immediate dentures offer numerous advantages, it's important to acknowledge that some studies have raised concerns regarding the potential for more issues compared to conventionally constructed dentures, which are made after a healing period [9]. Without adequate patient education and information regarding the complex clinical and laboratory procedures, the need for multiple adjustments, and the

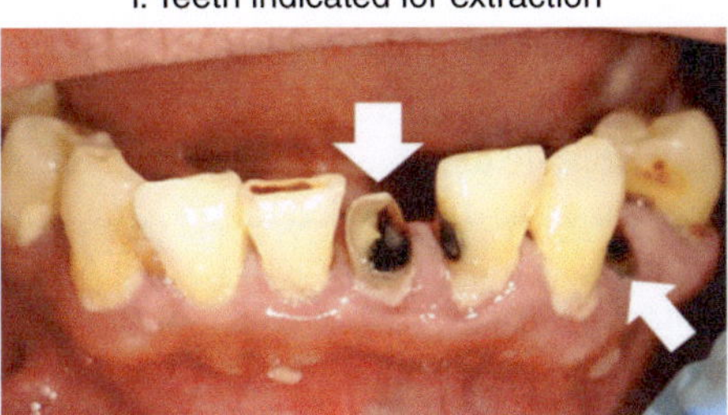

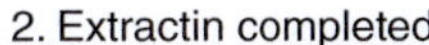

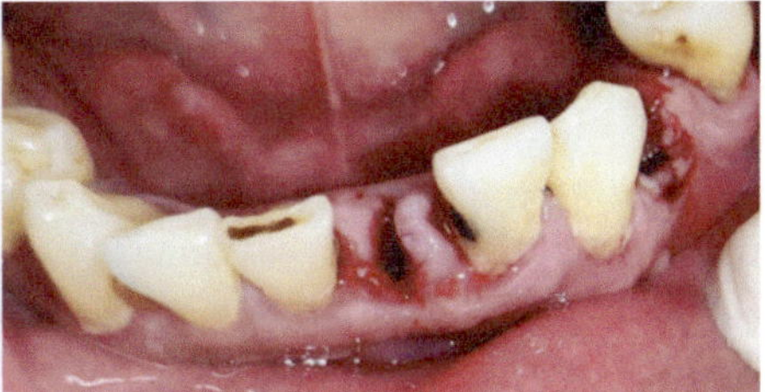

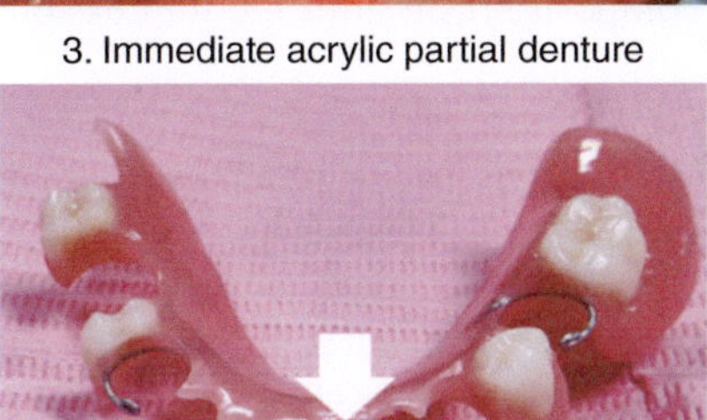

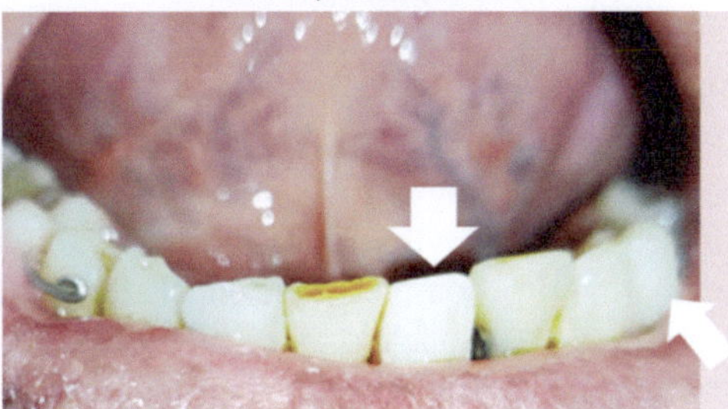

Fig. 7.2 Immediate acrylic partial denture case

financial considerations associated with immediate dentures, this facet of care may become a distressing experience for patients [10].

(a) **Unforeseen need for adjustments:** It's crucial to keep in mind that predicting the precise pattern of tissue changes following tooth extraction is challenging, and the fitting surfaces of dentures may inadvertently cause discomfort or trauma to healing sockets. However, it's reassuring to know that adjustments can be easily made during follow-up visits [10]. Explaining this to patients before treatment can help alleviate unnecessary worry and anxiety.

(b) **Increased cost and number of visits:** The construction of immediate dentures involves more extended periods of both laboratory work and chairside procedures, along with additional appointments for adjustments and relines. This is because both hard and soft tissues undergo changes after tooth loss. In the long run, a definitive denture will also need to be constructed, leading to increased costs for both the dentist and the patient. Informing patients about these stages can assist them in making appropriate financial preparations [10, 11].

(c) **Inability to assess aesthetics during the try-in stage:** When teeth are extracted simultaneously with the insertion of dentures, there is no opportunity for a prior aesthetic assessment. Consequently, there is a potential risk that patients may not be entirely satisfied with their appearance after the denture placement [8]. At best, the aim is to replicate the existing natural tooth arrangement if it is deemed satisfactory [4].

7.3 Clinical Tips

Managing Challenges in Impressions During the impression-making process, a common issue arises when dealing with highly mobile teeth, as impression material can become trapped in undercuts, potentially leading to unintended tooth extraction. To address this challenge, clinicians can employ a practical technique. They can block the undercuts temporarily with wax or temporary cement, which can be easily removed after completing the impressions. Alternatively, another approach is to temporarily stabilise the mobile teeth using composite resin until the impressions are successfully completed [11].

Preventing Seating Issues Seating problems frequently occur in clinical practice because the denture's fitting surface is created on a cast that undergoes modifications by removing teeth slated for extraction. To avoid this issue, a surgical stent made of clear acrylic can be fabricated on the modified cast and utilised during the extraction procedure. This surgical stent helps compress interfering areas and highlights them as blanched areas through the clear acrylic. This technique aids in performing necessary bone contouring and addressing unwanted undercuts before the denture insertion process [11].

Post-Insertion Patient Instructions It's essential to provide clear instructions to patients following denture insertion. Patients should be advised to wear the prosthesis continuously for the initial 24 to 48 hours, as most swelling occurs during this period. Additionally, patients should refrain from rinsing their mouth for several hours after extractions and avoid engaging in strenuous physical activities during this time [10, 11].

7.4 Essix Type Retainers with Tooth

In certain situations, patients may seek a temporary yet immediate solution to address their missing teeth, with the intention of pursuing a permanent restoration later. For instance, individuals undergoing conventional implant treatment typically face a waiting period of 3–6 months before moving to the prosthetic phase. During this waiting period, it is crucial to maintain the space and provide an aesthetically pleasing and functional interim solution. This is where a temporary immediate prosthesis, such as an Essix appliance, becomes a valuable consideration [12, 13].

The Essix appliance is crafted from a clear thermoplastic sheet, and it incorporates an acrylic tooth to effectively replace the missing tooth. One of the primary advantages of this appliance is that it relies on the existing teeth for support and exerts no pressure on the surgical site. It is particularly suitable for cases where there is limited interocclusal space or a deep anterior overbite [12]. However, it is important to note that this type of provisional restoration is not intended for prolonged use, as it may experience wear and could become uncomfortable for the patient due to its coverage of the remaining natural teeth (Fig. 7.3).

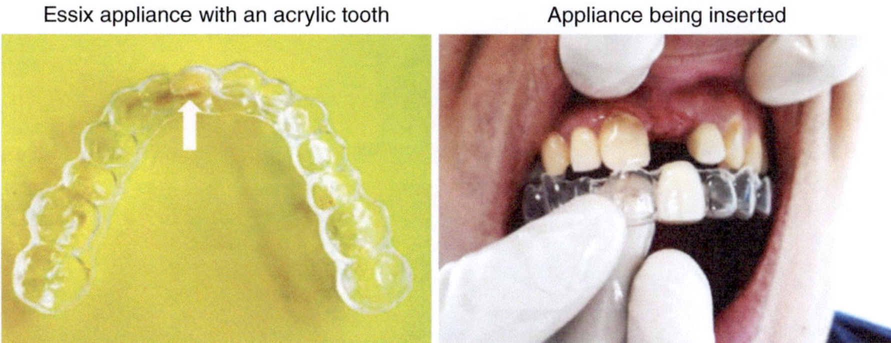

Fig. 7.3 Tooth replacement with Essix appliance

Maintenance Emphasising the importance of properly cleaning the appliance is important as the thermoplastic sheet can lodge bacteria and lead to malodour and discolouration [13]. Advise the patient to brush the retainer with a soft bristle brush and to use retainer cleaning tablets regularly.

7.5 Immediate Resin Bonded Bridge (IRBB)

Resin-retained bridges are now widely acknowledged as a practical alternative to conventional fixed partial dentures (FPD). An IRBB offers a minimally invasive solution for fixed tooth replacement while preserving the structural integrity of the abutment teeth [14] (Fig. 7.4). This option holds particular appeal for young patients grappling with early anterior tooth loss. In such cases, choosing a conventional FPD with extensive tooth preparation may introduce the risk of endodontic complications [14]. Without the IRBB alternative, patients might be faced with the prospect of wearing dentures for an extended period until they reach a stage where growth has ceased, making them eligible for implants or definitive bridges [15].

Furthermore, IRBB can be an excellent choice for patients who are unable to commit to multiple appointments but still desire teeth replacement to avoid aesthetic concerns. It's important to acknowledge that the primary cause of failure in this type of prosthesis is typically debonding, often driven by complex multidirectional stresses among abutments, especially in the case of thee-unit IRBBs [16]. To tackle this issue, the utilisation of two-unit cantilever IRBB has gained popularity. This approach minimises the generation of complex forces on the prosthesis and reduces stress on the single abutment, thus lowering the likelihood of debonding.

Preventing Debonding To prevent debonding, it is essential to secure extensive coverage of the lingual or palatal enamel with the retainer, incorporate a rigid connector with a minimum height of 4 mm, and adhere to a rigorous bonding protocol utilising a cement containing 10-MDP, such as Panavia V5 [17, 18].

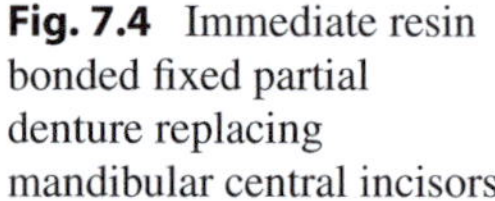

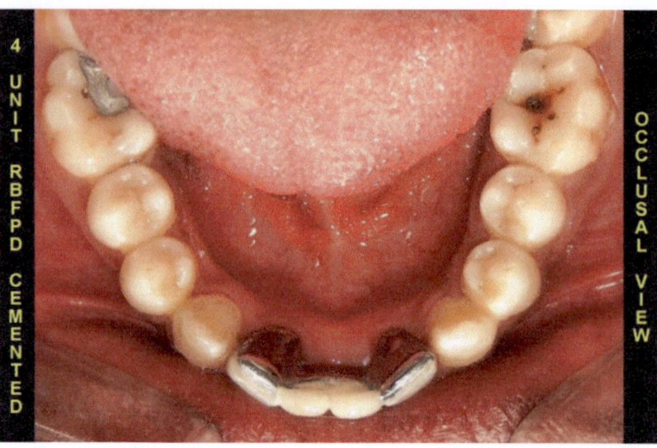

Fig. 7.4 Immediate resin bonded fixed partial denture replacing mandibular central incisors

Occlusal Considerations The effectiveness of this prosthesis hinges significantly on a thorough evaluation of both centric and eccentric occlusal relationships. It is imperative to consistently instruct the laboratory technician to utilise articulated casts and evaluate the palatal aspect to determine the interocclusal space available for the retainer wings and pontics. Ensuring that the pontic does not impede mandibular excursive movements is of utmost importance. If achieving this proves challenging, exploring the possibility of sharing guidance with adjacent natural teeth should be considered [17].

When to Seek Dental Attention In cases where a fixed-fixed IRBB has been utilised, it's imperative to warn patients about the risk of one retainer debonding. They should be encouraged to report any looseness in the bridge immediately. Failure to do so may result in caries developing beneath the debonded retainer, which could jeopardise the prognosis of the abutment tooth [17].

7.6 Immediate Fibre Reinforced Composite Bridge (IFRCB)

The IFRCB represents a minimal-invasive and immediate solution for situations, where one or more teeth require replacement. This prosthetic option is notably conservative, aesthetically pleasing, and cost-effective and offers a 'quick fix' for tooth replacement, achievable in a single session using the chairside direct method [3]. It serves as an excellent alternative for emergency tooth replacements, temporary replacements following implant placement, and for patients with budget constraints who cannot afford a conventional fixed partial denture [3, 19].

In IFRCBs, pontics can be crafted from natural extracted teeth, acrylic resin teeth, or composite resin. To secure the pontic to adjacent teeth, a bondable fibre-reinforced material is utilised. The success of IFRCBs hinges on good oral hygiene practices and maintaining a dry operating field [19].

Bonding to Metal or Porcelain When bonding fibres to porcelain or metal, it's important to be mindful of the potential for debonding. The use of metal and porcelain primers can enhance bond strength and improve the reliability of the attachment [19].

Occlusal Considerations Similar to IRBBs, occlusal considerations are of paramount importance for the success of IFRCBs. Ensuring adequate interocclusal space is essential prior to planning this prosthesis to guarantee its functionality and longevity [3].

7.7 Immediate Implant Placement

In the field of dentistry, a notable trend has emerged wherein dentists increasingly opt for immediate implant placement immediately following the extraction of a compromised tooth [20, 21]. This approach effectively bypasses the traditional waiting period of 4–6 months post-extraction, which is typically required for new bone formation. Moreover, immediate implant placement has demonstrated advantages, including reduced crestal bone loss compared to delayed implant procedures [21].

Furthermore, this method offers the benefits of swifter and more predictable healing, as osseointegration aligns seamlessly with the natural healing process [20, 21]. Importantly, the preserved anatomy of the extracted tooth socket necessitates minimal preparation during immediate implant placement, closely resembling the structure of root-form implants.

Patient Selection Thoughtful treatment planning is essential when considering immediate implant placement. Careful case selection is paramount. Patients lacking sufficient bone apical to the socket, those in close proximity to critical structures like the mandibular neurovascular bundle, maxillary sinus, or nasal cavity, and those with unfavourable anatomical configurations of the remaining bone should be considered contraindications for immediate implant placement [20].

Extraction Technique To ensure the success of immediate implant placement, the tooth must be extracted with utmost care and minimal trauma. This approach is vital for preserving the integrity of the buccal and lingual plates of the extraction socket [21].

Osteotomy Site Preparation Optimal implant primary stability can be achieved by engaging the apical 3 mm of virgin bone beneath the extraction socket. In cases where radiographs reveal periapical infection, it is advisable to perform socket curettage followed by immediate implant placement [20].

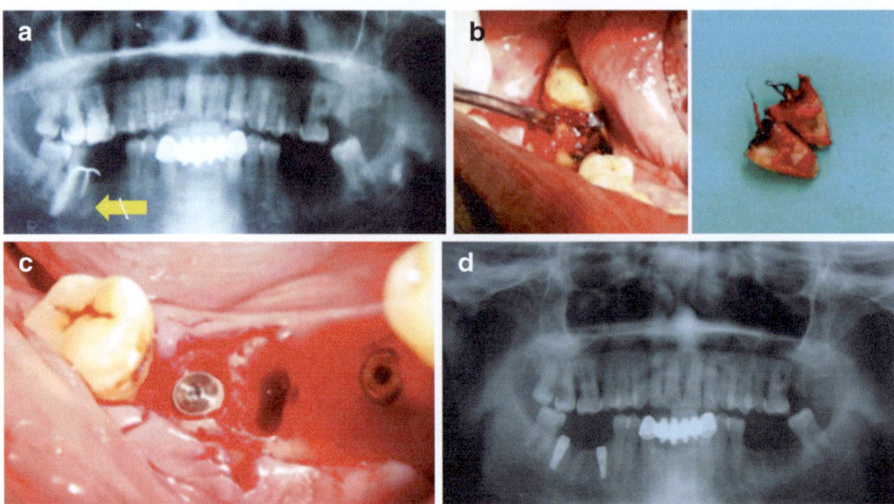

Fig. 7.5 A case of immediate implant placement. (**a**) Preoperative orthopantomogram (OPG) with arrow showing 46 indicated for extraction. (**b**) Extraction of the root stumps. (**c**) Immediate implant placement. (**d**) Post-operative OPG showing implant placement

Cost Considerations Patients should be informed of potential additional costs associated with the possibility of requiring graft placement. Transparent communication about these potential expenses is crucial to ensure patients are well-informed when making decisions about their treatment.

See Fig. 7.5.

7.8 Conclusion

This article explores several options for the immediate replacement of missing teeth. Through comprehensive patient assessments, well-considered treatment planning, and precise clinical techniques, these prosthetic choices can offer immediate solutions to restore both aesthetics and functionality effectively.

References

1. DDU. Guide to consent to dental treatment. 14 September 2022. https://www.theddu.com/guidance-and-advice/guides/quick-guide-to-consent (Accessed September 2023).
2. General Dental Council. Standards for the dental team. Principle Three: Obtain valid consent. 2013. Available at: https://standards.gdc-uk.org/pages/principle3/principle3.aspx (Accessed September 2023).
3. Perrin P, Meyer-Lueckel H, Wierichs RJ. Longevity of immediate rehabilitation with direct fiber reinforced composite fixed partial dentures after up to 9 years. J Dent. 2020; https://doi.org/10.1016/j.jdent.2020.103438.

4. St George G, Hussain S, Welfare R. Immediate dentures: 1. Treatment planning. Dent Update. 2010;37:82–91.
5. Johnson K. A three year study of the dimensional changes occurring in the maxilla following immediate denture treatment. Aust Dent J. 1967;12:152–9.
6. Johnson K. A study of the dimensional changes occurring in the maxilla following closed face immediate denture treatment. Aust Dent J. 1977;22:393–6.
7. Johnson K. A study of the dimensional changes occurring in the maxilla following open face immediate denture treatment. Aust Dent J. 1977;22:451–4.
8. Haeberle CB. Clinical considerations for delivery of immediate dentures. Decis Dent. 2019;5:36–41.
9. Beck CB, Bates JF, Basker RM, Gutteridge DL, Harrison A. A survey of the dissatisfied denture patient. Eur J Prosthodont Restor Dent. 1993;2:73–8.
10. Seals RR Jr, Kuebker WA, Stewart KL. Immediate complete dentures. Dent Clin N Am. 1996;40:151–67.
11. St George G, Lewis NJ, Malton C, Welfare R. Immediate dentures: 2. Clinical stages of construction. Dent Update. 2010;37:154–60.
12. Patel A, Prajapati P, Sethuraman R, Patel JR. Essix restoration: a novel approach for transitional teeth replacement. BMJ Case Rep. 2014; https://doi.org/10.1136/bcr-2013-200422 bcr2013200422.
13. Lally U. A simple technique for replacing extracted anterior teeth using a vacuum formed retainer. J Ir Dent Assoc. 2013;59:258–60.
14. Darbar UR, Hemmings KW, King PA. An immediate resin-bonded bridge using the natural tooth. Dent Update. 1995;22:288–90.
15. Al-Wahadni AM, Al-Omari WM. Immediate resin-bonded bridgework: results of a medium-term clinical follow-up study. J Oral Rehabil. 2004;31:90–4.
16. Prashanti E, Sajjan S, Kumar M. Comparison of stress patterns and displacement in conventional cantilever fixed partial denture with resin bonded cantilever fixed partial denture: a finite element analysis. Indian J Dent Res. 2010;21:59–62.
17. Durey KA, Nixon PJ, Robinson S, Chan MF. Resin bonded bridges: techniques for success. Br Dent J. 2011;211:113–8.
18. Carrilho E, Cardoso M, Marques Ferreira M, Marto CM, Paula A, Coelho AS. 10-MDP based dental adhesives: adhesive interface characterization and adhesive stability—a systematic review. Materials (Basel). 2019; https://doi.org/10.3390/ma12050790.
19. Van Rensburg JJ. Fibre-reinforced composite (FRC) bridge—a minimally destructive approach. Dent Update. 2015;42:360–6.
20. Ebenezer V, Balakrishnan K, Asir RV, Sragunar B. Immediate placement of endosseous implants into the extraction sockets. J Pharm Bioallied Sci. 2015; https://doi.org/10.4103/0975-7406.155926.
21. Lazzara RJ. Immediate implant placement into extraction sites: surgical and restorative advantages. Int J Periodontics Restorative Dent. 1989;9:332–43.

Practical Tips for Resin-Retained Bridge Construction

8

James Baker, Ewen McColl, and Christopher Tredwin

Learning Points

- Appreciate the key role management of the bonding substrate plays in resin-retained bridge provision.
- Understand the parameters of the framework design that will influence success.
- Understand how static and dynamic loads affect biomechanical success of the bridge.
- Recall the steps in the bonding process to optimise adhesion.
- Recognise the need for ongoing maintenance by the patient with the support of the dentist.

8.1 Introduction

In the rush to consider dental implants as replacements for missing teeth, resin-retained bridges (RRB) are often overlooked, but in the correct circumstances, they are often the treatment of choice. In this short paper, we will consider pre-operative considerations, site preparation, fit, cementation, and post-operative care and maintenance. These tried and tested top tips will hopefully facilitate successful outcomes for primary care practitioners utilising this effective treatment modality.

J. Baker
James Baker Dental Practice, London, UK

E. McColl (✉)
Peninsula Dental School, Plymouth, UK
e-mail: ewen.mccoll@plymouth.ac.uk

C. Tredwin
Institute of Dentistry, Queen Mary, University of London, The Royal London Dental Hospital, London, UK

E. McColl, A. Alani (eds.), *Practical Tips in Clinical Dentistry*, BDJ Clinician's Guides, https://doi.org/10.1007/978-3-031-90355-7_8

8.2 Pre-Operative Considerations

For any fixed prosthesis to be deemed successful, it should firstly be able to replicate the appearance of a natural tooth in relation to the gingival tissues, and secondly it must obviously remain attached to its abutments. Addressing this second point, since RRBs rely exclusively on the adhesive bond between the retainer and the abutment rather than traditional concepts of retention/resistance form, the primary concern when planning an RRB is the protection of this adhesive joint. Protection of the adhesive joint can be achieved by paying close attention to the following factors:

8.3 Bonding Substrate

(a) The abutment side of the joint should ideally be completely in enamel as the bond strength to etched enamel is superior to the bond to dentine. Where restorations are present in the part of the tooth to be covered by the retainer, it is advisable to replace these with new resin composite restorations, ideally placed under rubber dam.
(b) The retainer side of the joint should be to a material that can be roughened to provide micro-mechanical retention and one that forms a strong oxide layer (such as non-precious metal alloys) capable of forming a chemical bond to MDP, found in adhesive luting resin cements, notably Panavia.

8.4 Framework Design

(a) To prevent flexure that could cause fracture of the resin cement, the metal framework must be of sufficient thickness (ideally at least 1 mm) to be completely rigid. Connectors should be sufficiently thick to resist flexure in the direction that they will be loaded. In practical terms, this means bucco-palatally in the anterior region and occluso-gingivally in the posterior region.
(b) To increase the surface area for bonding, the retainer wing should cover all available enamel without unduly compromising the aesthetics through a labial show of the metal framework. This should involve extending the retainer wing into proximal areas, to the CEJ palatally, and up to (and, if the patient is willing, over) the incisal edge/cusp tip.

8.5 Loading

Compressive loading of the retainer-cement-abutment complex will not result in damage to the resin cement. Indeed, RRBs are routinely cemented in high, utilising the Dahl principle with no adverse effects. However, subjecting RRBs to excessive flexural loads will increase the risk of failure of the resin cement joint. To avoid this, eccentric occlusal contacts on pontics should be identified and removed whilst maintaining occlusal stops that prevent passive eruption of opposing teeth, which could lead to later unplanned eccentric contacts. Designing occlusal guidance on the wings, however, is perfectly acceptable, so long as the incline is not too steep, which can be said to equally apply to conventional crown and bridgework design.

8.6 Abutment Stability

When a fixed-fixed design is selected over a cantilever design, any differential movement will increase the strain on the resin cement joint, increasing the risk of luting failure. This risk will increase with the increasing mobility of the abutments. Wherever possible, cantilever designs should be chosen, and this is evidenced by improved survival in studies on RRBs. Paradoxically, when teeth are very mobile, fixed-fixed designs are often selected to provide periodontal splinting, but one needs to be especially vigilant of debonds in such cases.

Revisiting the aesthetic considerations of successful RRBs, they should in theory be as able to replicate the natural appearance of teeth as any other porcelain fused to metal (PFM) restoration, perhaps even more so, since there is no limit to the space available for the porcelain, unlike PFM crowns. Where RRBs do tend to fall short compared to implants is at the gum interface. Whereas implant supported crowns emerge through the gum, mimicking a natural tooth, RRB pontics often appear to float above the gum, casting a tell-tale shadow. This problem can be overcome in several ways ranging from immediate placement at extraction, sculpting of the soft tissues using ovate pontics on removable appliances, or by surgical methods, such as electrothermy (Fig. 8.1).

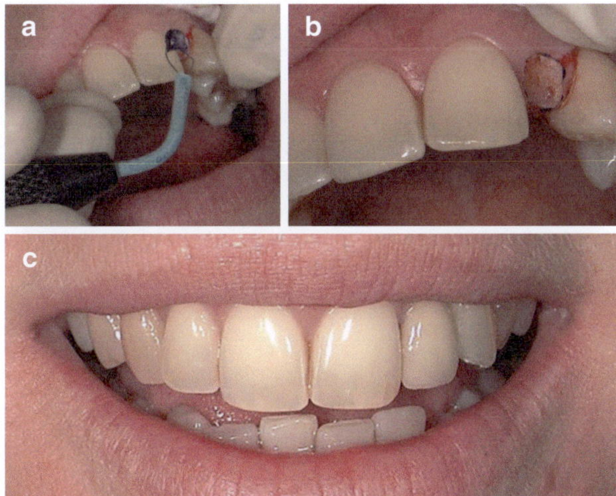

Fig. 8.1 (**a**) Soft-tissue sculpting of the gingiva with electrothermy. (**b**) Newly established soft tissue contour for ovate pontic. (**c**) The cemented bridges extra-orally

8.7 Optimising Preparation of the Site Prior to Impressions

The shade should be selected at the start of the impression appointment to avoid lightening of teeth due to dehydration. Since thin anterior teeth can result in a blue/grey appearance due to metal shining through translucent resin cements, opaque cements are usually advocated. However, this can come at the expense of incisal translucency, so it is sensible to mimic the opacity when selecting the shade. This can be achieved by holding a cotton wool roll palatal to the tooth, or even painting TempBond on the palatal surface (Fig. 8.2).

Since successful RRBs require an enamel substrate to bond to, tooth preparation is generally contraindicated. The only indication for preparing an RRB abutment is to increase the available surface area for bonding, such as the removal of a bulbosity that may limit the path of insertion of the framework. Occlusal reduction is unnecessary, since RRBs are routinely cemented in supra-occlusion. This results in intrusion of the abutment and opposing teeth and passive eruption of the remaining teeth. To increase the available bonding area further, the authors suggest packing two retraction cords and removing the most superficial one just prior to making the elastomeric impressions. Sometimes, more radical retraction may be indicated, such as electrothermy, to uncover more enamel in cases of delayed gingival maturation.

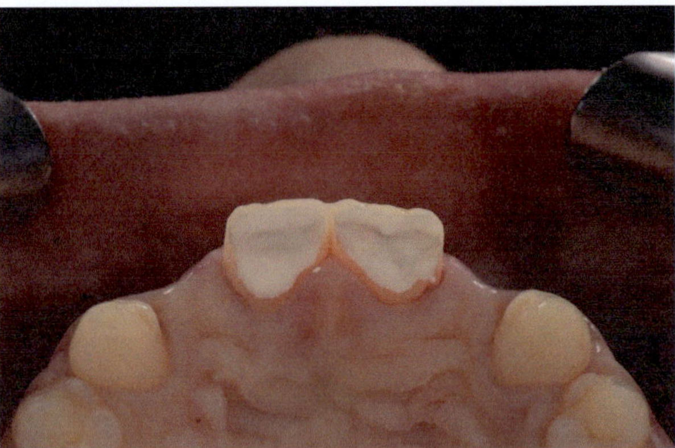

Fig. 8.2 Utilising temp bond during shade taking

8.8 Fit and Cementation

One example of a resin composite adhesive cementation system is Panavia V5 (Kuraray Noritake, Osaka, Japan), which is widely used for the cementation of RRBs and indeed for other restorations, which require to be bonded to dental hard tissue, such as lithium disilicate ceramics. Prior to its clinical use, it is essential to lay out the product and follow the instruction card, explaining to the patient that this is a highly technical cementation process. Asking your dental nurse to read out the instructions can act as a valuable checklist; good communication is key throughout. This material is often not used to its full potential, and it is important to remember that five distinct shades are available: white, brown, universal, clear, and opaque. In the aesthetic zone, although an opaque resin cement is frequently selected, it is advisable to utilise the try-in pastes, which are included in the kit to assess the effect of metal 'shine-through' prior to final bonding. This stage is one that can pay dividends, as the aesthetics of the definitive restoration can often be enhanced. Resin cements are often refrigerated to improve shelf-life, so it is important to allow them to reach room temperature before use or the set will be retarded. Prior to cementation, the surface of the tooth can be prepared by ultrasonic scaling, followed by application of a pumice slurry on a bristle brush or, even better, sandblasting. If the tooth surface has previously supported a RBB retainer or has been restored with resin composite, then sandblasting is essential. The surface should be particle air abraded with 50 μm alumina under rubber dam isolation prior to undertaking the bonding stages.

Because the bonding surface will have been contaminated with saliva during try-in, it is advisable to also sandblast the fit surface of the retainer wings immediately prior to cementation (Fig. 8.3).

Once mixed, the resin cement should be applied thinly to both the tooth and fit surface of the retainer wings to prevent air inclusions. Once seated, it is essential

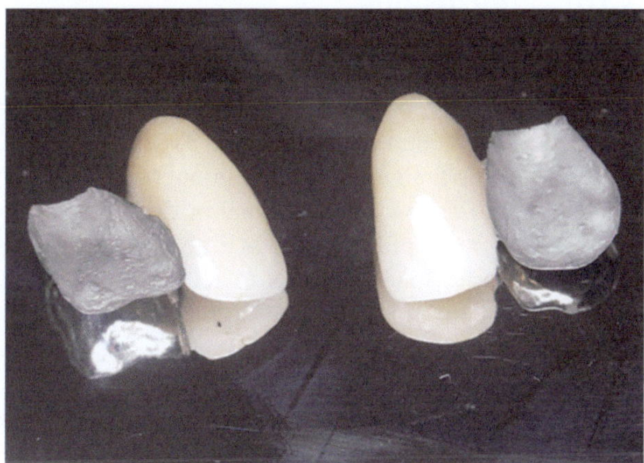

Fig. 8.3 Sandblasted fit surface prior to cementation

that the framework is loaded firmly so that it cannot move during the setting period, which can be as long as 5 min. Opaque cements are generally not dual cure, so immobility is crucial. To ensure complete curing, thew oxygen barrier, often supplied in the cement kit, should be used. To facilitate excess cement removal post-bonding, it is wise to place polytetrafluoroethylene (PTFE) tape interproximally between the abutment tooth and adjacent teeth and below the pontic.

Rotary instruments generate heat and vibrational movement, which can disrupt the bond, so adjustment should be avoided at the fit visit.

8.9 Post-Operative Care and Maintenance Are Key

Most RRBs will be bonded-in high, so there will be a period of several months before pre-operative occlusal contacts are re-established. During this period, orthodontic retainers and occlusal splints should not be worn, as this will prevent relative axial movement of the teeth. Since the interface with RRBs is generally in enamel, they tend to have less issues with microleakage and caries than conventional bridgework, where the preparation is into dentine. That said, the general advice on diet and oral hygiene measures still applies. Where fixed-fixed designs are used, the potential for partial debond poses a risk of caries beneath the retainer wings. Patients should be advised to attend regular recall appointments to check that all retainers are still completely bonded to tooth and to re-attend if they sense any increased movement of the bridge that might denote a partial debond. Should this occur, the pragmatic approach is usually to remove the debonded wing to convert the bridge to a cantilever. Should the bond fail on a cantilever RRB, it will be all too evident to the patient! Thankfully, resolving this is often very straightforward, simply requiring sandblasting of the tooth and retainer and then rebonding. However, if the cause of the debond is diagnosed to be a flexible retainer wing or connector, remaking the bridge after addressing the design faults is advisable.

8.10 Conclusions

RRBs are the ultimate in minimally invasive dentistry, where an entire tooth can be replaced with no removal of tooth tissue or the need to resort to surgery, as is the case for dental implants. They are less expensive, less biologically invasive, and less time consuming than either conventional bridges or dental implants. They are more resistant to caries than conventional bridges and less problematic than implants in periodontally susceptible patients, or those at risk of osteonecrosis. However, even though there are many reasons to recommend RRBs, they are the epitome of a technique-sensitive treatment. Designed and fitted poorly, they are a source of huge frustration for the dentist and patient alike. Executed correctly, however, RRBs provide an excellent solution to tooth loss from all causes, have predictable clinical survival, and, perhaps most importantly, have few negative effects should they fail.

Practical Tips for Implant Dentistry

9

G. E. Bryce and Ewen McColl

Learning Points

- Appreciate the importance of planning the provision of implant restorations and the various different stages and investigations that need to be provided.
- Understand the parameters of implant placement and the associated procedures that may be required.
- Recognise the need for function, aesthetics and cleansibility of the definitive restoration, and how this is achieved.
- Be aware of the need for long-term maintenance once the definitive restoration is provided.

9.1 Introduction

Dental implant placement and restoration is becoming increasingly common within primary care [1]. With this in mind, predictable implant therapy can only be achieved with appropriate assessment, case selection, treatment planning, and provision.

We are often asked by colleagues, 'how do I get started in implant dentistry?' In our view, you need to have a sound understanding of case assessment and diagnostic principles and be able to apply these appropriately, with the construction of a considered treatment plan. Whilst core surgical and restorative skills, achieved via experience within other dental disciplines, will greatly help with initial implant cases, ideally, the formative dental implant clinician should seek mentorship from an experienced colleague. Within this article, we will outline the key factors that we consider most important and discuss issues that we have experienced from our own

G. E. Bryce
Restorative Dentistry, Defence Centre for Rehabilitative Dentistry, Aldershot, UK

E. McColl (✉)
Peninsula Dental School, Plymouth, UK
e-mail: ewen.mccoll@plymouth.ac.uk

E. McColl, A. Alani (eds.), *Practical Tips in Clinical Dentistry*, BDJ Clinician's Guides, https://doi.org/10.1007/978-3-031-90355-7_9

clinical trial and error, questions that have been frequently posed, or observations of failing treatments that could have been avoided if cases had been appropriately planned.

9.2 Assessment and Case Selection

9.2.1 Assessment

1. Identifying the factors that will influence outcome is crucial to success [2]:
   (a) Patient factors: contraindicating medical history, smokers, poor compliance with oral hygiene—bleeding/plaque scores >10%, bruxists, or uncontrolled parafunction.
   (b) Soft tissue factors: high lip line, thin tissue biotype, lack of keratinised mucosa, high scalloped gingiva, and high susceptibility to periodontitis pose challenges for implant treatment, and consent and consideration of risks is crucial.
   (c) Hard tissue factors: tooth/root orientation, dento-alveolar defects (reduced bone volume), proximity of anatomical features (maxillary sinuses, incisive nerve foramen, IDN, lingual sulcus/shelf.

9.2.2 Imaging

We advise the taking of a limited volume CBCT scan for most placements [3] as this facilitates optimal insight/ planning of the implant in harmony with anatomical structures (such as the maxillary sinuses, IDN, and incisive canals and adjacent teeth) equating alveolar bone volume to implant length and platform width and integration with the prosthetic rehabilitation of the implant.

9.2.3 Case Selection

When setting out on your implant journey, choose simpler cases for implant placement, with mentorship. In our opinion, the ideal learning case is the single-bounded premolar site, with adequate keratinised mucosa, paralleled adjacent roots, and bone volume that provides a minimum of 7 mm interproximal, a bucco-palatal dimension of 7 mm, and sufficient height to place a 10 mm implant.

9.3 Treatment Planning

9.3.1 Prosthetic-Guided Implant Planning

The prosthetic rehabilitation should be foremost within the plan for implant placement [4]. The use of diagnostic wax-ups and computer planning software, alongside

CBCT volumes, enables the construct of a surgical plan to direct three-dimensional placement (bucco-lingual, mesial-distal, and vertical planes). The implant plan must account for the implant system's prosthetic interface (for instance, tissue or bone level systems) and whether additional abutments or platform-switching components are required, influencing the depth of placement necessary to achieve a natural mucosal emergence profile from implant to crown. Surgical guides, constructed from the treatment plan work-up, are recommended for all formative implant placements, with designs ranging from simple suck-down Essix-style appliances to fully guided 3D printed devices.

9.3.2 Placement Strategy

The plan should account for the rationales that underpin immediate, early and delayed implant strategies, with application as appropriate [5]. If extraction is required, ensure this is undertaken as atraumatically as possible (Luxators, periotomes) and consider alveolar ridge/socket preservation techniques, if immediate or early strategies not feasible (patient too young, extensive apical infection, or insufficient bone apical to the socket to facilitate primary stability of the implant). The decision on purchasing an implant system should also consider availability of company, educational and mentor support, validated implant outcome data, and manufacturer resilience (to ensure that components will be available throughout the anticipated lifespan of the implant).

9.3.3 Additional Surgical Measures

The plan should encompass the need for both pre-implant grafting (e.g. block-grafting of sinus floor elevation procedures) or grafting at the time of implant placement. It is crucial to stay within your competence zone given the significant complications that may ensue during and after such procedures [6, 7]. Appropriate referral in these cases is similarly essential in order to optimise outcomes for patients. Comprehensive training and mentorship is crucial to developing skills in this area.

9.3.4 Immediate Prosthetic Management

The immediate prosthetic replacement of the implant site should avoid mucosal loading of the implant site, to reduce the risks of mucosal recession or adverse healing. Options include the following: Essix retainer with pontic, flangeless acrylic RPD with extension onto the palatal surfaces of adjacent teeth to provide tooth support, resin-bonded bridge, cemented with glass ionomer cement (for ease of removal).

9.4 Surgical Placement

9.4.1 Core Surgical Skill Competence

(a) Soft tissue and flap management: In our opinion, experience with careful raising of mucoperisteal flaps and suturing should be gained within oral or, ideally, periodontal surgery procedures before considering implant surgery. In early cases, the planned flap design can be drawn on models or photographs to help pre-operative visualisation.
(b) Equipment: In our practice, a range of instruments are recommended to assist with precise surgical management of the soft tissue, including the following: round handled scalpels (allowing the scalpel to be finely manipulated, in a similar fashion to a pen), 15 c or microblade, papillae elevators—specific, flat plastic, Buser P5, and Castroviejo Suture holders. The surgical unit must have motor capable of controlling torque and speed settings to implant manufacturer guidelines and capability to provide sterile saline cooling of the surgical bur.

9.5 Prosthetic Rehabilitation

9.5.1 Provisional Restorations

Provisional restorations can play an important role in achieving optimal aesthetic and functional outcomes. Specific consideration should be given to the use of provisional restorations when there is the requirement to develop the mucosa/papilla within the aesthetic zone and restore multiple teeth/implants, altering or re-organising the occlusal scheme, within a phased treatment delivery strategy or when compliance relapses.

9.5.2 Definitive Restoration

(a) Emergence profile for aesthetics and cleansiblity. The close coordination of care with the dental laboratory technicians may help achieve an emergence profile of implant-retained crowns that optimises aesthetics and mucosal health. With regard to the latter, harmonising the emergence profile to the mucosal tissues may help prevent supracrestal tissue inflammation, which may be a precursor to peri-implantitis [8].
(b) Screw/cement retention. Screw-retained restorations eliminate the risks of soft tissue irritation created by excess cement that may be associated with cement-retained restorations. In addition, from a retrievability and maintenance perspective, screw-retained restorations are advantageous, when compared to cement retained counterparts [9]. However, the requirement to orientate the

conventional screw channel within the cingulum plateau of the anterior restoration is often not feasible, without extensive bone grafting or impairing the aesthetic emergence of the crown. The challenge of maintaining screw channel orientation is further increased when multiple implants are required to support the restoration.

(c) Advantages of angle correction systems. Angle correction systems may be employed at both the implant (commonly for single-unit restorations) and abutment level (for full arch implant-supported fixed prostheses) [10]. At the implant level, angle correction systems employ multidirectional screw-driver heads to allow torqueing of the restoration screw at angle up to 30° from the implant orientation. Subsequently, these systems offer the benefits of conventional screw retention retrievability whilst allowing the implant to be placed in the optimal site for osseointegration and restoration emergence.

9.6 Maintenance and Planning for Complications

9.6.1 Maintenance

Compliance with biofilm control around the implant/restoration interface is key to longer-term implant success and survival, with the importance of this highlighted to the patient during the consent process. Oral care of the implant must encompass both brushing and the use of adjuncts, such as TePe, or, our preferred method, of using floss (Super), wrapped around the implant and 'towelled' below the mucosal margin. Additional adjuncts such as Water/air flossers may be useful but should not replace mechanical plaque removal.

(a) Splint therapy is essential for implant prostheses' survival if patients have parafunctional habits.

9.6.2 Recall and Review

(a) The importance of recall should be emphasised as a component of the consent phase for implant therapy.
(b) Initial review of the implant restoration should be 3 months post-rehabilitation to reinforce oral hygiene compliance.
(c) Further review should be at 12 months for the taking of a six-point pocket chart [11, 12] and LCPA to assess peri-implant soft tissue and bone stability. CGDent Guidelines suggest a baseline radiograph be taken at the time of completion of the prosthodontic phase of treatment with views recommended after a further 12 months. Radiographs may then be taken at intervals of up to 5 years [3] with close monitoring of clinical parameters determining intervals.

9.7 Conclusions

As discussed above, planning, preparation, education, experience, and mentoring are, in our opinion, the keys to successful implant dentistry. The above tips can be considered a useful checklist of key elements to consider in implant dentistry in primary care.

References

1. Public Health England. National Dental Epidemiology Programme for England. Oral health survey of adults attending general dental practices 2018. 2020. Available https://assets.publishing.service.gov.uk/government/uploads/system/uploads/attachment_data/file/891208/AiP_survey_for_England_2018.pdf. Accessed 1 March 2022.
2. International Team for Implantology. SAC assessment tool. Step by step guidance to risk assessment in implant dentistry. Available https://www.iti.org/tools/sac-assessment-tool. Accessed 1 March 2022.
3. Horner K, Eaton KA, editors. Selection criteria for dental radiography. 3rd ed. London: FGDP; 2018.
4. Garber DA, Belser UC. Restoration-driven implant placement with restoration-generated site development. Compend Contin Educ Dent. 1995;16:796–8.
5. Buser D, Chappuis V, Belser UC, Chen S. Implant placement post extraction in esthetic single tooth sites: when immediate, when early, when late? Periodontol. 2000;2017(73):84–102.
6. Barone A, Santini S, Sbordone L, Crespi R, Covani U. A clinical study of the outcomes and complications associated with maxillary sinus augmentation. Int J Oral Maxillofac Implants. 2006;21:81–5.
7. Herford AS, Dean JS. Complications in bone grafting. Oral Maxillofac Surg Clin N Am. 2011;23:433–42.
8. Jepsen S, Berglundh T, Genco R, et al. Primary prevention of peri-implantitis: managing peri-implant mucositis. J Clin Periodontol. 2015;42(Suppl 16):S152–7.
9. Priest G. A current perspective on screw-retained single-implant restorations: a review of pertinent literature. J Esthet Restor Dent. 2017;29:161–71.
10. Cavallaro J, Greenstein G. Angled implant abutments: a practical application of available knowledge. J Am Dent Assoc. 2011;142:150–8.
11. Berglundh T, Jepsen S, Stadlinger B, Terheyden H. Peri-implantitis and its prevention. Clin Oral Implants Res. 2019;30:150–5.
12. British Society of Periodontology. The good practitioner's guide to periodontology. 2016. Available https://www.bsperio.org.uk/assets/downloads/good_practitioners_guide_2016.pdf. Accessed 1 March 2022.

Practical Tips for Managing Implant Complications in Primary Care

10

Neil Macbeth and Ewen McColl

Learning Points

- Recall the methods of preventing complications for implant restorations.
- Appreciate the importance of long-term implant maintenance.
- Understand the various ways in which complications can manifest and the potential techniques to manage them.

10.1 Introduction

Dental implant placement and restoration are becoming increasingly common in primary care [1]. With this in mind, predictable implant therapy can only be achieved with appropriate case assessment, treatment planning, and surgical provision. However, dental team members may be increasingly faced with addressing biological and prosthetic implant complications at the time of implant restoration or after delivery of the final restorative structure. Adler [2] outlines that biological and technical complications following implant placement can range from 32 to 52%. The range and complexity of these prosthetic and biological complications may be reasonably assessed and managed in primary care. In this short article, we discuss a range of frequently occurring complications, with a range of tips on how best to manage these complications in primary care.

A prosthetically driven surgical protocol, which uses an idealised final prosthetic tooth position to determine the correct three-dimensional (3D) spatial relationship for the implant fixture, supports the development of an optimal functional,

N. Macbeth
Defence Centre for Rehabilitative Dentistry, Defence Primary Health Care (DPHC), Dental Centre Aldershot, Hampshire, UK

E. McColl (✉)
Peninsula Dental School, Plymouth, UK
e-mail: ewen.mccoll@plymouth.ac.uk

E. McColl, A. Alani (eds.), *Practical Tips in Clinical Dentistry*, BDJ Clinician's Guides, https://doi.org/10.1007/978-3-031-90355-7_10

biomechanical, aesthetic peri-implant mucosal margin, improving the maintenance outcome for the patient.

Augmentation protocols have also been developed to promote retention of the original bone and soft tissue topographical contour (alveolar ridge preservation), minimise the inevitable post-extraction physiological bone resorption, and influence the bone and soft tissue modelling and remodelling process. The potential to improve the morphology of the healed alveolar ridge and to retain the volume of the alveolar bone foundation enables reconstruction of the ridge using an idealised prosthetic or implant-supported solutions.

10.2 Prevention

10.2.1 Maintenance and Planning for Complications

10.2.1.1 Periodontal health

Healthy peri-implant tissue is characterised by the absence of inflammation and swelling around the implant, no evidence of redness or bleeding on probing (BOP), and the lack of suppuration at the implant-mucosal margin. A stable zone of keratinised mucosa is also seen as being beneficial to the long-term health of the peri-implant tissue, as it prevents tissue displacement during function, aids patient comfort, and facilitates plaque removal.

10.2.1.2 Maintenance

Compliance with biofilm control around the implant/restoration interface is key to longer-term implant success and survival, with the importance of this highlighted to the patient during the consent process. Oral care of the implant must encompass mechanical cleaning through brushing and the use of interproximal cleaning aids (TePe) or, our preferred method, of using floss (Super), wrapped around the implant and 'towelled' below the mucosal margin. Additional adjuncts such as water and air flossers and antiseptic mouthwashes may be useful but should not replace mechanical plaque removal.

10.2.1.3 Biomechanical Complications

Control of occlusal overloading of the implant structure is considered important in order to reduce the risks of implant crown fracture, screw loosening/fracture, retention of the implant retained prosthesis, and an increased potential for marginal bone loss. Screw loosening is one of the commonest causes of implant complications. Screw loosening occurs when the tensile force of the tightened screw is overloaded, leading to loss of the clamping force. Localised bacterial infection can result, leading to per-implant mucosal inflammation, sinus formation, and abnormal loading of the implant. Whilst screw loosening risks can be influenced by implant positioning, type of implant, implant diameter and abutment connection and type of implant appliance, early identification of biomechanical complications is important.

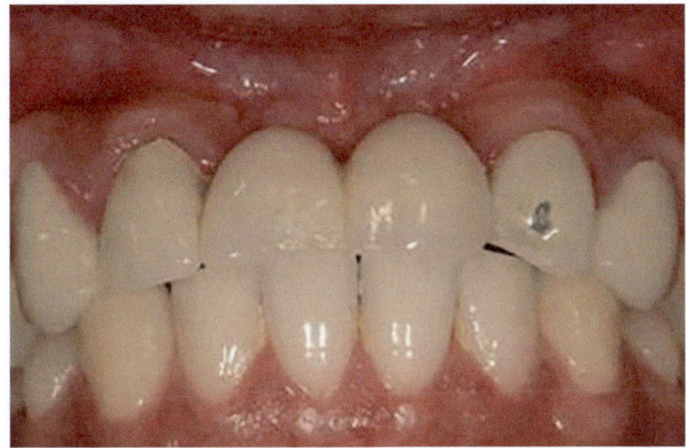

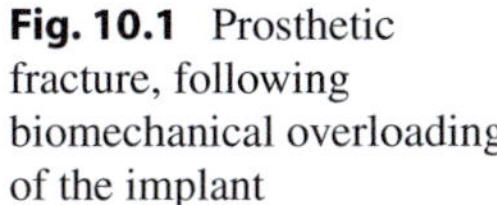

Fig. 10.1 Prosthetic fracture, following biomechanical overloading of the implant

Prosthetic structures should be designed to share both static and dynamic loading with the remaining dentition or implant fixtures configured to distribute the tensile and compressive forces over a wide surface area of the occlusal surface. Adequate consideration should be given to the size of the occlusal surface, the size abutment, accuracy of fit in the implant abutment connection, angle correction, cantilever design, and prosthetic retrievability. The design of the superstructure should also ensure adequate support to porcelain surfaces.

Figure 10.1 shows a prosthetic fracture following biomechanical overloading of the implant.

10.2.1.4 Implant Identification

Replacement of the implant-supported restoration can be undertaken when biomechanical complications occur. However, before remedial treatment is undertaken, it is important to ensure the correct identification of the implant system and abutment components utilised. Identification of implant system can be achieved by review of past patient documentation or models, the calculation of implant dimensions, assessment of external morphology and internal connection characteristics, utilisation of implant identification websites or apps, use of artificial intelligence recognition systems, correspondence with dental implant manufacturer companies (radiograph and intra-oral images), and discussions with professional peer-review groups. Once the implant systems and restorative components have been identified, the replacement crown or bridge prosthetic structure should be adapted to account for the cause factors of the precipitation failure of the appliance. The newly designed appliance should be designed to prevent further mechanical, aesthetic, and phonetic complications.

10.2.1.5 Protection of Prosthetic Structures

Whilst case selection helps to identify risks, post-treatment splint therapy is considered essential to prevent occlusal overloading associated with parafunctional habits such as bruxism and local adaptive habits (nail biting).

10.3 Recall and Review

(a) The importance of recall should be emphasised as a component of the consent phase for implant therapy.
(b) Initial review of the implant restoration should be 3 months post-rehabilitation, to reinforce oral hygiene compliance.
(c) Further review should be at 12 months for the taking of a six-point pocket chart [3] and LCPA to assess peri-implant soft tissue and bone stability. CGDent Guidelines suggest a baseline radiograph be taken at the time of completion of the prosthodontic phase of treatment with views recommended after a further 12 months. Radiographs may then be taken at intervals of up to 5 years [4] with close monitoring of clinical parameters determining intervals.

10.4 Complications

10.4.1 Implant Complications Associated with Systemic Disease

Medical systemic disorders can have longer-term complications for implant patients, making their management more complex. Case selection and risk parameters are important to consider when formalising treatment plans, with careful management of drug usage and patient physiological health considered essential. Conditions that may directly impact implant treatment include myocardial infarction or cerebrovascular disease, bleeding disorders, immunosuppression, diabetes, bisphosphonate medication, psychiatric care, and active cancer treatment. Patients with poorly controlled diabetes mellitus may also suffer from impaired bone formation, an increased risk of peri-mucositis, and peri-implantitis after fixture placement and require elongated treatment times. The overall influence on implant survival is, however, recorded as being negligible [5].

10.4.2 Mucosal Disease

Oral diseases, such as vesicular bullous disease, lupus, and lichen planus, may result in chronic inflammation of the peri-implant tissue, affecting the patient's ability to clean around the crown-implant interface. This local restriction may predispose the patient to a higher level of per-mucositis and peri-implantitis.

10.4.3 Allergic Reaction

Most implants are made of titanium alloy. Even though extremely rare, some patients have been known to present with a hypersensitivity to titanium or another metal. This type IV sensitivity can present as an altered taste, tingling, and inflammation or swelling in the area. Allergy to a resin or acrylic-based prosthetic supper structure is also a possibility and can present as localised discomfort, presenting as a burning sensation, itching, local gingival inflammation, or swelling around the prosthetic structure. If the patient has a potential metal or resin hypersensitivity, allergy testing can be undertaken prior to treatment. In cases with a known allergy, an alternative restorative material can be used, to mitigate against implant removal.

10.4.4 Anatomical and Sensory Risks

Damage to the mental and inferior alveolar nerve is a rare occurrence but can occur during implant placement, resulting in temporary, or permanent sensory impairment. Symptoms may include pain, numbness, hot or cold stimuli, itching, a tingling sensation in the mucosal tissue, or discomfort on occlusal pressure. Early changes not caused by direct nerve damage can include sensory change due to reversible compression of the tissue because of oedema, haematoma, stretching of the flap, and anatomical tissue. Persistent sensory change will require radiographic assessment, onward referral, and accurate recording of oral mechanoceptive, thermal, and chemical tests. Early referral may assist in pharmacological, physical therapy, and monitoring of the patient. Issues associated with implant placement into the maxillary sinus may also require careful patient review and appropriate referral. Chronic sinus pathology (sinusitis), due to perforation of the Schneiderian membrane and bacterial infection, will again require referral and treatment with antibiotics, chlorhexidine mouthwashes, nasal irrigation, and the use of decongestants. If symptoms persist, removal of the implant fixture is required.

10.4.5 Peri-implant Mucositis

The clinical characteristics of peri-implant mucositis include bleeding on probing, erythema, tissue swelling, and/or suppuration. An increase in probing depth is detected clinically due to a loss of tissue integrity and probing resistance. Treatment options include mechanical debridement of the implant restorative interface using hand curettes, ultrasonic instrumentation, air abrasive systems, and occasional adjunctive antimicrobials or antiseptics. Local bacterial infection can sometimes occur due to cementation protocols, incorrect seating of the crown, impaction of deposits into the mucosal tissue, or graft particle sequestra, following guided bone regeneration at implant placement. The sources of abutment-level bacterial infection can sometimes result in the development of a peri-implant abscess. Removal of the healing abutment or prosthetic crown, followed by elimination of any displaced or sequestered graft particle and local debridement, in conjunction with antiseptic irrigation of the tissues, may result in the removal of the initiating factor, allowing tissue healing. Replacement of the implant-supported restoration will be required in the majority of these cases. Persistent chronic infection may require a local tissue flap to be raised to allow the removal of embedded particulates and placement of a local connective tissue where thinning of the mucosal tissue is present.

Figure 10.2 shows abutment level infection, with sinus formation.

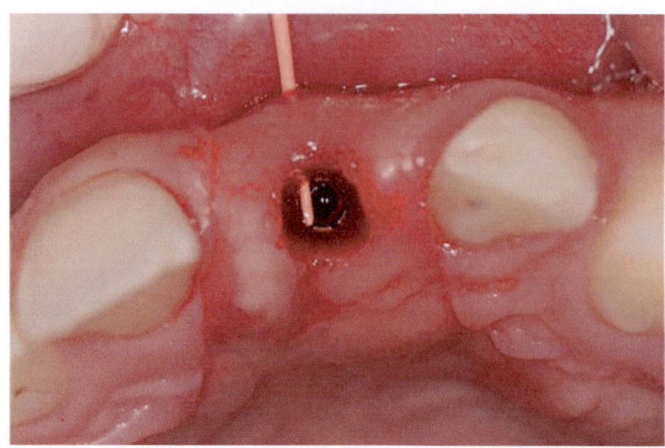

Fig. 10.2 Abutment level infection, with sinus formation

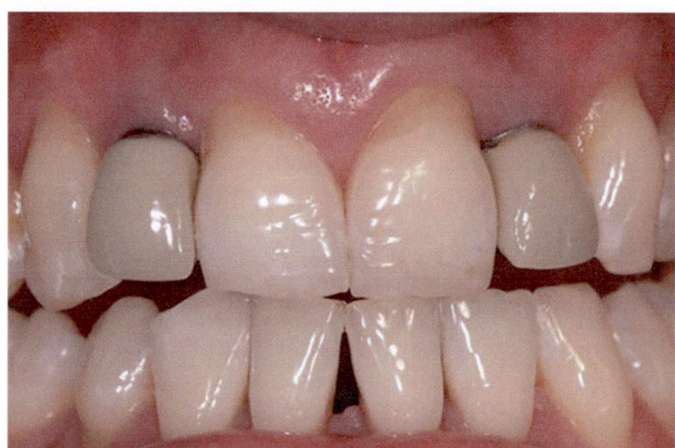

Fig. 10.3 Peri-implant soft tissue recession, following peri-mucositis in a patient with past poor oral hygiene and a thin peri-implant phenotype

10.4.6 Peri-implantitis

Peri-implantitis is a plaque-associated pathological condition, which is the most common complication in implant dentistry. It is characterised by inflammation in the peri-implant mucosa and subsequent progressive loss of supporting bone, following initial implant healing. Increased probing depths are also seen at the implant site. Radiographic bone loss of ≥3 mm, in combination with BOP, and probing depths of ≥6 mm are indicative of peri-implantitis. Suppuration and recession of the mucosal margin are frequently seen.

Figure 10.3 shows peri-implant soft tissue recession, following peri-mucositis in a patient with past poor oral hygiene and a thin peri-implant phenotype.

Risk factors for disease progression include plaque, smoking, history of periodontitis, abutment angle and surface roughness, lifetime of the restoration, and systemic disease (diabetes). Nonsurgical therapy of peri-implantitis cases usually involves mechanical debridement of the implant surface using curettes, ultrasonic devices, air-abrasive devices, or lasers, with or without the adjunctive use of local antibiotics or antiseptics, antimicrobial photodynamic therapy (aPDT), or

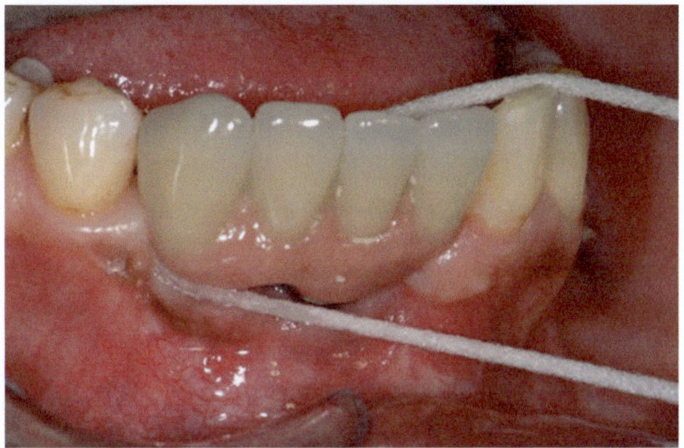

Fig. 10.4 Control of peri-implantitis under an implant bridge using oral health aids

alternative measures (air-abrasive devices, galvanic treatment). Surface chemical and galvanic decontamination of the implant surface alone may not be successful in treating the disease, with surgical pocket elimination, bone recontouring, implantoplasty, and regenerative techniques (bone grafts, guided bone regeneration) often required. Whilst successful treatment of the site requires concurrent plaque control and biofilm disruption, evidence suggests that the regenerative approach can be unpredictable [6].

Figure 10.4 demonstrates control of peri-implantitis under an implant bridge using oral health aids.

10.5 Conclusions

Implant complications are not uncommon and, in most cases, can be managed both by a suitable preventative programme and careful monitoring of the implant and associated restoration.

You can reduce your chance of complications with dental implants by:

- Comprehensive patient assessment prior to implant treatment
- Control of the patient's risk of periodontal disease
- Adoption of a biological approach to implant placement to reduce peri-implant mucosal complications
- Early management of mucosal tissue complication
- Interproximal cleaning reinforcement
- Design of abutment and restorative margins to facilitate plaque control
- Advice on the impact of smoking and tobacco products
- Control of systemic disease risk factors
- Regular visits with your dental professional
- Properly caring for your dental restorations.
- Consider providing your patient with a mouthguard at night to reduce the risk of occlusal trauma and tissue damage

References

1. Public Health England. National Dental Epidemiology Programme for England. Oral health survey of adults attending general dental practices 2018. 2020. Available https://assets.publishing.service.gov.uk/government/uploads/system/uploads/attachment_data/file/891208/AiP_survey_for_England_2018.pdf. Accessed 1 March 2022.
2. Adler L, Buhlin K, Jansson L. Survival and complications: a 9- to 15-year retrospective follow-up of dental implant therapy. J Oral Rehabil. 2020;47:67–77.
3. British Society of Periodontology. The good practitioner's guide to periodontology. 2016. Available https://www.bsperio.org.uk/assets/downloads/good_practitioners_guide_2016.pdf. Accessed 1 February 2023.
4. Horner K, Eaton KA. Selection criteria for dental radiography. 3rd ed. London: FGDP; 2018.
5. Donos N, Calciolari E. Dental implants in patients affected by systemic disease. Br Dent J. 2014;217:425–30.
6. Berglundh T, Jepsen S, Stadlinger B, Terheyden H. Peri-implantitis and its prevention. Clin Oral Implants Res. 2019;30:150–5.

Digital Dentistry for Primary Care 11

Eimear O'Connell, Simon Fieldhouse, G. E. Bryce,
Ewen McColl, and David Claridge

Learning Points

- Identify the various aspects of digital dentistry that can be applied in your clinical environment and how to balance costs and benefits.
- Understand the differences between open and closed systems and the merits of deciding on either for your practice.
- Appreciate the need to design a digital workflow for the delivery of treatment.

11.1 Introduction

As digital dentistry becomes increasingly commonly used in primary care [1], we share some tips that we feel will save time and improve efficiency across primary care. The tips will also facilitate those considering incorporating digital dentistry into their clinical workflow.

E. O'Connell
Dentist at Bite Dentistry, Edinburgh, UK

S. Fieldhouse
The Dutch Barton Dental Practice, Bradford on Avon, UK

G. E. Bryce
Restorative Dentistry, Defence Centre for Rehabilitative Dentistry, Aldershot, UK

E. McColl (✉)
Peninsula Dental School, Plymouth, UK
e-mail: ewen.mccoll@plymouth.ac.uk

D. Claridge
ALS Dental Laboratories, London, UK

E. McColl, A. Alani (eds.), *Practical Tips in Clinical Dentistry*, BDJ Clinician's Guides, https://doi.org/10.1007/978-3-031-90355-7_11

11.2 Getting Started

When integrating digital processes into your practice, it is essential to plan what outcomes you want to achieve from the outset. A digital intra-oral scanner (DIOS), if purchased and used appropriately, enables the delivery of dentistry successfully and more consistently. For example, if you envisage having a scanner as part of an in-house integrated manufacturing process to deliver crowns and bridges, very different workflows and equipment are required when compared to a workflow that is for the construction of orthodontic aligners or externally contracted laboratory work.

Once you have decided on your workflow or digital care pathway, research which scanners are best suited to meet this requirement. This, of course, must be balanced against costs and both hardware and software ease of use. Given the cost of DIOS, practice collaborations to split the cost of the hardware may improve the business case justification for purchase. The user should also consider some of the hidden costs, such as consumables (replacement scanner tips), servicing, and software updates. Dependent on what you need a scanner for, your budget, and how much time you will give to undertaking training for yourself and your team will necessarily help inform your decision. Similarly, so will talking to other clinicians already using digital workflows to find out their personal experience. If possible, attend trade shows and try before you buy. The technique of intra-oral scanning is not an innate skill, it's a learned habit, so familiarise yourself by in vivo scanning in your clinic. Involve all members of your team, as they are stakeholders in the adoption of disruptive technology. This is a capital purchase, and whilst it can be offset against your tax bill, the investment must pay for itself in due course.

11.3 Deciding on a DIOS System

11.3.1 Closed Platform Versus Open Platform System

Open platform saves images as an .stl file dataset (in greyscale) or as a .ply file dataset (which is in colour) for viewing and manipulation and can be transferred and utilised between any manufacturer/laboratory or system operator that employs open platform software. A closed platform, in contrast, limits the user to a single manufacturer/provider. Most platforms have now moved to be able to share openly, and this is a trend that is set to continue.

Each scanner has its own specific 'best' scanning strategy that will optimise capture and stitching of the data to achieve trueness and accuracy. The size of the camera head does equate to the ability to capture a larger field of view, and full arch scanning is easier for the user with some DIOS than others. Again, this emphasises the need to try in vivo scanning before committing to purchase.

The depth of field, the size of the camera, the bulk of the scanning wand, and the ease of handling are different and can affect the outcomes of the digital capture accuracy [2–5].

Full arch implant prosthesis manufacture versus a single crown on a prepared tooth may require differing parameters for delivery of successful outcome, so again, understanding what you want to be able to achieve is paramount to successfully integrating scanning into your practice. For implant scanning, for example, it is important to discuss with your laboratory that their CAD software can read the intra-oral scan bodies provided by your chosen implant manufacturer. After all, scanning is one part of the workflow, and your laboratory must be able to import, read, and design from your scans/scan bodies. Listen to clinicians about why they have the scanner they use and what they can do with it.

11.4 Treatment Planning

A DIOS dataset can be an excellent tool for planning both restorative and orthodontic procedures [6].

Proposed treatments can be digitally 'waxed-up' more simply and cost-efficiently than conventional waxed stone models, with multiple approaches being feasible. This can be especially useful in cases that involve smile aesthetics or changes to the vertical dimension. Time spent with the technician team to ensure harmony of the interface between the DIOS dataset and subsequent CAD/CAM outputs will reduce error and improve the clinical outcome. Another benefit is that proposed treatment plan/s can be easily translated to the patient and, if employed appropriately, can greatly aid the consent process. The ability for patients to visualise 3D images of their teeth and proposed treatment/s is probably the most underrated but powerful tool offered by digital workflows. It builds trust by enhancing understanding.

11.5 Treatment Delivery

The dataset images also allow the clinician to plan key clinical steps either by improving pre-operative visualisation, such as tooth preparation for crowns, or by the construction of precision-guided stents, such as 3D printed implant guides. Subsequently, patient-facing time can be reduced, improving the efficient use of clinical time.

Many of the principles of restorative dentistry (maintaining a dry field, retraction of soft tissues, good preparations, analysis of occlusion) are as applicable to digital workflow as conventional treatment. Practice with your new system is crucial as it takes time to learn both an efficient scanning technique and to become proficient with the software. Subsequently, it is important to plan this learning curve into your diary to afford the necessary time for both you and your team to become proficient users.

A good starting case would involve planning and delivery of a single unit tooth supported implant crown, and progressing from there may be a good option. Prior to this first case, practice scanning with colleagues so that a level of proficiency is already gained, rather than learning with a patient, and the potential added stress this may cause.

11.6 Care Pathways

DIOS datasets can be easily archived and retrieved for future viewing. This can enable novel means of precisely monitoring chronic conditions, such as tooth substance loss. Used appropriately, DIOS can be integrated into at-risk patients' periodic dental inspections to allow both the clinician and patient to accurately visualise dental changes.

Through investment in more equipment and training of the whole team clinicians can carry out full-mouth comprehensive functional and aesthetic dentistry. We use photography, CBCT, intra-oral scanning, in-house production when necessary, and desirable to plan outcomes with our technicians, our team, and the patient. Communication with your team, your patient, and your laboratory is so much better with digital workflows [7], whether they be digital impressions or a full, in-house workflow ending with an in-house restoration made in one visit.

Before starting a procedure, know the desired outcome and how you are going to achieve that using restorative dentistry, orthodontics, or implant dentistry. Guides can be made to help deliver outcomes more predictably. Making sure the hardware and software are set up to work together accurately so that no inadvertent errors are introduced during planning is very important.

The most exciting and rewarding part of the journey is better communication with your in-house team, your laboratory team, and the patients. Your scans can be in your laboratory, wherever they are located, in a couple of minutes. This benefit delivers the opportunity of almost immediate communication, whilst the patient is still in the chair. In fact, your laboratory can dial in remotely and watch you scanning in real time, if required. The laboratory can 'sign off' that they have everything they need for that case. This doesn't just mean the scans. Several DIOS offer shade taking, margin marking, undercut checking tools, occlusal clearance measuring, colour HD photos, multiple bite registrations, extra scans for the case, lateral excursions captured in video, etc.

Patients who can understand what we can deliver and how we can help them in a very efficient and pain-free way are more likely to choose treatment. Patients are actively seeking digital dentistry. The perception is that it is less intrusive and an overall more pleasant experience, which is a powerful motivator. Additionally, seeing a 3D image of your crown preparations is a very effective way of ensuring these are optimal.

Don't forget the potential environmental benefits of digital dentistry. No impression materials, no models, no courier or postal service as required for impressions, and fewer patient visits are all important when considering the environmental impact we have as clinicians.

Dentistry becomes desirable to achieve health, and the patient can see the outcomes. What we do in dentistry is seen as a black art to most people, and this lack of understanding devalues what we do. Digital tools increase trust between patients and clinical teams, and never has that been in shorter supply, so investing in digital integration will enhance your work in ways you never imagined!

11.7 Conclusions

The implementation of digital technology represents an opportunity to improve all aspects of restorative dentistry pathways through removing logistical bottlenecks, improving efficiency and accuracy. The progression to a digital workflow is likely to be onerous initially but rewarding in the long term.

References

1. GFDI. Atlas Dental Study. European markets. Structures, challenges and scenarios. Cologne: Rebmann Research. 2018. Available https://www.gfdi.de/ids-2019/Atlas_Dentalstudie_2018_EN.pdf. Accessed September 2022.
2. Scherer MD. The invention of 3D printing and its impact on dentistry: an interview with check hull. Compend Contin Educ Dent. 2020;41:504–7.
3. Diker B, Tak Ö. Comparing the accuracy of six intra-oral scanners on prepared teeth and effect of scanning sequence. J Adv Prosthodont. 2020;12:299–306.
4. Ender A, Zimmermann M, Mehl A. Accuracy of complete and partial arch impressions of actual intraoral scanning systems in vitro. Int J Comput Dent. 2019;22:11–9.
5. Nedelcu R, Olsson P, Nyström I, et al. Accuracy and precision of three intraoral scanners and accuracy of conventional impressions: a novel in vivo analysis method. J Dent. 2018;69:110–8
6. Sfondrini MF, Gandini P, Malfatto M, et al. Computerised casts for orthodontic purposes using powder free intraoral scanners: accuracy, execution time and patient feedback. Biomed Res Int. 2018;2018:4103232. https://doi.org/10.1155/2018/4103232.
7. Jahangiri L, Akiva G, Lakhia S, Turkyilmaz I. Understanding the complexities of digital dentistry integration in high-volume dental institutions. Br Dent J. 2020;229:166–8.

Part II

Endodontics

12 Practical Tips for Managing Enamel Infractions, Cracks, and Fractures. Part 1: Diagnosis

R. J. R. Smith, Ewen McColl, and G. E. Bryce

Learning Points

- Understand how infractions, cracks, and fractures can develop and the risk factors associated with aetiology.
- Recognise the pathophysiological signs and symptoms and how they relate to the clinical presentation.
- Recall the various techniques for assessment and diagnosis of discontinuities in teeth.

12.1 Introduction

Tooth infractions, cracks, and fractures (ICF) represent mechanically induced discontinuities within the dental hard tissues. Such findings are commonly observed in clinical practice and, whilst often asymptomatic, may be associated with a range of symptoms and/or aesthetic issues. In part 1 of this two-part series, we offer top tips for the assessment and diagnosis of these problems.

R. J. R. Smith
Defence Centre for Rehabilitative Dentistry, Aldershot, UK

E. McColl (✉)
Peninsula Dental School, Plymouth, UK
e-mail: ewen.mccoll@plymouth.ac.uk

G. E. Bryce
Restorative Dentistry, Defence Centre for Rehabilitative Dentistry, Aldershot, UK

E. McColl, A. Alani (eds.), *Practical Tips in Clinical Dentistry*, BDJ Clinician's Guides, https://doi.org/10.1007/978-3-031-90355-7_12

12.1.1 Terminology

(a) Key definitions are shown in Table 12.1. Definitions are adapted from Abbot and Leow [1].
(b) Patients with cracked and fractured teeth may present with a range of symptoms including the following: no symptoms, pain on biting (or release), temperature sensitivity, or (if pulpitis) spontaneous pain. Such symptoms in cracked teeth are often collectively referred to as 'cracked tooth syndrome'. However, this terminology is erroneous because the word 'syndrome' relates to a 'disease', whereas a crack is a clinical finding, not a disease [1].

12.1.2 Aetiology

(a) The high inorganic content of enamel makes it hard but inflexible, with a flexural modulus variously reported to be within the range 10–130 GPa [2].

Table 12.1 Definitions of tooth infractions, cracks, and fractures

	Definition
Enamel infraction	Micro-cracks confined to enamel (Fig. 12.1)
Crack[a]	Defect where there is a break between two parts of a tooth, *without separation of the fragments* (Fig. 12.2) May involve dentine +/− enamel +/− cementum +/− direct communication with pulp
Fracture[a]	Defect where there is a break between two parts of a tooth *and the fragments have separated* (Fig. 12.2) May involve one or more of the following hard tissues: Enamel, dentine, or cementum +/− direct communication with pulp

[a] The terms 'crack' and 'fracture', whilst often used interchangeably, represent distinct clinical situations

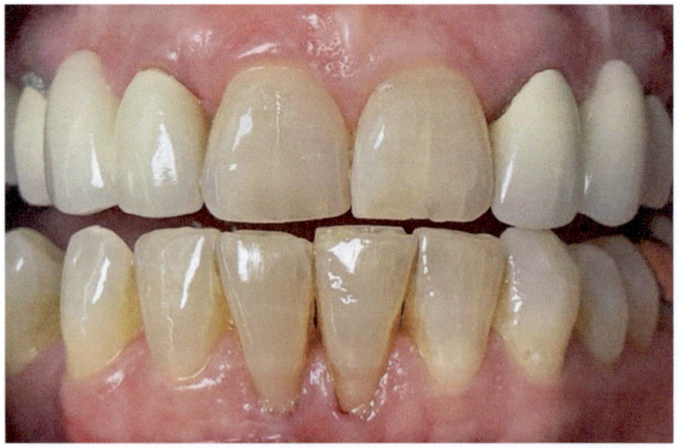

Fig. 12.1 Enamel infractions in anterior teeth

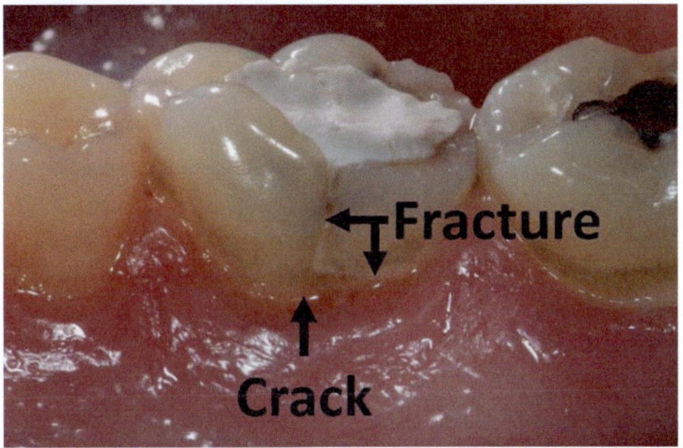

Fig. 12.2 LR6 with vertical crack-line in mid-lingual aspect and fracture of the disto-lingual cusp

However, the relative flexibility of dentine (flexural modulus within the range 10–20 GPa) [3], periodontal (suspensory) ligament, and (to a much lesser extent) alveolar bone, combined with neuromuscular occlusal force feedback mechanisms, reduces the risk of overloading of teeth. However, where the flexural strength of tooth tissue is exceeded, crack initiation may occur and, if the crack propagates, fracture with separation of the fragments may ultimately occur.

(b) ICFs may be caused by acute dental trauma related to events, such as accidents, physical assault, and sporting mishaps. Such incidents should be screened for during the history taking.

(c) The muscles of mastication can generate large occlusal forces. One study reported a patient who could generate a biting force of 575N within the molar/premolar region [4]. Frequent or sustained occlusal forces (associated with parafunctional activity) can be problematic, and a correlation between bruxism and cracks and fractures in teeth has been reported [5]. Parafunction can take several forms, and it is useful to screen for the following habits: clenching/holding teeth together, tapping teeth together, grinding, fingernail chewing, and cheek chewing).

(d) Hard diets (e.g. nuts/bone/ice) may cause ICFs.

(e) Unfavourable inter-occlusal relationships (e.g. non-working side interferences, edge-to-edge incisors/canine relationship, and cusps that occlude with the opposing marginal ridges) can predispose to ICFs. In addition to clinical examination to identify these features, a history of repeated failure of restoration(s) should signal that unfavourable occlusal relationships/forces may be at play.

(f) ICFs may unfortunately also be induced iatrogenically. Awareness of the potential for this to occur, and undertaking mitigating action, should reduce the incidence of this. Areas for consideration include the following: ultrasonics (use lowest power suitable to the task), rubber dam clamp selection (plastic vs metal, or alternatively use of elastic rubber dam stabilising cord), avoidance of excessive wedging forces during compaction of root canal fillings and amalgam, and avoiding use of dentine pins and threaded posts.

12.1.3 Pathophysiology

(a) Dentinal pain, characterised by 'sharp'/intense/short-lasting pain upon application of suitable stimulus (e.g. thermal/sweet/drying/mechanical), may arise in vital teeth with exposed dentine (+/− porosities in enamel) +/− cracks or fractures. The hydrodynamic theory of dentine sensitivity postulates that dentinal pain is related to the induction of transient fluid movement within dentinal tubules (caused by application of a suitable stimulus, which in turn stimulates Aδ nociceptors within the pulp/dentine complex [6]). If, upon removal of the stimulus, the symptoms cease immediately, this suggests that, at that time, the problem is confined to dentine and that significant pulpal inflammation has not yet occurred.

(b) Coronal cracks/fractures may act as a portal for bacteria and their by-products to infiltrate the dentine and pulpal complex, with complications including the following: tertiary dentine formation/calcific metamorphosis (causing yellow discolouration of the crown) (Figs. 12.3, 12.4, and 12.5) and pulpitis (reversible or irreversible) that may ultimately lead to pulpal necrosis and apical disease.

(c) Cracks extending into the root may initiate additional complications within the periodontal ligament complex. For example, periodontal tissues adjacent to an infected crack or fracture will undergo inflammatory events, which classically result in periodontal attachment loss that vertically aligns with the crack, forming a deep narrow periodontal pocket. With further crack propagation to the apex (especially in the case of root fractures), more extensive periodontal destruction may ensue, resulting in the radiographic appearance of crater or (classically) 'J-shaped' bone loss. A further (unusual) presentation of note is an apico-coronal root fracture in a tooth testing 'vital', which can present with a peri-apical radiolucency +/− symptoms of apical periodontitis (typically presenting in maxillary second molars with 'spindly' roots).

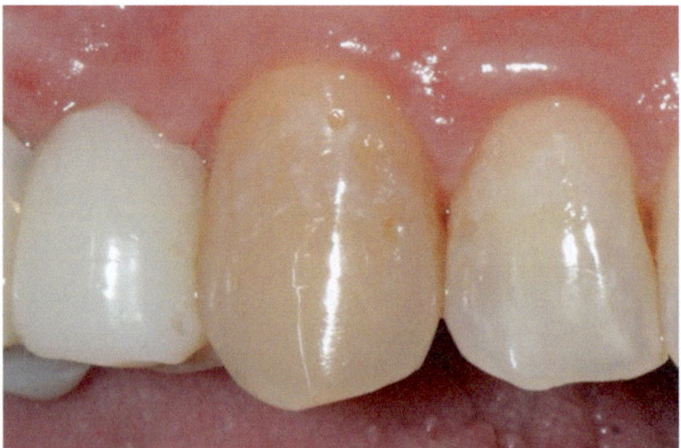

Figs. 12.3 Labial view of an UR3 with yellow discolouration. The tooth had been traumatised 5 years previously

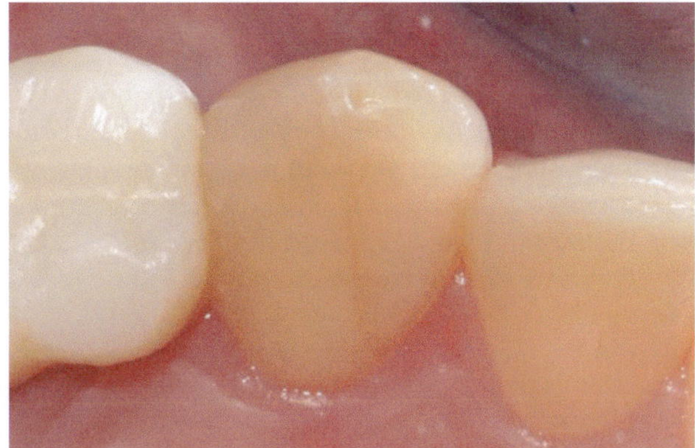

Fig. 12.4 Palatal examination revealed a crack-line. The tooth was asymptomatic and tested positive with electric pulp test (but negative with cold testing)

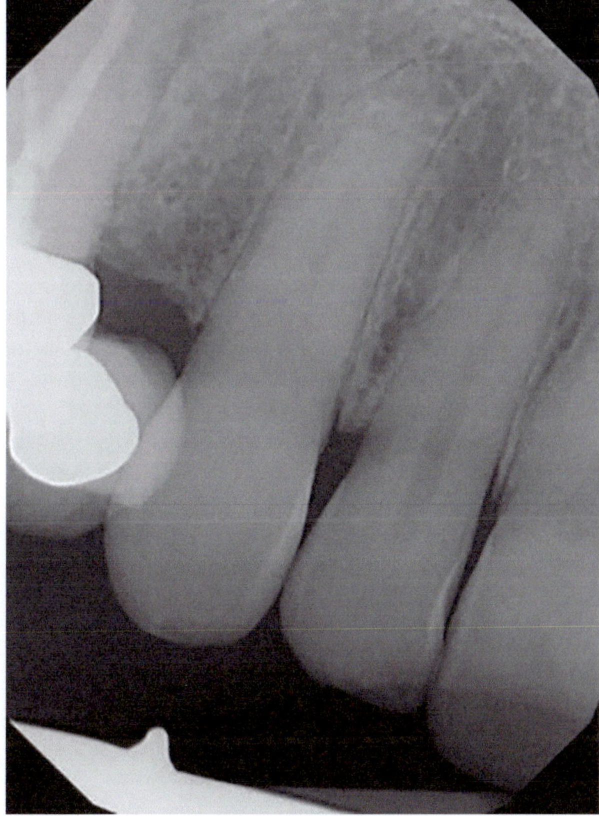

Fig. 12.5 A long cone peri-apical radiograph demonstrated *calcific metamorphosis* and an intact periodontal ligament space. No treatment was deemed necessary, and the tooth was placed under long-term clinical and radiographic review

12.1.4 Practical Tips for Assessment

(a) The aspiration is to either directly visualise the ICF or, in symptomatic cases, achieve ICF localisation by precise replication of the patient-reported symptoms.
(b) Teeth should be dried (with a 3:1 syringe) and examined under good lighting conditions with magnification (loupes or microscope).
(c) Pulp testing with both cold (e.g. Endo-Frost, Coltène/Whaledent, Langenau, Germany) and electric pulp test (EPT) provides a surrogate measure for pulp vitality.
(d) Rubber dam held in place with fingers (or rubber dam clamp) can be readily used to individually isolate suspect and 'control' teeth, prior to application of stimuli relevant to the patient's pain history. For example:
   (i) Cold or warm water can be syringed into the dam to form a pool around the tooth and left for several seconds before being aspirated out.
   (ii) Air may be blown over the tooth using a 3:1 syringe.
(e) The character of pain (e.g. sharp/aching/throbbing. etc), intensity of pain (using a visual analogue scale 1–10), and duration (fleeting or lingering) should be determined. Taken together, these findings can help localise the *source* of pain and the structure(s) involved (e.g. specific tooth/cusp and whether dentine/pulp +/− peri-apical tissues). It should be noted that sometimes pulpless teeth with vertical root fractures may sometimes give a false positive test with a hot/cold stimulus due to fluid percolation through the fracture line to the periodontal ligament.
(f) Transillumination of teeth may demonstrate cracks/fractures by virtue of the refraction phenomenon at the crack/fracture boundary (Fig. 12.6). However, the effectiveness of transillumination is reduced in teeth with restorations and not possible in teeth with full-coverage restorations. Where (direct/indirect) restorations are removed as part of a restorability assessment, it is useful to carry out transillumination (again) once the tooth structure is revealed.

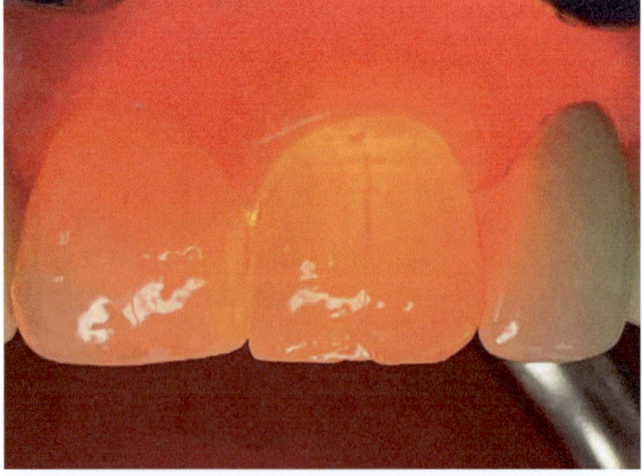

Fig. 12.6 Same case as shown in Fig. 12.1, with transillumination of the upper left central incisor tooth highlighting enamel infractions

(g) A Tooth Slooth (Professional Results, Laguna Niguel, USA) is a plastic device for identifying teeth/specific cusps eliciting pain on biting (or, following biting, upon release). The device should be used methodically, placing it on one specific cusp at a time and asking the patient to bite onto it. The patients reported pain experience (if any) should be recorded for each tooth/ cusp of interest.
(h) Deep narrow periodontal defects associated with cracks or fractures may be subtle and can easily be missed. A UNC15 probe is well-suited for periodontal assessment and should be carefully 'walked around' the tooth/teeth of interest—noting the pocketing profile. Where inflammation is present, the patient may signal particular discomfort on periodontal probing, and an underestimation of pocket depth may be made. In such cases, we would advise the administration of infiltrations of local anaesthesia prior to re-probing. It should also be noted that whereas the buccal and palatal/ lingual aspects are usually readily accessible for periodontal probing, where a proximal tooth contact exists, access to probing in that area will be compromised. In such cases, where a class II restoration is present and requires removal, the gingival sulcus at the proximal surface(s) should be re-probed after removal of the restoration.
(i) Dyes, such as methylene blue, may also be used in the detection of cracks in teeth.
(j) Two-dimensional radiographs will not directly demonstrate fractures unless the X-ray beam is within 4° of the plane of fracture [7]. However, appropriate intraoral radiographs may be indicated if there is no previous or recent imaging available in order to screen for caries/defective restorative margins/crestal bone levels/peri-radicular pathology.
(k) Three-dimensional radiographic imaging (e.g. cone beam computerised tomography) has been shown to able to predictably detect root fractures in the lab-based setting [8]. However, in the clinical situation, the reliability of CBCT for the detection of root fractures is limited by voxel size (linked to the need to keep radiation dose as low as reasonably practicable) and the degree of separation of the fractured portions potentially being below the limit of resolution. Additionally, where the tooth has been previously root-filled, imaging artefacts caused by gutta-percha can frustrating attempts to screen for root fractures [9]. However, as previously mentioned, the finding of deep localised or 'J-shaped' radiolucency (on either 2D or 3D radiographs) is characteristic of the pattern of bone loss associated with cracked or fractured roots (Figs. 12.7 and 12.8).

12.1.5 Practical Tips for Diagnosis

(a) Following assessment, relevant provisional or (ideally) definitive diagnoses are made based on triangulation of findings.
(b) Causes of signs and symptoms other than cracks/fractures must be identified (and managed) including the following: dentine sensitivity secondary to gingival recession, caries, non-carious tooth surface loss, or defective restorations.

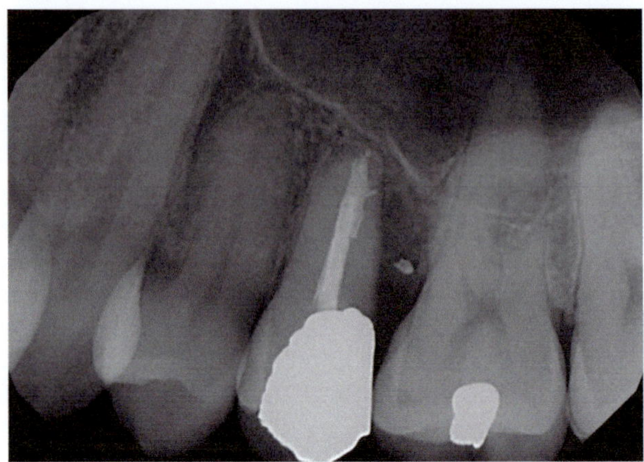

Fig. 12.7 Localised infrabony defect distal to a root-filled upper UL5 tooth

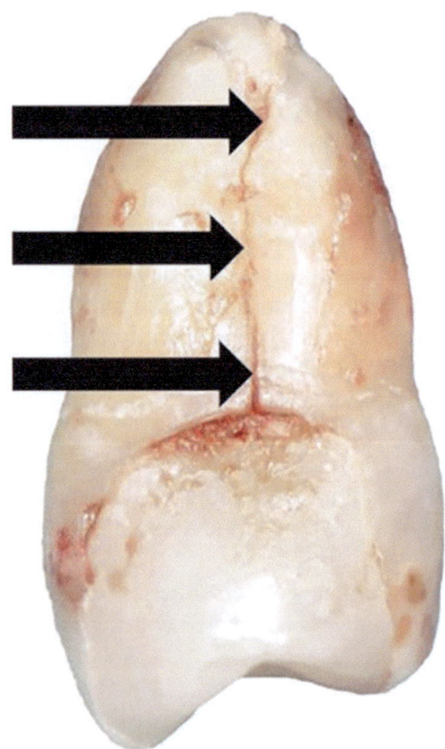

Fig. 12.8 A restorability assessment of the UL5 tooth (shown in Fig. 12.7) revealed that the root was cracked, deemed not predictably restorable, and extracted. Crack-line is arrowed

(c) The following diagnoses may be appropriate within the context of cracked or fractured *vital* teeth:
  (i) Enamel infraction
  (ii) Enamel or enamel-dentine fracture +/− pulp exposure (e.g. complicated or uncomplicated)
  (iii) (Apico-coronal) root fracture +/− (clinical symptoms of) pulpitis
  (iv) Dentine sensitivity secondary to crack/fracture
  (v) Reversible pulpitis secondary to crack/fracture
  (vi) Irreversible pulpitis secondary to crack/fracture
(d) The following diagnoses may be appropriate within the context of cracked or fractured *non-vital* teeth:
  (i) Apical periodontitis (acute or chronic) secondary to crack/fracture
  (ii) Perio-endo lesion secondary to crack/fracture of root

12.2 Conclusion

Discontinuities in teeth are a complex challenge as they can provide a diagnostic conundrum for both patient and clinician. Understanding the aetiological basis for disease development is key for subsequent management and treatment.

References

1. Abbott P, Leow N. Predictable management of cracked teeth with reversible pulpitis. Aust Dent J. 2009;54:306–15.
2. Lu C, Nakamua T, Korach C. Effective property of tooth enamel: monoclinic behaviour. J Biomech. 2012;45:1437–43.
3. Kinney J, Balooch M, Marshall G, Marshall S. A micromechanics model of the elastic properties of human dentine. Arch Oral Biol. 1999;44:813–22.
4. Edmonds H, Glowacka H. The ontogeny of maximum bite force in humans. J Anat. 2020;237:529–42.
5. Lobbezoo F, Manfredini D, Bracci A. Bruxism. BMJ Best Practice. 2022; Available at: https://bestpractice.bmj.com/topics/en-gb/708. Accessed May 2023.
6. Brännström M. A hydrodynamic mechanism in the transmission of pain-producing stimuli through the dentine. In: Anderson D, editor. Sensory mechanisms in dentine. Oxford: Pergamon Press; 1963. p. 73–9.
7. Rud J, Omnell K. Root fractures due to corrosion. Diagnostic aspects. Scand J Dent Res. 1970;78:397–403.
8. Guo XL, Li G, Zheng JQ, et al. Accuracy of detecting vertical root fractures in non-root filled teeth using cone beam computed tomography: effect of voxel size and fracture width. Int Endod J. 2019;52:887–98.
9. Patel S, Brady E, Wilson R, Brown J, Mannocci F. The detection of vertical root fractures in root filled teeth with periapical radiographs and CBCT scans. Int Endod J. 2013;46:1140–52.

Practical Tips for Managing Enamel Infractions, Cracks, and Fractures. Part 2: Management

13

R. J. R. Smith, Ewen McColl, and G. E. Bryce

Learning Points
- Understand the principles of preventing discontinuities in teeth.
- Appreciate the challenges in restorative management of these issues.
- Recognise the various stages in definitive restoration delivery.

13.1 Introduction

In this chapter, we will be looking at treatment strategies for infractions, cracks, and fractures. Restorative intervention must be preceded by a comprehensive assessment and (at least a provisional) diagnosis as this provides the basis for the aims and objectives of treatment.

13.1.1 Patient Discussions Related to Management of ICF

(a) The prognosis for teeth with ICFs is largely dependent on the location and extent of break(s) and whether or not the defect(s) extend below the attachment level. However, there is often uncertainty about the absolute depth of any given ICF and whether its further propagation can be ultimately arrested.

R. J. R. Smith
Defence Centre for Rehabilitative Dentistry, Aldershot, UK

E. McColl (✉)
Peninsula Dental School, Plymouth, UK
e-mail: ewen.mccoll@plymouth.ac.uk

G. E. Bryce
Restorative Dentistry, Defence Centre for Rehabilitative Dentistry, Aldershot, UK

E. McColl, A. Alani (eds.), *Practical Tips in Clinical Dentistry*, BDJ Clinician's Guides, https://doi.org/10.1007/978-3-031-90355-7_13

(b) The consent process should include discussion about the following: the uncertain outcome for cracked/fractured teeth, potential for pulpal complications (if these are not already manifesting), potential need for root canal treatment (RCT), or need for extraction if symptoms do not settle/tooth splits (and is deemed non-restorable).

13.1.2 Practical Tips for Prevention

(a) Following the identification of ICF and associated aetiological factors, bespoke preventative advice should be delivered, which may include recommendations to:
   (i) Avoid clenching/grinding/tapping/or holding teeth together.
   (ii) Avoid chewing fingernails/inside of cheeks/pens or using teeth as ‘tools’ (e.g. cutting tape/opening bottles/stripping wire, etc.).
   (iii) Avoid chewing on particularly hard or abrasive foods, such as nuts/bone/ice, etc.

(b) Additionally, where relevant, the patient should be provided with:
   (i) An occlusal splint for wear during sleep. In the absence of confirmed (nocturnal) bruxism, for diagnostic purposes, the ‘occlusal’ surface of the splint may be lightly abraded with 50-micron alumina powder, producing a matt finish—subsequently after a period of wear, shiny marks are left on the splint in any areas of repeated contact with opposing teeth. The patient and splint should be reviewed 4–6 weeks after fitting to assess compliance with splint wearing and review the splint itself for evidence of damage associated with parafunctional activity.
   (ii) A mouth protector for use during contact sports.

13.2 Practical Tips for Restorative Management

13.2.1 Enamel Infractions

See Figs. 13.1 and 13.2.

(a) These defects do not usually require any treatment. However, micro-cracks provide an entry point for diet and tobacco-derived chromophores to penetrate the enamel, which may cause staining. Beyond dietary modification and tobacco cessation advice (as applicable), management of this situation should begin with mechanical removal of surface stains. Further to this, a course of bleaching may be undertaken to break down and remove subsurface staining compounds.

(b) Bleached teeth with enamel infractions remain liable to ‘rebound’ staining unless the enamel surface is subsequently sealed (e.g. with an adhesively bonded composite resin layer). The long-term maintenance implications of placing such restorations (e.g. need to periodically polish and ultimately replace) should be discussed within the consent process.

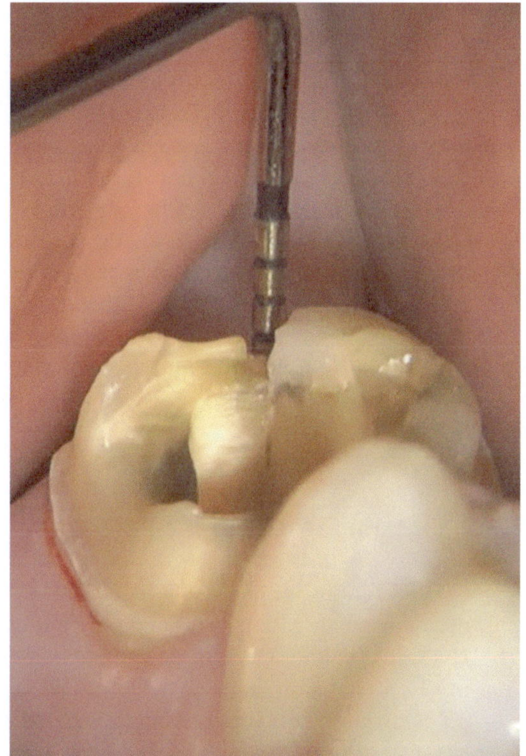

Fig. 13.1 Restorability assessment confirmed a stained crack-line running mesio-distally through this LR6 tooth. A localised 7 mm probing defect was detected at the distal aspect, adjacent to the crack-line, indicating extension of the crack into the root. The tooth was deemed to be not predictably restorable and extracted

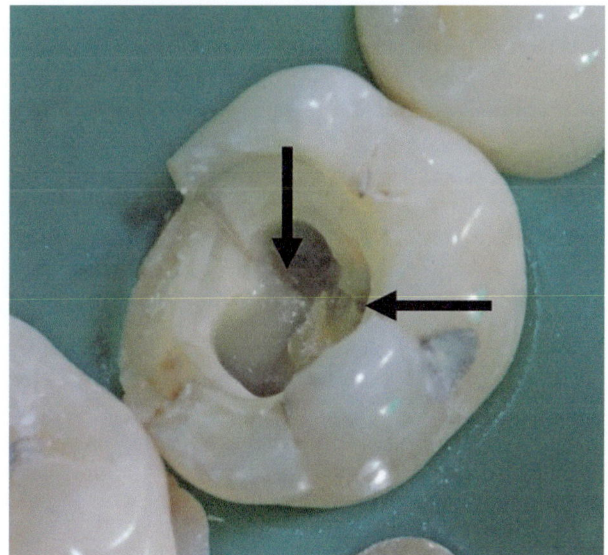

Fig. 13.2 Restorability of another LR6 (the same case as shown in Fig. 13.2 of Chapter 12) revealed stained crack-lines extending into the mesial root canal orifices. The tooth was deemed to be not predictably restorable and extracted

13.2.2 Restorability Assessment

(a) Pre-existing restorations (where present) and defective tooth tissue (caries/unsupported enamel/cracked/fractured cusps) should be removed. The use of magnification and transillumination is recommended within this stage. After taking into account the quantity, quality, and distribution of tooth tissue for ferrule effect (+/− crown lengthening surgery), a decision is made as to whether, and how, the tooth can be predictably restored.
(b) Where the tooth is deemed to be predictably restorable (and where time allows within the appointment), a definitive direct composite resin restoration (cuspal-coverage in case of posterior tooth) may be placed, or otherwise a provisional restoration should be placed (see Sect. 13.2.4).
(c) Management for tooth deemed to not be predictably restorable is summarised in Sect. 13.2.7.

13.2.3 Management of the Pulp

(a) Considerations influencing the decision of whether to try and preserve the pulp of a vital tooth with a traumatic pulp exposure are shown in Table 13.1.
(b) Hydraulic calcium silicate cements (HCSCs) have been recommended for use in VPT in both immature [2] and permanent teeth [3] with traumatically exposed pulps. Both mineral trioxide aggregate (MTA) and biodentine (Septodont, Saint Maur des Fosses, France) are HCSCs, which may be used within pulp capping and pulpotomy procedures, but as such, there is limited evidence as to whether one is biologically superior to the other in these situations [1]. However, one factor that influences HCSC selection is that MTA causes grey staining of tooth tissue (unlike biodentine) [4]. Therefore, when an HCSC is indicated for use within the clinical crown or coronal-third of root, biodentine is the material of choice.

Table 13.1 Considerations influencing the decision of whether to try and preserve the pulp of a vital tooth with a traumatic pulp exposure

Favouring VPT (e.g. pulp cap or pulpotomy)	Favouring RCT
Asymptomatic	Symptoms of (irreversible) pulpitis
Immature root/open apex	Root development complete/closed apex
Small pulp exposure (≤1 mm) [1]	Large pulp exposure (>1 mm)
Early presentation (within hours)	Delayed presentation
>50% of clinical crown remaining, supra-gingival cavity margins, and margins in enamel	<50% of clinical crown remaining, and requirement to use pulp chamber/root canal to retain core or post/core

(c) VPT and RCT must both be carried out within an aseptic field, achieved via measures including:
   (i) Isolation with rubber dam.
   (ii) Disinfection of the tooth (following isolation) with a cotton wool pledget soaked in a 1–3% sodium hypochlorite solution).
(d) Where there is a need to dress the pulp/root canal prior to definitive endodontic management, suitable non-setting intra-canal medicaments should be used, such as:
   (i) Non-setting calcium hydroxide, which is both antibacterial and non-staining.
   (ii) Ledermix (Aspen Pharmacare Australia, Dandenong South, Australia). This paste has both anti-inflammatory and anti-bacterial properties, which makes it particularly suitable for use in cases of symptomatic pulpitis. However, Ledermix can cause stained tooth tissue [5], so it ideally should not be placed above the level of the cemento-enamel junction.
(e) In general, the authors suggest that where a cracked or fractured tooth has associated symptoms of irreversible pulpitis, the definitive endodontic management is most predictably managed via RCT.

13.2.4 Provisionalisation

(a) Where definitive restorative management of the tooth cannot be completed within a single appointment, a provisional restoration is required to provide the following: mechanical protection/bracing for thin/cracked tooth tissue, antibacterial seal over dentine/pulp, +/− sedative effect for inflamed pulp.
(b) In posterior teeth, reduction of guiding cusps by 2 mm and balancing cusps by 1.5 mm is recommended to provide space for placement of adequate bulk of restorative material as a protective overlay.
(c) Options for intermediate restorative materials:
   (i) *Glass ionomer cement (GIC)* can be quickly placed/shaped/polished and has the advantages of inherent adhesion to tooth tissue and reasonable aesthetics (suitable for anterior and posterior teeth).
   (ii) *Zinc oxide eugenol (ZOE) cement* (e.g. IRM, Dentsply Caulk, Milford, USA) combines the advantages of an antibacterial seal (if optimally placed when still 'sticky') and sedative effect on pulp via its eugenol content [6]. However, the eugenol component may negatively affect the quality of any subsequent attempts for resin bonding within the same cavity [7]. Additionally, whilst the sedative effect of ZOE can be helpful in relieving symptoms in the short term, the authors have noted that symptoms can return upon removal of the dressing and placement of a non-eugenol-containing restoration. A final consideration is that IRM is bright white in colour, and this may pose an aesthetic issue (albeit as a short-term restoration).

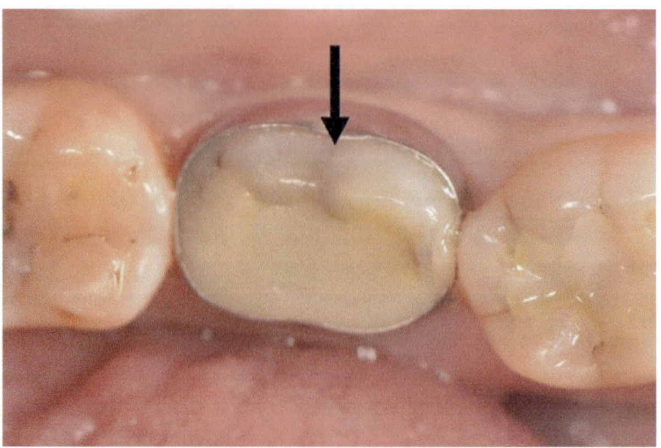

Fig. 13.3 LL7 with crack (arrowed), stabilised with orthodontic band prior to definitive management

(d) A posterior tooth may also be stabilised via its encirclement with a suitable-sized/adapted orthodontic band (Fig. 13.3):
   (i) In general, bands are usually only placed in situations where ultimately it is considered that the tooth in question is to be restored with a cast cuspal-coverage restoration. Therefore, where contact points are tight, inter-proximal space for the band may be created by the use of interdental polishing strips or where the tooth has been previously restored with class II restorations, a flame-shaped high-speed diamond bur may be used to create space.
   (ii) An orthodontic band is chosen from a commercially available selection box. A suitably sized band should fit snuggly over the tooth and, after trying-in, can be removed with an excavator.
   (iii) To cement the band, the tooth should be isolated and dried; GIC should be liberally applied circumferentially to the internal aspect of the band and the band placed over the tooth and pushed down into position using an orthodontic 'band pusher' (or alternatively cotton wool roll)—asking the patient to bite down to provide the force required for seating. After allowing the material to set (+/− light curing in the case of a resin-modified GIC), excess cement and metal protruding above the occlusal table is removed/polished with a suitable high-speed diamond or white stone. Excess cement at the inter-proximal and gingival aspect of the band can be removed with an ultrasonic scaler.
   (iv) The patient should be asked to confirm that there are not sharp areas detectable with the tongue, and where present, these should be addressed to prevent soft tissue irritation/injury.
   (v) At a future appointment, when the band is to be removed, it can simply be sectioned with a high-speed bur, loosened with an ultrasonic (if necessary), and removed with tweezers. Remnants of GIC can be polished off or removed with an ultrasonic scaler.

13.2.5 Definitive Restoration

(a) Recommendations for restoration of cracked/fractured posterior teeth:
  (i) Provision of cuspal-coverage.
  (ii) Preferably indirect restoration (e.g. casting) for molars.
  (iii) Conservative preparation for indirect restorations (e.g. onlay vs 3/4 crown, vs full-coverage crown).
  (iv) Direct (e.g. composite resin overlay) or indirect restoration for premolars. Select direct restoration if insufficient tooth tissue for ferrule.
(b) Recommendations for the restoration of cracked/fractured anterior teeth:
  (i) Composite resin restoration if >50% of tissue of the clinical crown remains, and margins can be placed in enamel.
  (ii) Crown if <50% of coronal tooth tissue has been lost.
  (iii) RCT and post/core placement required if insufficient tooth tissue for core (to retain casting).
(c) For discoloured teeth, consider vital or non-vital bleaching (as indicated) prior to definitive restoration.

13.2.6 Vertical Root Fracture

(a) Where a vertical root fracture is diagnosed in a multi-rooted tooth, it may be possible (following RCT) to undertake resection of the affected root whilst preserving the remaining roots [8], so facilitating continued function of the tooth. Otherwise, teeth with vertical root fractures are considered to have a hopeless prognosis.

13.2.7 Tooth Deemed Not Predictably Restorable

(a) Following a restorability assessment, where a tooth is deemed to be not predictably restorable, arrangements should be made for extraction +/− prosthetic replacement as indicated.
(b) Where the tooth to be extracted is in the aesthetic zone and/or a dental implant supported restoration is being considered as the prosthetic replacement (and immediate implant placement is deemed not to be feasible), consideration should be given to using alveolar ridge preservation techniques at the time of extraction. The rationale for this is to minimise the amount of post-extraction bone loss and gingival recession, so as to optimise the site for prosthetic replacement [9].

13.2.8 Follow-Up

It is important to provide long-term follow-up for teeth with ICFs to assess and deliver timely management for any for endodontic, periodontal, or other complications.

13.3 Conclusion

In this chapter, we have appreciated the various challenges in managing tooth discontinuities, especially when trying to maintain pulp vitality and supporting the surrounding tooth tissue from propagating further apart, resulting in further issues. Assessment of the extent of the discontinuity provides the indication on how best to manage the tooth, through provisionalisation, definitive restoration, or tooth removal in cases of a hopeless prognosis.

References

1. Bjørndal L, Simon S, Tomson P, Duncan H. Management of deep caries and the exposed pulp. Int Endod J. 2019;52:949–73.
2. Bogen G, Chandler N. Pulp preservation in immature permanent teeth. Endod Topics. 2012;23:131–52.
3. Krastl G, Weiger R, Filippi A, et al. European Society of Endodontology position statement: endodontic management of traumatized permanent teeth. Int Endod J. 2021;54:1473–81.
4. Camilleri J, Atmeh A, Li X, Meschi N. Present status and future directions: hydraulic materials for endodontic use. Int Endod J. 2022;55:710–77.
5. Kim ST, Abbott PV, McGinley P. The effects of Ledermix paste on discolouration of mature teeth. Int Endod J. 2000;33:227–32.
6. Abbott P, Leow N. Predictable management of cracked teeth with reversible pulpitis. Aust Dent J. 2009;54:306–15.
7. Carvalho C, de Oliveira BJ, Loguercio A, Reis A. Effect of ZOE temporary restoration on resin-dentin bond strength using different adhesive strategies. J Esthet Restor Dent. 2007;19:144–52.
8. Patel S, Bhuva B, Bose R. Present status and future directions: vertical root fractures in root filled teeth. Int Endod J. 2022;55:804–26.
9. Macbeth N, Trullenque-Eriksson A, Donos N, Mardas N. Hard and soft tissue changes following alveolar ridge preservation: a systematic review. Clin Oral Implants Res. 2017;28:982–1004.

Identifying Endodontic Case Complexity: Part 1

14

Saiba Ghafoor, Matthew Philip Sarstedt, and Julie K. Kilgariff

Learning Points

- Identify the main patient-related factors that may influence endodontic complexity.
- Understand the features of a radiograph that relate to the complexity of the proposed endodontic treatment.
- Recall how the utilisation of CBCT can identify the source of pain in cases of non-odontogenic origin.

14.1 Introduction

Increased tooth retention in an ageing population [1] poses challenges for specialist endodontic services. Older adults may have more complex medical histories that impact dental care, such as frailty, dementia, and multi-morbidity (two or more chronic conditions, including respiratory or coronary heart disease and type 2 diabetes) [2]. Due to the coexistence of multiple long-term conditions, patients increasingly experience polypharmacy, with 44% of patients over 65 taking five or more medications [3]. In addition, tooth-related challenges in an ageing population can present difficulties: treating the increased prevalence of root caries increases the risk

S. Ghafoor
Leeds Dental Institute, Leeds, UK

M. P. Sarstedt
University of Sheffield, School of Clinical Dentistry, Sheffield, UK

J. K. Kilgariff (✉)
Dundee Dental Hospital & Research School, Dundee, UK
e-mail: julie.kilgariff@nhs.scot

E. McColl, A. Alani (eds.), *Practical Tips in Clinical Dentistry*, BDJ Clinician's Guides, https://doi.org/10.1007/978-3-031-90355-7_14

of pulpal exposure [4]; secondary and tertiary dentine deposits can make root canals more tortuous to negotiate [4]; and restorative cycles result in multiple pulpal insults, reducing the pulp's regenerative capacity [5].

Today, it is desirable to retain one's natural dentition in a comfortable, functional, and aesthetically acceptable state to allow engagement in normal, everyday activities [6]. This demands clinicians provide more complex endodontic treatment, frequently including dismantling indirect restorations, root canal retreatment, and periradicular surgery.

This article discusses tips for identifying more complex cases and discusses tools available to guide assessment and identification of complex cases, which may benefit from referral.

14.2 Referral of Endodontic Cases

There is variation between UK health boards on what is considered suitable for specialist services and/or secondary care, complicating the issue of when to treat or refer. Thorough, structured dental assessment allows clinicians and patients to make decisions about teeth regarding benefits, risks, predictability and cost-effectiveness of treatment, and whether referral is warranted and beneficial to achieve a predictable outcome, minimising treatment risk and harm. The outcome of endodontic treatment is known to be influenced by the dentist's skill [7], and thus, pre-treatment identification of endodontic case complexity is essential. Difficult endodontic cases pose an increased risk of iatrogenic error, which can directly reduce treatment success [8].

14.3 Assessing Endodontic Case Complexity: Patient Factors

Patient factors can affect tooth prognosis. For example, cases with restricted mouth opening, patients who cannot lie supine, or who have a tremor tend to increase the complexity of care. Individuals who cannot or will not tolerate a dental dam make endodontic treatment an impossibility due to safety risks such as the inhalation or ingestion of irrigants or files. Reduced endodontic outcomes are associated with microbial contamination of the root canal system from saliva if a dental dam is not used. In addition, some studies suggest medical conditions, such as diabetes, may reduce endodontic treatment success [9], thought due to the alterations in immune functions and gingival crevicular fluid [10].

Furthermore, the use of medications such as bisphosphonates, antiplatelet or anticoagulants, or a pre-existing bleeding condition may influence the decision on whether to try retaining a tooth in order to avoid risking the development of medication-related osteonecrosis of the jaw (MRONJ) or risk of post-operative bleeding following extraction [11]. It is noteworthy that the placement of subgingival rubber dam clamps is considered invasive dental procedures for those patient cases at risk of infective endocarditis [12].

14.4 Assessing Endodontic Case Complexity: Radiographic Interpretation

An up-to-date, appropriate radiograph is an essential part of the pre-operative endodontic assessment. The gold standard view for diagnosing and treatment planning endodontic cases is a paralleling periapical [2, 13]. This should clearly show the radiographic apex of the root(s) and at least 2–3 mm of surrounding periradicular tissues, allowing analysis of pathology and root morphology [14]. This is the image of choice due to high sensitivity identifying periradicular pathology (being almost twice that of panoramic radiographs) and specificity is similarly high, indicating a high probability of a true negative rate [15].

Two-dimensional imaging allows visualisation in a mesiodistal plane only, and diagnostic yield may be improved by taking two periapical views of the same tooth, at different angles (using parallax shift) [13]. Both horizontal and vertical parallax shifts can be useful. Using this, the more distant object appears to move in the same direction as the tube shift, while the closer object appears to move in the opposite direction. Figure 14.1 shows examples of the benefit of using horizontal and vertical parallax shifts in assessing endodontic cases.

Table 14.1 summarises key features usually identifiable from paralleling periapical views that impact endodontic case complexity and therefore treatment planning.

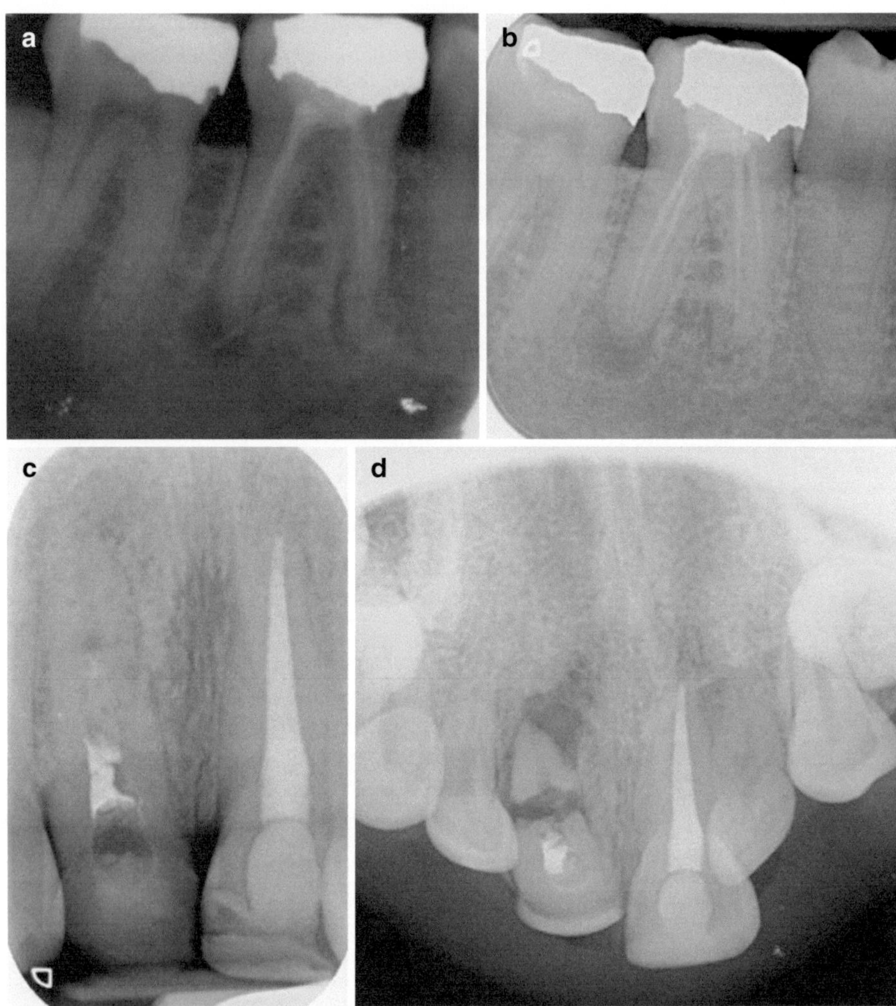

Fig. 14.1 Images **a** and **b** show an example of horizontal parallax shift during assessment of a patient referred with pain from previously root canal treated tooth 46. The X-ray tube head is more mesially positioned in image **b**, which reveals there are four previously obturated canals, not the three suggested in image **a**. Image **c** is of tooth 11 referred by the patient's GDP stating a perforation and internal root resorption in tooth 11 was identified when root canal treatment was commenced. The patient relates a history of trauma and describes a lateral luxation of tooth 11. A maxillary occlusal radiograph (Image **d**) sheds light on a different diagnosis: an unhealed mid-third horizontal root fracture and periradicular changes are seen. This is an example of a vertical parallax shift, which shows the horizontal root fracture more clearly than the periapical image (**c**), clarifying the diagnosis and steering treatment planning

Table 14.1 Relevant radiographic features for endodontic treatment planning

Caries and coronal restoration(s)	Caries, if present, should be removed to allow assessment of tooth restorability and facilitate placement of a good quality coronal seal for the duration of endodontic treatment. For predictable restorability, a tooth requires 1.5–2 mm supragingival height supragingivally and 1 mm width of dentine [16] Providing endodontic treatment through existing restorations can help retain the rubber dam clamp but may hinder visibility and decrease restoration retention [16]. Furthermore, access through crowns can cause the operator to lose orientation (as shown in Fig. 14.2), increasing the risk of iatrogenic error. The possibility of detecting caries, cracks, or marginal breakdown is reportedly enhanced with restoration removal [17]
Pulp stones	Figure 14.3 shows calcifications known as pulp stones, often seen radiographically, which vary in size and can be attached, embedded, or free in the pulp [18]. Endodontic management can be more complex if canal orifices are concealed or blocked by pulp stones [19]. Loose pulp stones can be inadvertently displaced into root canals, blocking access and increasing treatment complexity
Canal calcification/ pulpal obliteration	Root canal size reduces with ageing [20] and pulpal obliteration (clinically, manifesting with a yellowing of the clinical crown) is a known complication of dental trauma luxation injuries [21]. Root canal systems hard to discern radiographically, because of significant size reduction, will generally be harder to locate and prepare clinically, increasing risks of iatrogenic errors and therefore increasing treatment complexity
Root canal morphology and tooth position	A good working knowledge of the expected number of canals for each tooth type is advisable [18, 22]. Radiographic 'fast-breaks' (Fig. 14.4) indicate division of the canal. Canal division increases endodontic case complexity because of the technical challenges successfully navigating bends, divisions and merges in root canals [18] There are several common anatomical variations, many increasing complexity; these include additional canals, 'c' or 's' shaped canals, and dens invaginatus [23]. Individual teeth have variable morphology; for example, Fig. 14.5 shows two canals in a mandibular incisor. Carrotte [22] (2004) highlights that 58% of mandibular central and lateral incisors have one canal, whilst 42% have two canals Pre-operative radiographs allow an opportunity to identify canal morphology and measure estimated working lengths. Particularly long roots are more challenging to prepare and fill and therefore may require referral. In addition, radiographs may highlight excessively angled or rotated teeth, sometimes disguised clinically by extra-coronal restorations. Such teeth have a higher chance of iatrogenic error, particularly perforations, when cutting access into the root canal system. Root canal re-treatments are generally accepted as being more complex than primary cases, although the standard of previous treatment and presence of iatrogenic errors will influence this. Various iatrogenic errors can be identified radiographically, as shown in Fig. 14.6

(continued)

Table 14.1 (continued)

Severity of canal curvature(s)	Generally, the more severe the canal curvature, the more challenging root canal treatment will be because iatrogenic errors, such as blockages, ledges, and potentially perforations, are more likely to occur. 'S' or 'C' shaped curves (Fig. 14.7) particularly complicate endodontic treatment. Curvatures are not always visible radiographically, depending on their direction and because of superimposition, although taking parallax views may help identify these. When identified pre-treatment, the technical challenge these present for successful instrumentation and obturation should be noted and onward referral considered for particularly severe curvatures, if necessary [18]
Radiographic root end/apex	The anatomical apex (i.e. 'true' working length) is often 1–2 mm from the radiographic apex [13]. Open apices are more challenging to endodontically manage, and referral for specialist input is encouraged. The shape of the radiographic apex/root end may be affected by root end resorption, for example, stemming from chronic inflammation or orthodontic tooth movement, which can result in blunting of the apex [24]. If a significant length of root end has been lost, a pseudo-open apex may be present, increasing endodontic complexity, and, if sizeable, may need to be managed as an open apex case. Generally, if a file or gutta-percha tip of a size 50 does not bind (friction fit) at the working length, the case can be considered as an open apex, and obturation using a mineral trioxide-based material is preferable. This may necessitate referral for placement of such material under magnification
Periradicular radiolucencies	The inflammatory response following pulp necrosis takes time to show radiographically and is ultimately seen as a widened periodontal ligament and apical radiolucency [25]. It is notoriously difficult to determine the histopathology of a lesion from its radiographic appearance; however, the larger a radioluency is, the more likely it is to be cystic. This increases the complexity of cases, and therefore radiolucencies approaching, or in excess of 1 cm diameter, should be considered for referral to a specialist in the first instance. Fig. 14.8 illustrates such a case. Cysts can be associated with resorption and displacement of roots, and those showing these factors are less likely to be a radicular cyst [25]
Root fractures	Vertical root fractures are generally only seen radiographically when the tooth root has split, as illustrated in Fig. 14.9. Horizontal root fractures can often be diagnosed with the use of a periapical and occlusal film, but these too can be challenging to visualise. Cone-beam CT scans are helpful if it is essential to clarify if a fracture is present Radiographic features of root fractures vary and include the following: Widening of the periodontal ligament, separation of root fragments, presence of a 'radiographic halo' on each side of the root (Fig. 14.10), 'J' shaped radioluency (Fig. 14.11), and bifurcation radiolucency [26]
Resorption	Several types of root resorption may be seen radiographically. Only some impact on endodontic treatment planning by increasing treatment complexity. Those which can increase complexity are: • Resorption related to pulpal degeneration or necrosis (external and internal infection-related resorption). • Cervical root resorption. • Those which create a pseudo-open apex due to loss of the apical constriction in a tooth which is non-vital. • Replacement resorption, most often as a consequence of significant periodontal ligament damage, for example, following avulsion or intrusion dental trauma injuries.

Table 14.1 (continued)

Anomalies	Various anomalies affecting root canal treatment can occur. For example: **Dens invaginatus** This developmental malformation, an example of which is shown in Fig. 14.12, is a folding of enamel into dentine, most commonly affecting maxillary lateral incisors and affecting 0.3–10% of the population [27]. Where this anomaly is identified, it is advisable to check the contralateral tooth. Treating such teeth endodontically is more complex, and as such, referral is advocated **Clinically:** The crown may appear normal or be dilated, peg [28] or barrel-shaped, or have a deep foramen coecum **Radiographically:** A pear-shaped invagination of enamel and dentine is seen **Taurodont teeth** **Clinically:** Taurodont teeth are associated with syndromes such as down's and Klinefelter's syndromes and ectodermal dysplasia [28]. Teeth have large pulp chambers, a long 'trunk' (cervical area) with the root bifurcation or trifurcation placed apically **Radiographically:** An extended length cervical area is seen, and as root canal orifices are more apically placed, this complicates identification and instrumentation for root canal treatment. **Additional cusps or projections, for example, talon cusps** **Clinically:** Talon cusps protrude from the tooth with enamel covering a dentine core that usually contains pulp tissue and a slender pulp horn [28] **Radiographically:** A pulp horn is seen [28] For endodontic treatment, it is important that the pulp tissue present in the additional cusp or projection is accessed and removed
Previous endodontic management: Non-surgical	Endodontic re-treatment outcome is influenced by the presence of a pre-operative periapical lesion, apical extent of root filling, and quality of coronal seal [29] Iatrogenic errors, although not always identified radiographically, are known to decrease treatment outcome [9, 30]. Errors that may be identified radiographically are: • **Short root fillings** may be the result of a blocked canal (when dentine and pulp debris are packed into the canals 'apical third, resulting in loss of working length). Blockages can be avoided using copious irrigation and recapitulation with small files [31]. • **Excessive overfills** of obturation materials tend to be problematic if the material is an irritant to the periradicular tissues, if microbes/biofilm is carried on the material(s) from within the root canal system into the extraradicular tissues, or if the overfilled material affects an adjacent structure, such as a neurovascular bundle. In each of these cases, various signs and symptoms can ensue, and if symptomatic, further treatment is likely to be required. This treatment will be of a more complex nature and referral is recommended. • **Ledging** may be avoided by pre-curving instruments, avoiding forcing instruments into the canal, using nickel titanium files or, if using stainless steel hand files, using a step-back preparation technique [31]. • **Perforations** can result from ledges or transportation of a canal when, for example, a large, stiff file is used in a curved canal, causing zipping. Incorrect orientation of the access cavity can also result in perforation [31]. • **Instrument separation/fracture** within the canal or beyond the canal confines can be avoided by using appropriate techniques such as establishing a guide path using a size ten stainless steel hand file in the canal prior to entering it with rotary files, always using files in a wet canal, examining files prior to and during treatment to insure each is intact, and using magnification [32].

(continued)

Table 14.1 (continued)

Previous endodontic management: Surgical	Previous periradicular surgery identified clinically or radiographically will have an impact on treatment planning if the tooth is symptomatic and requires further treatment to retain it Modern materials and techniques for periradicular microsurgery are associated with high success rates [33]. The different surgical techniques used can impact endodontic treatment planning, and any tooth to have had surgery in the past is more complex to manage and referral to a specialist for surgical revision using microsurgical techniques prudent. The radiographic appearance of a tooth to have been surgically managed using modern techniques is usually different from that done as a traditional 'apicectomy' (Fig. 14.13). Identifying this difference is relevant for endodontic treatment planning because symptomatic cases treated using traditional techniques (associated with low success rates) may be re-treatable using modern, microsurgical methods and therefore referral may be of benefit. Cases previously treated using modern microsurgical techniques and materials can also have surgical re-treatment/revision if needed, but success rates are lower than that for 'first time' root-end microsurgery

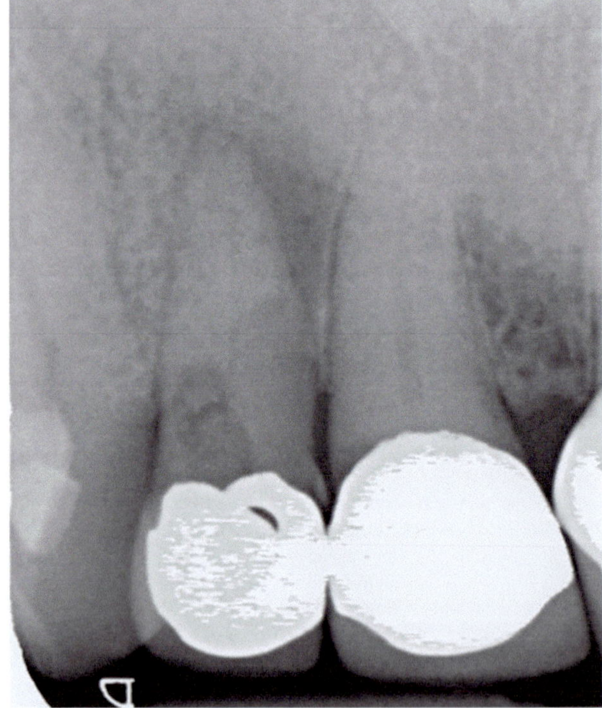

Fig. 14.2 Radiograph of a referred case where access to the root canal system through an existing metal-ceramic crown was attempted, but the root canal system was not found. The radiograph demonstrates loss of orientation when searching for the root canal system and associated significant dentine removal

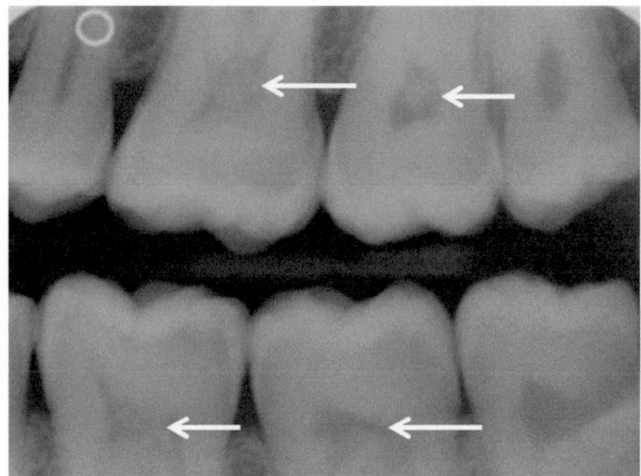

Fig. 14.3 A bitewing radiograph shows evidence of calcific change and pulp stones in several teeth

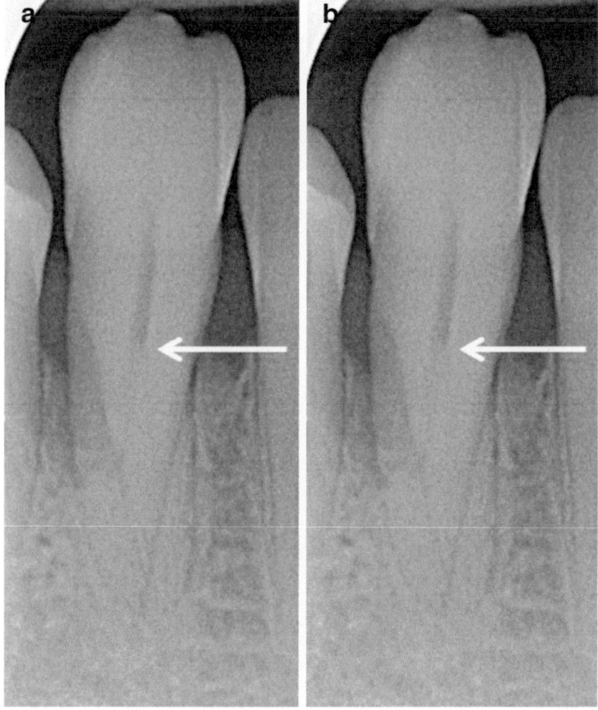

Fig. 14.4 Two examples of radiographic 'fast breaks' are shown. This is where the root canal system is clearly visible for some of the way along the root length and then abruptly becomes harder to discern. This appearance indicates the division of the main root canal into two or more branches. Image A: a premolar tooth where one canal splits into two. Image B: a less commonly seen case of a mandibular canine with two separate roots, each with one canal

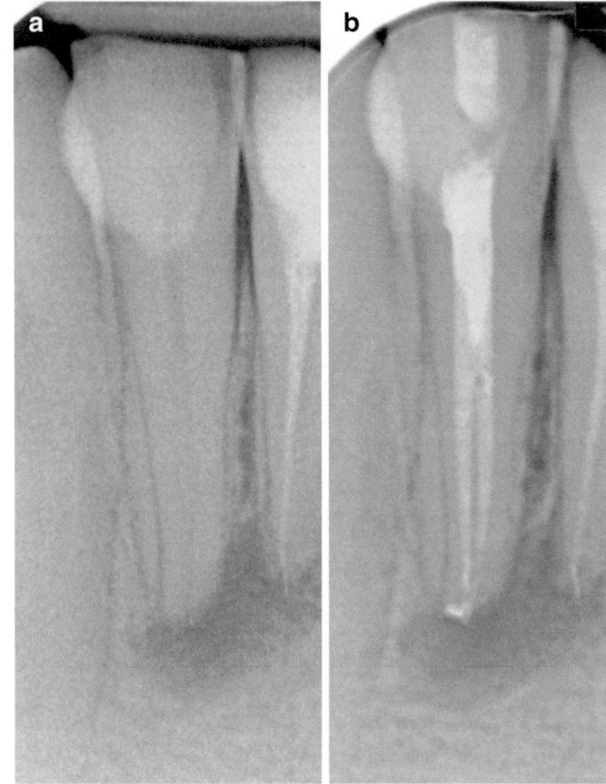

Fig. 14.5 A fast-break is seen in tooth 42. The referring dentist located the root canal system but encountered a 'blockage' a few millimetres into the root canal. This 'blockage' was the point of canal bifurcation. Precurving small stainless steel hand files is of help in successfully negotiating such anatomy

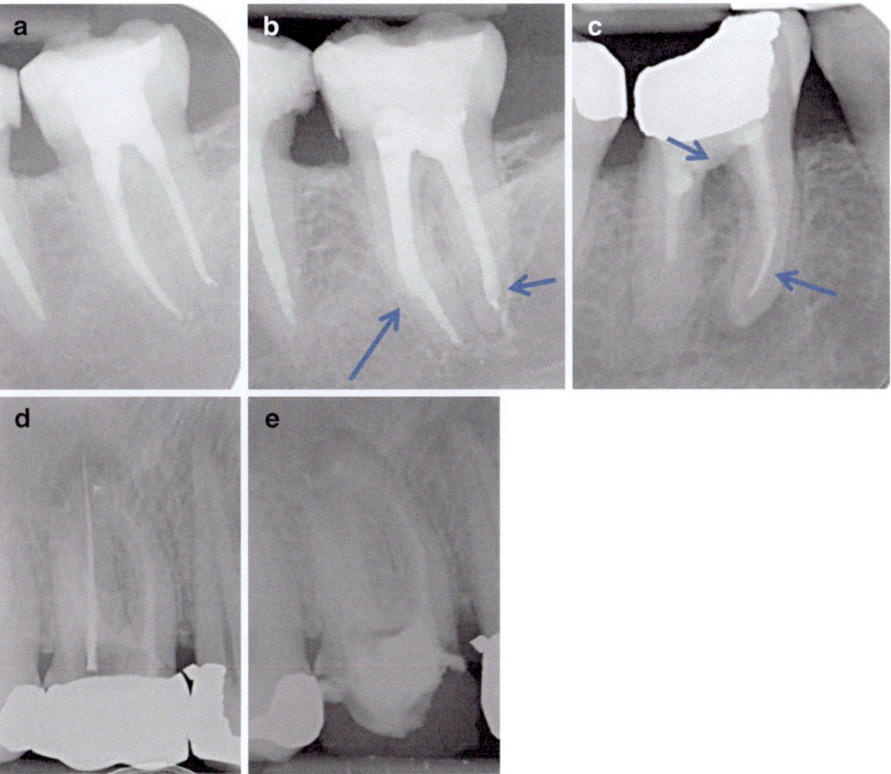

Fig. 14.6 Iatrogenic errors identifiable radiographically. (**a**): A patient with low-grade symptoms and no overt periradicular pathology opts to embark on root canal re-treatment. (**b**): Root canal re-treatment of the case in image A results in ledging and failure to reach working length in the distal canal (arrowed). A mesial canal is transported and ledged (arrowed). Symptoms are unchanged, and the likelihood of treatment success is now reduced. (**c**): A compromised tooth with evidence of a furcal perforation, associated intraradicular radiolucency (arrowed), and a separated file fragment in the mid-apical third of a mesial canal (arrowed). The distal canal is short of the radiographic apex by >2 mm. This tooth has a very poor, if not hopeless, outlook. (**d** and **e**): Tooth 16 has a 16 mm length separated rotary file in the palatal canal. This iatrogenic error was correctable (**e**)

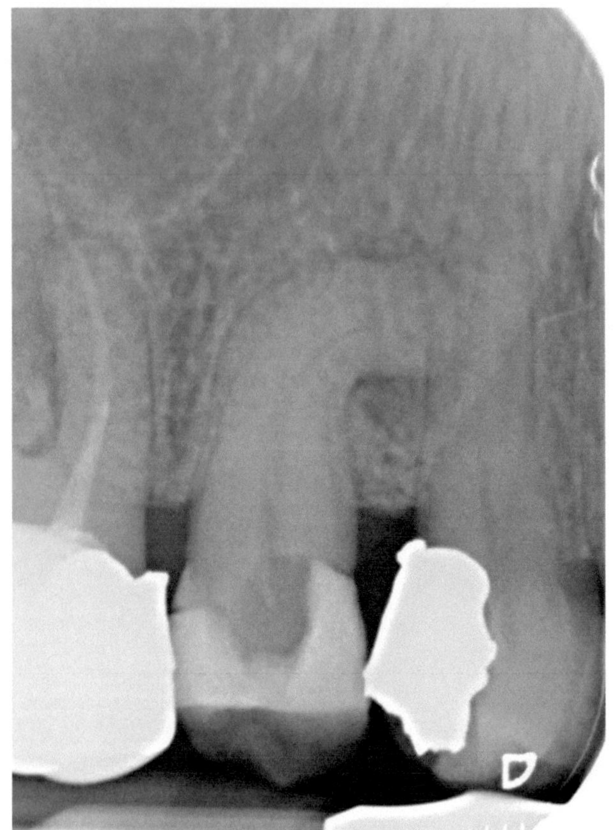

Fig. 14.7 Extreme canal curvatures increase the likelihood of ledging, perforation, and file separation. Tooth 15 was referred because full working length could not be reached. This is an extremely complex case and would have benefitted from referral to a specialist in the first instance because ledging of the canal was very likely and indeed occurred prior to referral. The patient opted to extract the tooth

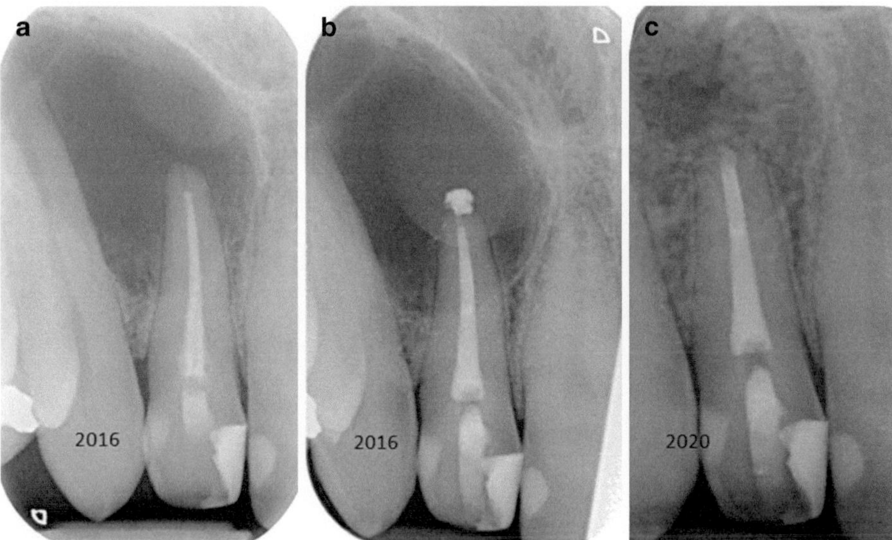

Fig. 14.8 Particularly large periradicular radiolucencies are more likely to be cystic. If a radicular cyst is suspected, extraction or non-surgical endodontic management is indicated in the first instance. Those cases not showing a resolution in signs or symptoms, or reduction in periradicular pathology within 6–12 months of root canal treatment completion, may need to be tackled surgically. (**a**) Radiograph from 2016 was sent with a referral because of ongoing symptoms from root canal treated tooth 12. (**b**) Completion of root canal re-treatment (sealer overfill) in first instance. Symptoms did not resolve during multi-visit root canal re-treatment; therefore, periradicular microsurgery was planned and undertaken in 2016. (**c**) 4 year review following periradicular microsurgery shows significant resolution of lesion and no clinical signs or symptoms are present. The lesion removed during endodontic surgery was sent for processing, and histopathology confirmed a benign odontogenic cyst

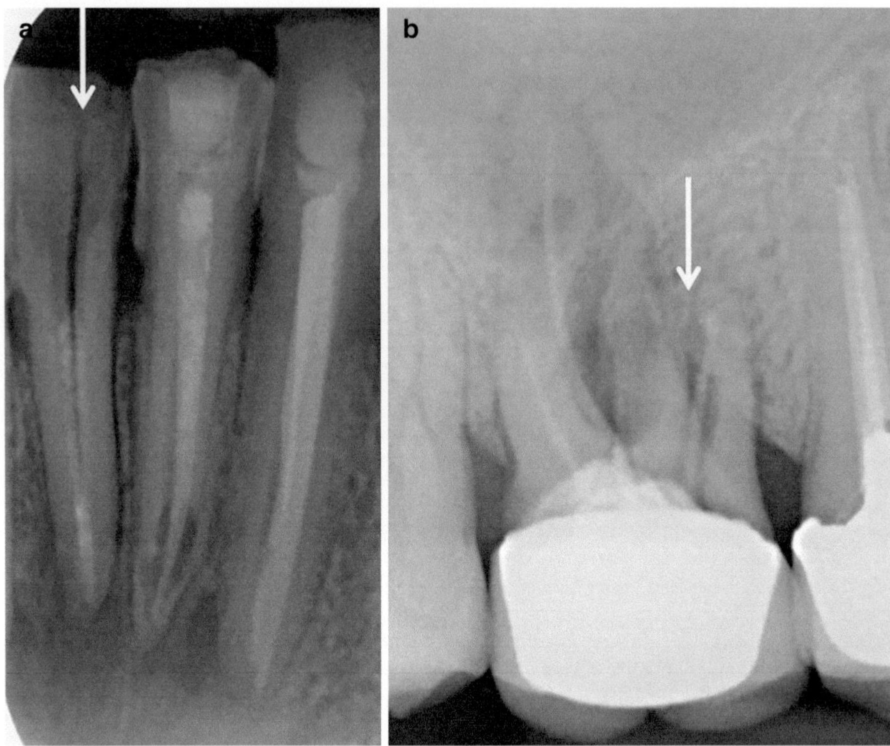

Fig. 14.9 Vertical root fractures are not often seen on radiographs until the tooth has split. A lower central incisor has split (arrowed), as has the mesio-buccal root of the maxillary right first molar (arrowed). Both bases had associated periodontal pocketing clinically, and tooth fragments could be seen without magnification moving independently. Each has a hopeless outlook

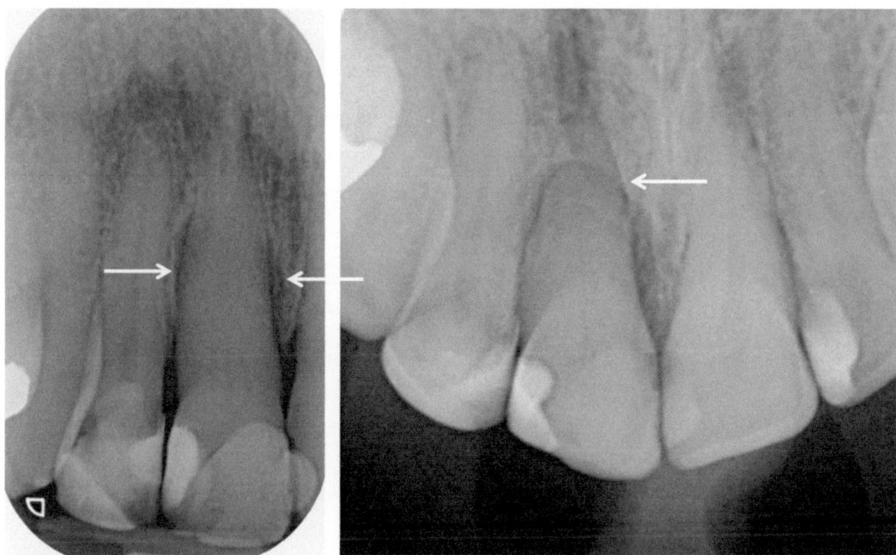

Fig. 14.10 A patient with symptoms from tooth 11 relates a history of trauma over 20 years ago. The periapical radiograph shows alveolar changes at each side of the root, suggesting a crack may be present. A maxillary occlusal film confirms a horizontal root fracture

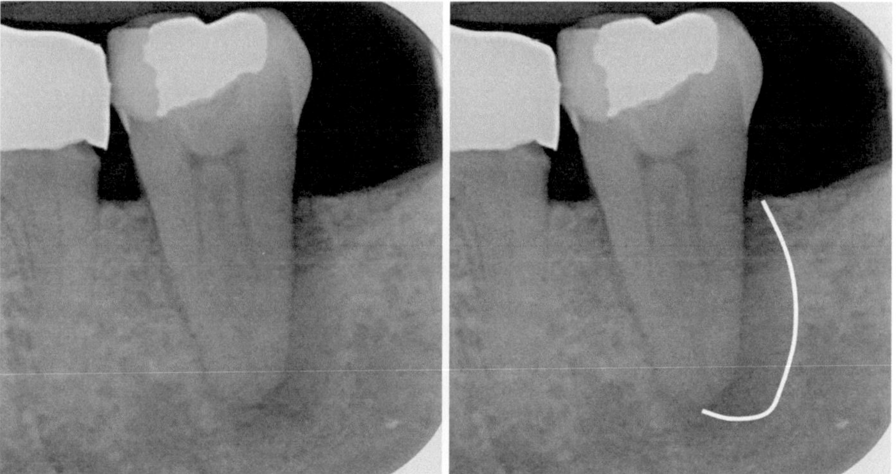

Fig. 14.11 Tooth 37 is a functional molar with an extensive multi-surface restoration in situ. The shape of the radiolucency, loss of the mesial-marginal ridge, and functional demands on this tooth highlight it as a tooth that could fracture irretrievably. Root canal treatment was started and after several visits, with no reduction in systems, referred. Magnification revealed a crack distally. A 'J-shaped' radiolucency can be indicative of a longitudinal root crack

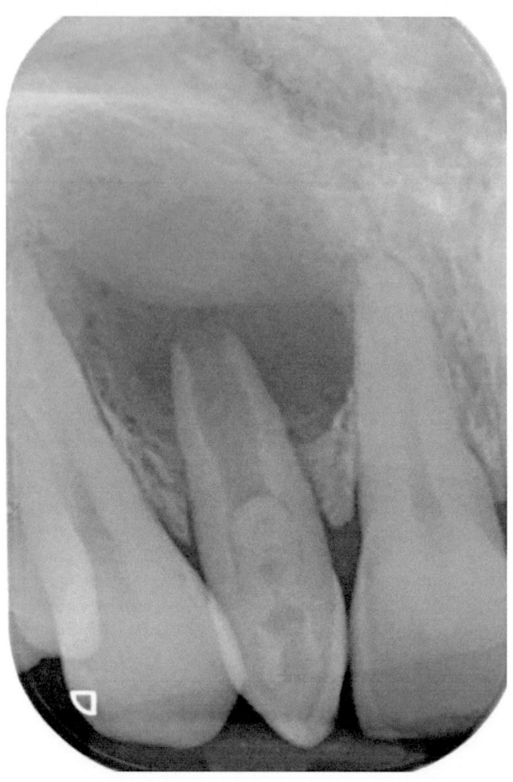

Fig. 14.12 Dens in dente affecting tooth 12

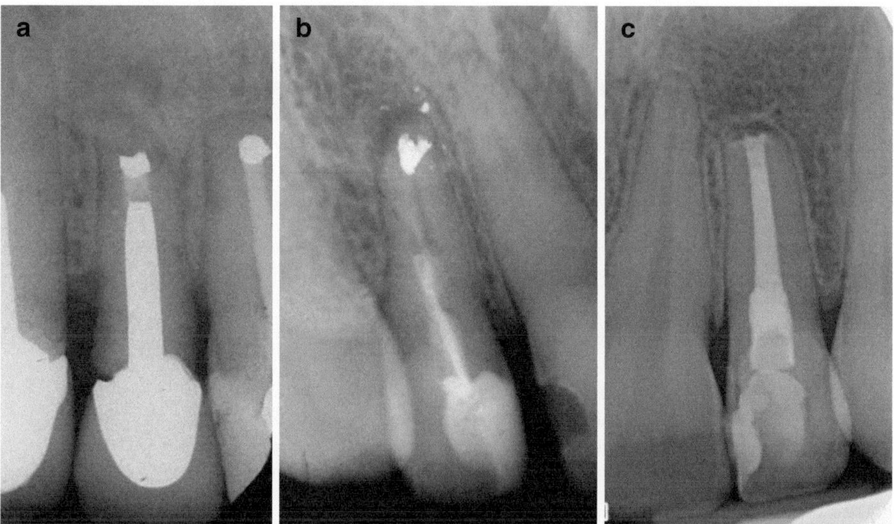

Fig. 14.13 Radiographs highlighting differences between traditional and modern techniques and materials associated with periradicular surgery. (**a**) Tooth 12 has an amalgam root end filling in situ. Approximately 2 mm of root length remains apical to the root end filling. This suggests that the root end may not have been entirely resected or that a large bevel has been prepared on the root surface during surgery. The adjacent tooth (partially seen) shows an amalgam root end filling, which has been placed into a cavity created by a round bur. (**b**) An amalgam root end filling has been placed, and amalgam particles are seen in the periradicular tissues. It is unclear if the root end filling is in the canal. The root length continues apical to the root end filling, again suggesting insufficient root resection or creation of bevel. (**c**) Tooth 22 has been treated using modern, micro-surgical techniques and materials. The root end is entirely resected with minimal or no bevel. A root end cavity preparation to a depth of 3 mm in the long axis/within the root canal has been prepared and filled to a depth of 3 mm using mineral trioxide aggregate

14.5 Cone-Beam Computed Tomography Systems (CBCT)

In recent years, advantages of CBCT for endodontic treatment planning have emerged, for example, in cases of possible non-odontogenic pain when conventional radiography has been insufficient in identifying pathology, which could account for symptoms. However, the radiation dose is generally higher with CBCT than with conventional radiography [34], although the advent of limited volume (where the field of view is limited to the area of interest), high-resolution CBCT reduces the effective dose of radiation to the patient [34].Limited volume CBCT can be of use in the assessment of dental trauma, complex root canal morphology, resorption, endodontic complications, and planning for surgical endodontic management [34]. However, significant radiographic artefacts from metallic restorations and even gutta-percha can compromise the detail gained [13].

14.6 Conclusion

Several patient-related, clinical, and radiographic factors impact endodontic treatment planning and case complexity. In the next part, the assessment tools available and their benefits and limitations for guiding endodontic case complexity will be considered.

References

1. The Health and Social Care Information Centre. Adult dental Health survey. London: NHS Digital; 2010.
2. Carrotte P. Endodontics: part 2 diagnosis and treatment planning. Br Dent J. 2004;197:231–8.
3. Morin L, Johnell K, Laroche M-L, Fastbom J, Wastesson JW. The epidemiology of polypharmacy in older adults: register-based prospective cohort study. Clin Epidemiol. 2018;10:289–98.
4. Jablonski RY, Barber MW. Restorative dentistry for the older patient cohort. Br Dent J. 2015;218:337–42.
5. Bernick S, Nedelman C. Effect of aging on the human pulp. J Endod. 1975;1:88–94.
6. Fiske J, Davis D, Frances C, Gelbier S. The emotional effects of tooth loss in edentulous people. Br Dent J. 1998;184:90–3.
7. Ingle JI, Beveridge EE, Glick DH, Weichman JA. Modern endodontic therapy. In: Ingle JI, Bakland LK, editors. Endodontics. 4th ed. Baltimore: Williams & Wilkins; 1994. p. 27–53.
8. Gorni FG, Gagliani MM. The outcome of endodontic re-treatment: a 2-yr follow-up. J Endod. 2004;30:1–4.
9. Ng YL, Mann V, Gulabivala K. A prospective study of the factors affecting outcomes of non-surgical root canal treatment: part 1: periapical health. Int Endod J. 2011;44:583–609.
10. Fouad AF, Burleson J. The effect of diabetes mellitus on endodontic treatment outcome: data from an electronic patient record. J Am Dent Assoc. 2003;134:43–51.
11. SDCEP. Oral health management of patients at risk of medication-related osteonecrosis of the jaw. Dundee: SDCEP; 2017.
12. SDCEP. Antibiotic prophylaxis against infective endocarditis: implementation advice for National Institute for Health and Care Excellence (NICE) clinical guideline 64 prophylaxis against infective endocarditis. Dundee: SDCEP; 2018.
13. FGDP. Selection criteria for dental radiography. 3rd ed. London: FGDP; 2018. Available at: https://cgdent.uk/wp-content/uploads/2021/08/FGDP-SCDR-ALL-Web.pdf. Accessed 14 Jan 2022.
14. European Society of Endodontology. Quality guidelines for endodontic treatment: consensus report of the European Society of Endodontology. Int Endod J. 2006;39:921–30.
15. Estrela C, Bueno M, Leles C, Azevedo B, Azevedo J. Accuracy of cone beam computed tomography and panoramic and periapical radiography for detection of apical periodontitis. J Endod. 2008;34:273–9.
16. Eliyas S, Jalili J, Martin N. Restoration of the root canal treated tooth. Br Dent J. 2015;218:53–62.
17. Abbott PV. Assessing restored teeth with pulp and periapical diseases for the presence of cracks, caries and marginal breakdown. Aust Dent J. 2004;49:33–9.
18. Vertucci F. Root canal morphology and its relationship to endodontic procedures. Endod Topics. 2005;10:3–29.
19. Patel S, Rhodes J. A practical guide to endodontic access cavity preparation in molar teeth. Br Dent J. 2007;203:133–40.
20. Johnstone M, Parashos P. Endodontics and the ageing patient. Aust Dent J. 2015;60:20–7.
21. McCabe P, Dummer P. Pulp canal obliteration: an endodontic diagnosis and treatment challenge. Int Endod J. 2011;45:177–97.

22. Carrotte P. Endodontics: part 4 morphology of the root canal system. Br Dent J. 2004;197:379–83.
23. Ahmed HMA, Dummer PM. A new system for classifying tooth, root and canal anomalies. Int Endod J. 2018;51:389–404.
24. Barker C, Parvizi F, Weiland F, Sandy J, Ireland A. Orthodontics and root resorption part 1. Orthodontic Update. 2010;3:102–6.
25. Chapman MN, Nadgir RN, Akman AS, et al. Periapical lucency around the tooth: radiologic evaluation and differential diagnosis. Radiographics. 2013;33:E15. https://doi.org/10.1148/rg.331125172.
26. Khasnis SA, Kidiyoor KH, Patil AB, Kenganal SB. Vertical root fractures and their management. J Conserv Dent. 2014;17:103–10.
27. Hülsmann M. Dens invaginatus: aetiology, classification, prevalence, diagnosis, and treatment considerations. Int Endod J. 1997;30:79–90.
28. Shrestha A, Marla V, Shrestha S, Maharjan IK. Developmental anomalies affecting the morphology of teeth—a review. RSBO Revista Sul-Brasileira de Odontologia. 2015;12:68–78.
29. Ng YL, Mann V, Gulabivala K. Outcome of secondary root canal treatment: a systematic review of the literature. Int Endod J. 2008;41:1026–46.
30. Tsesis I, Rosenberg E, Faivishevsky V, Kfir A, Katz M, Rosen E. Prevalence and associated periodontal status of teeth with root perforation: a retrospective study of 2,002 patients' medical records. J Endod. 2010;36:797–800.
31. Carrotte P. Endodontics: part 7 preparing the root canal. Br Dent J. 2004;197:603–13.
32. Dummer PMH. The quality of root canal treatment provided by general dental practitioners working within the General Dental Services of England and Wales: part 2. J Practice Board of England and Wales. 1998:8–10.
33. Del Fabbro M, Taschieri S, Testori T, Francetti L, Weinstein RL. Surgical versus non-surgical endodontic re-treatment for periradicular lesions. Cochrane Database Syst Rev. 2007:CD005511.
34. Patel S, Durack C, Abella F, et al. European Society of Endodontology position statement: the use of CBCT in endodontics. Int Endod J. 2014;47:502–4.

Identifying Endodontic Case Complexity: Part 2

15

Matthew Philip Sarstedt, Saiba Ghafoor,
and Julie K. Kilgariff

Learning Points

- Recall the various indices and tools available in assessing endodontic complexity prior to considering endodontics.
- Appreciate the differing factors each of these tools put emphasis on when assessing the endodontically involved unit.
- Understand the relative advantages and disadvantages of these tools in practice.

15.1 Introduction

This chapter discusses the various tools and guides that can be utilised in assessing endodontic complexity.

15.2 Tools Available to Guide Assessing Endodontic Case Complexity

There are various published tools that help with endodontic clinical decision-making and treatment planning, providing information on likely risks and their impact on treatment outcome [1]. Using these can help focus patient discussions, enhancing understanding of complexities, risks, and benefits, enabling informed consent and the decision as to whether to refer [2]. Additionally, the use of tools and assessments, when recorded in patient records, may provide benefit medico-legally.

M. P. Sarstedt
University of Sheffield, School of Clinical Dentistry, Sheffield, UK

S. Ghafoor · J. K. Kilgariff (✉)
Dundee Dental Hospital & Research School, Dundee, UK
e-mail: julie.kilgariff@nhs.scot

E. McColl, A. Alani (eds.), *Practical Tips in Clinical Dentistry*, BDJ Clinician's Guides, https://doi.org/10.1007/978-3-031-90355-7_15

Endodontic diagnosis and treatment planning are based upon clinical and radiographic findings. Studies suggest that general dental practitioners tend to underestimate the complexity of endodontic cases [3]. Screening-type tools focus assessment and particularly consider relevant pre-operative radiographs factors. Their use is helpful because dentists' radiographic interpretation of relevant factors is improved by repetition and training [4, 5].

Regular use of structured assessment tools can enhance complexity identification, recommending the use of objective criteria for case assessment and treatment planning [6].

There are a number of published indices to aid endodontic assessment:

- Case Difficulty Assessment form (AAECAF) [7]
- Restorative Index of Treatment Need (RIOTN) [8]
- Dutch Endodontic Treatment Index (DETI) leading to the Endodontic Treatment Classification (ETC) [9]
- EndoApp [10]
- The Dental Practicality Index [11].

The diagnostic criteria for these tools are compared and summarised in Table 15.1.

Table 15.1 Summary comparison of endodontic complexity tools available for use

	AAECAF	RIOTN	DETI	EndoApp	DPI
Difficult diagnosis	✓		✓		
Medical history	✓	✓	✓	✓	✓
Trauma	✓		✓	✓	✓
Mouth opening/access	✓	✓		✓	
Co-operation/special care needs	✓		✓	✓	✓
Structural integrity					✓
Periodontal condition/endodontic-periodontal lesion	✓	✓	✓	✓	✓
Canal curvature/root morphology	✓	✓	✓	✓	✓
Resorption	✓	✓	✓	✓	✓
Gag reflex	✓	✓		✓	
Retreatment	✓	✓	✓	✓	✓
Iatrogenic damage/perforation	✓	✓	✓	✓	✓
Root development/open apex	✓	✓	✓	✓	✓
Obstruction		✓	✓	✓	✓
Difficulty isolating/pre-treatment required for isolation	✓		✓	✓	
Facial/neuropathic pain	✓	✓			

15.3 Case Difficulty Assessment Form, *American Association of Endodontics (2005)*

The first version (1997) of the American Association of Endodontists guidelines for 'Evaluating Endodontic Treatment Risk Factors' [12] was revised and re-released as the 'Case Difficulty Assessment Form' (AAECAF) in 2005 [7].

Originally devised in an educational setting to inform case suitability for students or trainees, the tool considers patient, diagnosis, and treatment factors in deciding case difficulty.

Cases are scored and categorised as:

- Minimal difficulty: Treatment is appropriate for a general practitioner.
- Moderate difficulty: May warrant referral, depending on skill and experience of clinician.
- High difficulty: Meriting consideration of a referral to a dentist with advanced skills in endodontics or a specialist.

Although there is no evidence regarding its utilisation in primary care settings across the UK, there is some uptake amongst GDPs in the USA. Research into the validity of this system is needed [13].

15.4 Restorative Index of Treatment Need (RIOTN), *Royal College of Surgeons of England (2001)*

In the UK, a Restorative Index of Treatment Need (RIOTN) was developed by the Royal College of Surgeons of England [8] using three complexity codes:

- 1: Treatment able to be performed by any dental graduate
- 2: Treatment able to be performed by any experienced dentist
- 3: Treatment able to be performed by any dentist with skills developed following specialist training.

It can be used for assessing the complexity of periodontal, endodontic, and fixed and removable prosthodontic cases. Since the RIOTN was developed, there have been huge advances, in particular within microsurgical endodontics, and therefore, for some aspects of endodontics, this recommended scoring no longer reflects up-to-date evidence. It is also reportedly too simplistic, incomplete, and with poor reproducibility for endodontic case difficulty assessment [14].

15.5 Dutch Endodontic Treatment Index (DETI) and Endodontic Treatment Classification (ETC), *Ree, Tinnerman, & Wesselink (2003)*

Ree and colleagues (2003) [9] surveyed GDPs in the Netherlands to produce a shortened screening tool for assessing risk and difficulty, named the Dutch Endodontic Treatment Index (DETI). The DETI is quicker and easier to use, potentially overcoming the proposed time-consuming shortcomings of AAECAF [13].

DETI indicates the difficulty of a case, and if found to be potentially difficult, a further index is used—the Endodontic Treatment Classification (ETC)—to provide further information. ETC was well received by practitioners in the Netherlands, with the majority finding it helpful in determining if referral is indicated. Endodontic assessments using DETI carried out by both GDPs and specialists also, reassuringly, show high correlations [13], which is encouraging, considering the lack of agreement between GDPs and endodontists about which teeth should be referred in other studies (with the exception of periradicular surgery cases) [3].

15.6 EndoApp, *British Endodontic Society (2018)*

The EndoApp is a structured web-based tool available for use online or download for endodontic evaluation and triage in primary and secondary care [10]. It aims to overcome the limitations of other tools, for example, the absence of a quantification system with RIOTN and the absence of some variables in AAECAF [10]. The tool calculates a case difficulty score from a series of questions answered by the user and recommends which type of dental practitioner is best suited to managing the case. Small-scale studies suggest the app is relatively quick to use and preferred by users to AAECAF [10].

15.7 Dental Practicality Index, *Dawood & Patel (2017)*

A further recently published tool that takes into account the tooth's restorative state in relation to the patient's dentition, needs, expectations, and medical and dental history is the Dental Practicality Index [11]. This has three restorative categories and a 'context' category (i.e. general oral and patient factors), which are scored out of six, where zero means that no treatment is required and six indicates that the tooth is not practical to restore and extraction should be considered. The scores between these extremes guide as to what level of endodontic skill/training is needed to treat the case. Scores can also be totalled; a score of 1–2 implying the case can be simply and predictably treated. An increasing score indicates more complex care is needed, with a score ≥ 6 indicating the tooth is impractical to treat.

Since the DPI's inception, a number of studies have attempted validation. The first [15] retrospectively assessed the DPI from notes, study models, and radiographs for 137 teeth and correlated this with the root canal treatment outcome. A moderate level of agreement between the two independent assessing endodontists was found, demonstrating the tool's subjectivity; however, several advantages of using the DPI were recognised: the DPI encourages the consideration of patient cases holistically and for root canal retreatments, and using the DPI has good outcome prediction [16]. Al-Nuaimi et al. (2020) [16] used a similar retrospective method and two assessing endodontists. One hundred and forty-four teeth had DPI scores calculated and followed up to identify what happened to the tooth 4 years later. Teeth with a DPI score of >6 were found to have significantly less chance of survival than teeth with lower scores. This study concluded that the DPI can predict which teeth, if endodontically retreated, are likely to be extracted. A recent *BDJ Student* article [17] highlighted confusion regarding whether a tooth *can* be restored versus whether it is *practical* to restore it. This paper reported ease of use with the DPI, increasing clinician confidence in assessing tooth restorability.

15.8 Discussion

Endodontic treatment outcomes are affected by the complexity of the case, the presence/creation of iatrogenic errors, and the skill level of the clinician carrying out the treatment. Assessing case complexity prior to embarking on treatment will help guide appropriate referral, particularly when directed to NHS funded specialist services, and impact endodontic treatment outcome for patients.

Structured, freely available tools are useful aids for assessing endodontic case complexity and can be retained as part of the dental records and guide as to when a referral might be considered. However, clinical reasoning and decision-making is complex and multifactorial, and the use of indices does not eliminate subjectivity, specifically with regard to the accuracy of radiographic understanding. Repeated use of case complexity guides increases the speed at which these can be completed [9], and regular use may improve endodontic care quality through improved identification of possible problems/challenges before starting treatment; after treatment is started, iatrogenic errors are not always correctable. Using such guides may help structure clinical decisions, treatment planning, and discussions and aid evidence for inclusion in dental records. Of the tools available, there is no consensus on which assessment tool is superior.

The European Society for Endodontology [18] provides undergraduate endodontic guidelines stating that students should be competent at identifying treatment complexity and suggests the DETI or AAECAF may be helpful. Speculatively, the use of such structured assessment tools might favourably impact the suboptimal quality of endodontic treatment identified as being carried out in the UK [19], which in turn may impact endodontic-related medico-legal litigation. Consistency, understanding, and agreement between GDPs and those receiving referrals are in the best interests of patients because identifying cases that may be better treated by a specialist clinician and referring appropriately improves treatment outcomes [1].

15.9 Conclusion

There are several factors to consider when assessing the complexity of an endodontic case, and clinicians must also take into account their own experience and skill and the patient's wishes. There are a number of assessment tools freely available to help guide assessing endodontic case complexity, and whilst there is no current consensus on which assessment tool is superior, each provides some benefit in structuring and steering assessment, which can aid discussions, informed consent processes, and when to refer.

References

1. Messer HH. Clinical judgement and decision making in endodontics. Aust Endod J. 1999;25:124–32.
2. Webber J. Risk management in clinical practice. Part 4: endodontics. Br Dent J. 2010;209:161–70.
3. Caplan DJ, Reams G, Weintraub JA. Recommendations for endodontic referral among practitioners in a dental HMO. J Endodont. 1999;25:369–75.
4. Lanning SK, Pelok SD, Williams BC, et al. Variation in periodontal diagnosis and treatment planning among clinical instructors. J Dent Educ. 2005;69:325–237.
5. Suthiprapoporn P, Taguchi A, Nakamoto T, et al. Diagnostic performance of general dental practitioners after lecture in identifying post-menopausal women with low mineral density by panoramic radiographs. Dentomaxillofac Radiol. 2006;35:249–52.
6. Bader JD, Shugars DA. Agreement among dentists' recommendations for restorative treatment. J Dent Res. 1993;72:891–6.
7. American Association of Endodontists. AAE Endodontic Case Difficulty Assessment Form and Guidelines. 2005. https://endomishra.co.uk/wp-content/uploads/2021/04/Difficulty-assessment-form.pdf. Accessed Aug 2022.
8. Falcon HC, Richardson P, Shaw MJ, Bulman JS, Smith BG. Developing an index of restorative dental treatment need. Br Dent J. 2001;190:479–86.
9. Ree MH, Timmerman MF, Wesselink PR. Evaluation of the usefulness of two endodontic case assessment forms by general dentists. Int Endod J. 2003;36:545–55.
10. Shah PK, Chong BS. A web-based endodontic case difficulty assessment tool. Clin Oral Investig. 2018;22:2381–8.
11. Dawood A, Patel S. The dental practicality index—assessing the restorability of teeth. Br Dent J. 2017;222:755–8.
12. American Association of Endodontists. Evaluating Endodontic Treatment Risk Factors 1997. https://f3f142zs0k2w1kg84k5p9i1o-wpengine.netdna-ssl.com/specialty/wp-content/uploads/sites/2/2017/05/ss97ecfe.pdf. Accessed 6 June 2022.
13. Curry MC. The utilization of case difficulty assessment when determining endodontic referral [masters]. University of North Carolina at Chapel Hill; 2010.
14. Muthukrishnan A, Owens J, Bryant S, Drummer PM. Evaluation of a system for grading the complexity of root canal treatment. Br Dent J. 2007;202:E26.
15. Tifooni A, Al-Nuaimi N, Dawood A, Mannocci F, Patel S. Validation of the effectiveness of the dental practicality index in predicting the outcome of root canal retreatments. Int Endod J. 2019;52:1403–9.
16. Al-Nuaimi N, Ciapryna S, Chia M, Patel S, Mannocci. A prospective study on the effect of coronal tooth structure loss on the 4-year clinical survival of root canal retreated teeth and retrospective validation of the dental practicality index. Int Endod J. 2020;53:1040–9.

17. Cottham-Cartledge C. What is the dental practicality index? BDJ Student. 2022; https://doi.org/10.1038/s41406-021-0266-7.
18. De Moor R, Hülsmann M, Kirkevang L, Tanalp J, Whitworth J. Undergraduate curriculum guidelines for endodontology. Int Endod J. 2013;46:1105–14.
19. Dummer PMH. The quality of root canal treatment provided by general dental practitioners working within the general dental Services of England and Wales: part 2. J Dent Pract Board Eng Wales. 1998;19:8–10.

Practical Tips for Endodontic Access 16

R. J. R. Smith, Ewen McColl, and G. E. Bryce

Learning Points
- Recall the need to assess and prepare prior to beginning endodontic access.
- Recognise the need to understand the trajectory and orientation for endodontic access.
- Once the pulp chamber has been breached, understand the stepwise process for identifying the canals and subsequent provisionalisation/temporisation.

16.1 Introduction

Orthograde root canal treatment (RCT) or root canal treatment (RCReTx) is a multi-step process for the treatment or prevention of apical periodontitis. Securing adequate access to the root canal system is one of several factors that influence the overall success of these procedures. In this chapter, we offer practical tips for effectively and efficiently securing endodontic access.

16.2 Clinical Objectives for Endodontic Access

(a) Removal of all diseased tooth tissue and identification of poor prognostic factors (cracks/fractures)

R. J. R. Smith
Defence Centre for Rehabilitative Dentistry, Aldershot, UK

E. McColl (✉)
Peninsula Dental School, Plymouth, UK
e-mail: ewen.mccoll@plymouth.ac.uk

G. E. Bryce
Restorative Dentistry, Defence Centre for Rehabilitative Dentistry, Aldershot, UK

E. McColl, A. Alani (eds.), *Practical Tips in Clinical Dentistry*, BDJ Clinician's Guides, https://doi.org/10.1007/978-3-031-90355-7_16

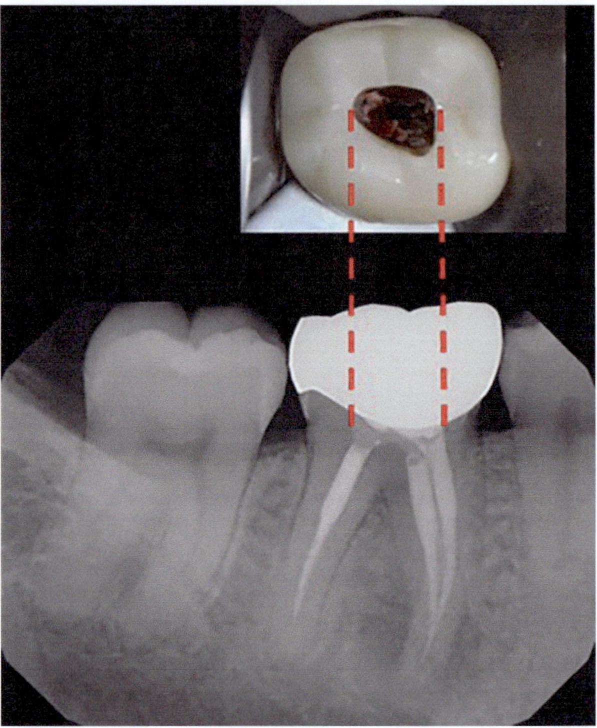

Fig. 16.1 Conservative endodontic access cavity prepared through a recently placed zirconia crown, prior to RCReTx

(b) Direct (ideally straight-line) access to the root canal orifice(s) (Fig. 16.1)
(c) Conservation of dentine (as far as is practicable)
(d) A four-walled cavity that facilitates controlled provision of the RCT
(e) Temporisation that reduces the risk of (further) bacterial ingress and tooth fracture

16.3 Armamentarium

(a) Dental loupes with a direct light source are recommended for use in RCT/RCReTx, as well as an operating microscope (if available). However, magnification may affect spatial awareness, and the operator must take care to orientate their handpiece correctly to avoid adverse angulation of the cavity and the subsequent risks of excessive removal of tooth structure and perforation.
(b) Front surface reflecting dental mirrors are preferred as they eliminate the 'double image' produced with rear surfaced mirrors.
(c) Further recommended equipment is listed in Table 16.1.

Table 16.1 Further recommended equipment for endodontic access

Instrument	Photo	Comments
DG-16 probe	Fig. a	Double-ended probe with long sharp tips. Useful for identifying root canal orifices and determining the angulation of the coronal aspect of the canal with respect to the pulp chamber floor. Can be used to 'pick' away material from the walls and floor of the access cavity
Long-tapered, round-ended course diamond bur (e.g. 770.8C bur from Two-Striper, Abrasive Technology, Lewis Center, Ohio, USA)	Fig. b	Length of bur enhances ability to orientate and improve visibility. Round-end avoids creation of step defects. Course diamond coating provides efficient tooth preparation. Useful for removal of restorative material[a] within the restorability assessment and for gaining initial access to the pulp chamber
Long-tapered, safe-ended, tungsten carbide bur (e.g. Endo-Z, Dentsply Maillefer, Ballaigues, Switzerland)	Fig. c	The non-cutting tip will follow the outline of the floor of the access cavity (or walls of the root canal in teeth with single wide canals). The tip can then be moved laterally like a 'milling machine' to de-roof the pulp chamber and create smooth flowing axial walls into the root canal(s)
Pulp chamber bur (Hager & Meisinger GmbH, Neuss, Germany)	Fig. d	Long shank enhances visibility. Round end cuts dentine without leaving steps (and does not 'smear' dentine like ultrasonic instruments can). Available in different sizes 120 (1.2 mm)–180 (1.8 mm). Useful for removing calcifications to uncover the pulp chamber floor
Ultrasonic instruments (e.g. Start-X, Dentsply Maillefer, Ballaigues, Switzerland)	Fig. e	Ultrasonic instruments of various designs can be used to refine and finish the preparation of the access cavity walls and remove calcification from the floor of the pulp chamber of the access cavity. Using ultrasonics dry (e.g. without water coolant) enhances visibility but will heat the dentine, necessitating intermittent alternate irrigation to cool the dentine. Caution should be exercised that 'false canals' are not inadvertently prepared when using pointed tipped ultrasonic instruments

[a] Where a metallic restoration needs to be cut through, a tungsten-carbide bur may be more efficient than a diamond-coated bur

16.4 Restorative Assessment

(a) Teeth requiring RCT/RCReTx should be assessed for restorability, with all caries and existing restorations removed prior to endodontic access [1] (unless the restoration has been recently placed and is deemed to be satisfactory).
(b) Direct visualisation and assessment of the remaining sound dentine enables the clinician to formulate a restorative prognosis for the patient's tooth [2–4] and allows planning of the definitive restoration (Figs. 16.2, 16.3 and 16.4).

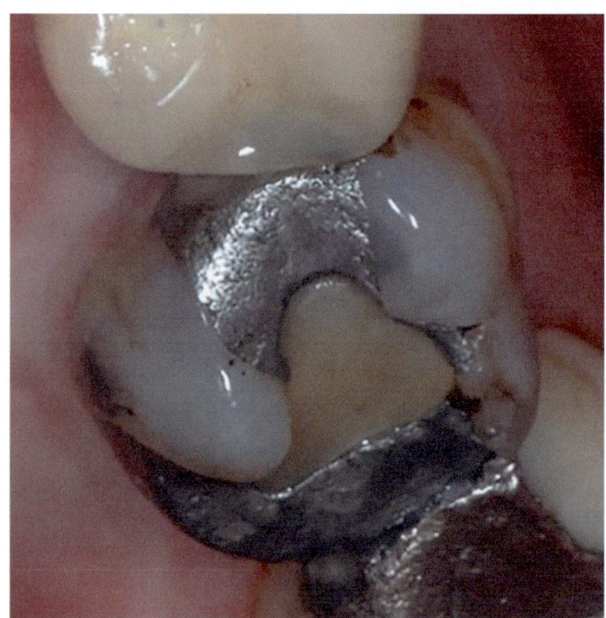

Fig. 16.2 Maxillary left first molar with previous aborted attempt to gain endodontic access through existing metallic (amalgam) restoration

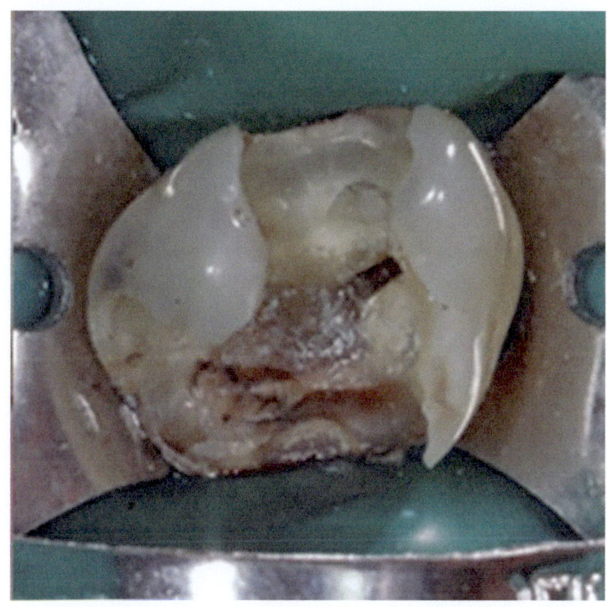

Fig. 16.3 Removal of restorations revealed secondary caries and that the pulp chamber floor was obscured by calcification

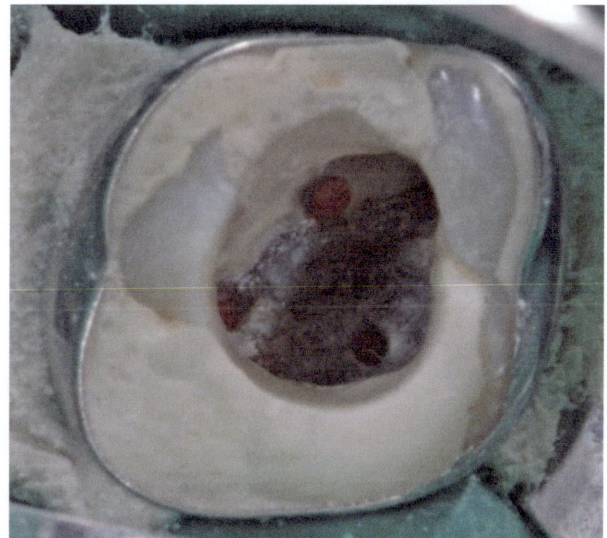

Fig. 16.4 Following removal of the caries and calcifications, missing axial walls were replaced with temporary restorative material, the access cavity refined, and RCT completed

16.5 Orientation and Initial Access

(a) Prior to access cavity preparation, the expected boundaries of the pulp chamber (roof, walls, and floor) and root canal orifice(s) should be mentally visualised, aided by:
   - Knowledge of anatomical trends in the position of pulp chambers and root canals, based on tooth type (Fig. 16.5)
   - Clinical assessment to determine the orientation of the tooth in the arch (e.g. proclination/retroclination, or rotation) (Fig. 16.6), which may be disguised by restorative materials
   - Two-dimensional (2D) radiographic assessment with long cone periapical (LCPA) radiograph (supplemented by a second LCPA at a different angle as required), to assess for:
     - Presence and extent of existing restorative materials and caries.

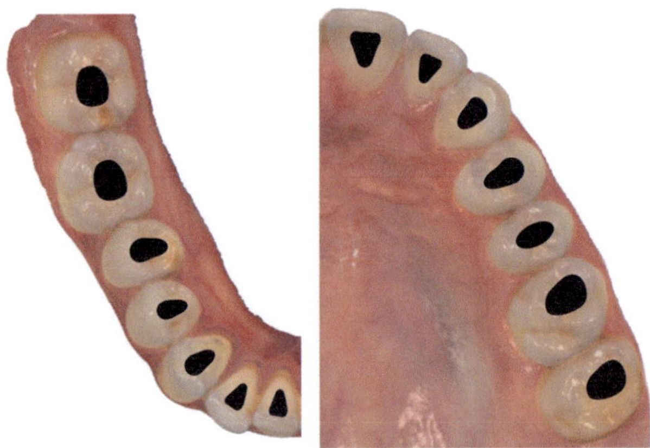

Fig. 16.5 Expected position of pulp chambers in mandibular and maxillary teeth (with the exception of third molars, in which the anatomy is particularly variable)

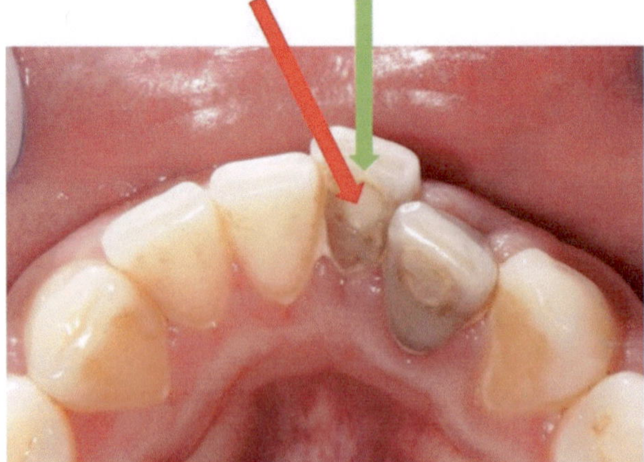

Fig. 16.6 Misaligned access cavity in the 41. Red arrow indicates the direction of tunnelling (which resulted in root perforation on the labial aspect). Green arrow indicates the correct orientation of the bur for initial access cavity preparation in this tooth

  - Position of pulp chamber/pulp horns. Measurement of the distance between the occlusal table (or incisal edge), and the roof of the pulp chamber can help guide the point of initial entry to the pulp chamber. Equally, especially where there has been extensive calcific metamorphosis within the pulp chamber, the expected position of the floor of the pulp chamber can also be estimated from the LCPA.
  - Position and number of root canals.
- Three-dimensional cone radiographic assessment with cone beam computed tomography (CBCT) scan can be a useful adjunct to 2D imaging. However, the use of CBCT should be balanced against the risks of additional radiation exposure, as well as awareness of the limitations in image quality associated with artefacts due to metallic restorations and root fillings [5]. Situations where CBCT may be helpful within the assessment include:
  - Complex anatomy, including dens invaginatus
  - RCReTx where there is suspected untreated root canal anatomy
  - Assessment and planning for management of iatrogenic issues (Figs. 16.7 and 16.8).

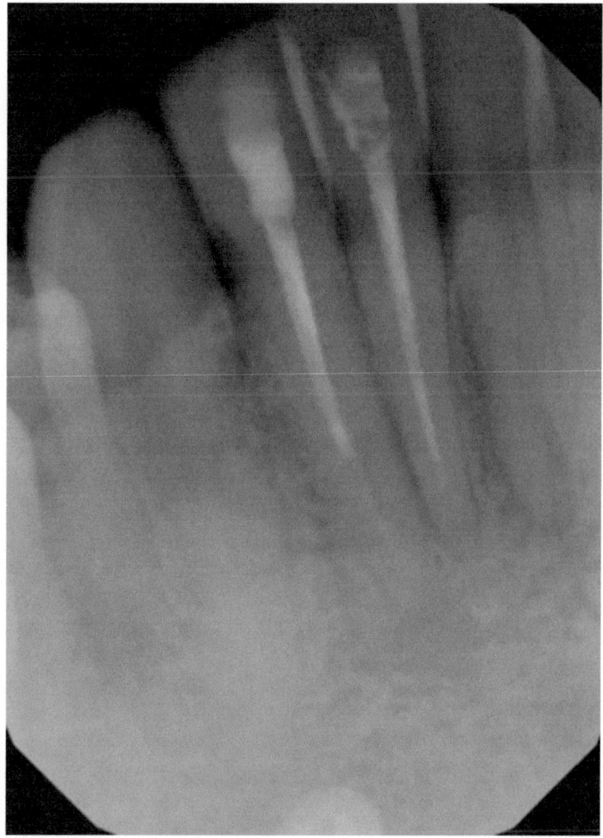

Fig. 16.7 LCPA radiograph of 41, 42, and 43 (as shown clinically in Fig. 16.6). Although not demonstrated in this 2D image, from the history and examination, a labial root perforation was suspected

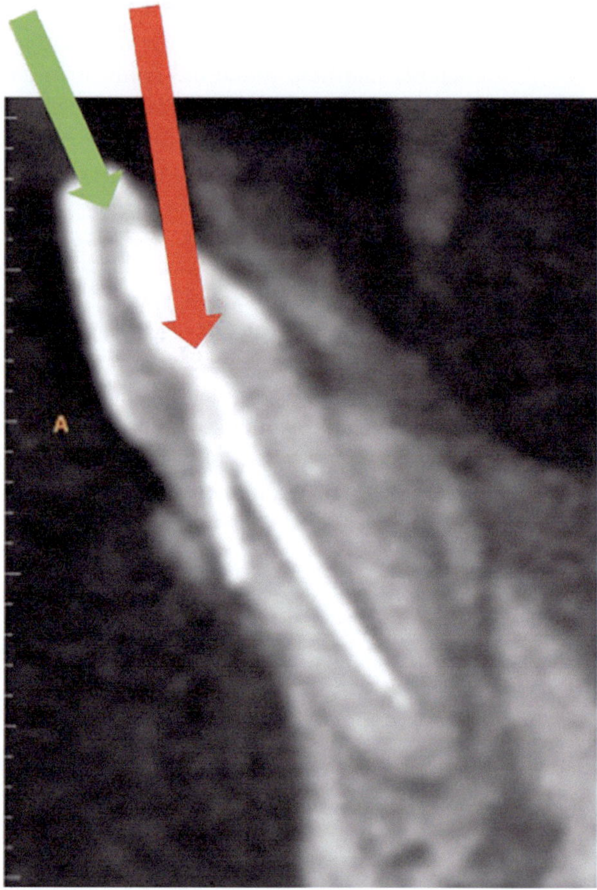

Fig. 16.8 Sagittal slice from CBCT showing 41 with misaligned access cavity (red arrow) and iatrogenic perforation within the mid-third of root at the labial aspect. Straight-line access to the root canal(s) was subsequently achieved by extending the access cavity just into the incisal edge, with the bur angulated to the long axis of the tooth (direction indicated by green arrow)

(b) The drilling sequence for access cavity preparation should commence in the centre of the outline of the planned access cavity, using a long-tapered diamond bur, heading initially for the point of the maximum height of the pulp chamber (as identified on a pre-operative radiograph). Once the roof of pulp chamber is breached and floor identified, the access cavity can be extended laterally, using a safe-ended side-cutting bur, and refined (as far as possible) to meet the requirements of the objectives of access cavity preparation listed in Sect. 16.2

(c) The cavity should allow direct (ideally) or indirect access to the pulp horns for debridement and disinfection, as remaining pulpal tissue may compromise the disinfection and result in unsightly staining of the tooth [6]. There should be an absence of overhangs or ledges above the root canal orifices that may inhibit easy placement of files or obturating materials

(d) Upon preparation of the access cavity, the walls and floor of the pulp chamber should be screened for cracks and fractures, which if present, may influence the restorability of the tooth.

16.6 Rubber Dam

(a) Rubber dam isolation is considered the standard of care within the delivery of RCT/RCReTx [7]. However, if rubber dam is placed prior to access cavity preparation, this will obscure key anatomical landmarks, increasing the risk of misalignment, compromising identification and instrumentation of the root canals, and weakening the tooth +/− perforation. Therefore, less experienced operators may find it pragmatic to initiate access cavity preparation without a rubber dam in place but to isolate with rubber dam immediately after the initial access has been secured.
(b) Once rubber dam is in situ +/− placement of caulking agent (e.g. OraSeal Caulking, Ultradent Products, South Jordan, Utah, USA) to enhance the seal, the following surfaces should be disinfected by wiping them over with a cotton wool pledget soaked in 1–5% sodium hypochlorite irrigant (concentration as per operator preference): external surface of the tooth/teeth to be treated, rubber dam adjacent to the tooth/teeth, as well as the clamp (as applicable). The access cavity should then be flushed with the same irrigant and refined, as necessary, prior to initiating chemomechanical preparation of the root canals.

16.7 Identification of the Pulp Chamber Floor and Root Canal Orifice(s)

(a) In teeth with multiple root canals, the root canal orifices naturally lie in the floor of the pulp chamber. The exception to this is if there has been significant instrumentation (dentine removal) from the pulp chamber floor, which can result in the transportation of the orifice(s) to the wall(s) of the pulp chamber.
(b) In teeth subject to ageing/cracks/caries/restoration, the pulp chamber may be significantly reduced in size, or even completely obliterated, due to the presence of calcification or restorative materials related to previous treatment. Such situations can present significant challenges to root canal identification. However, fortunately, there are a number of anatomical landmarks that can aid in the identification of the pulp chamber floor and root canal orifice(s), which were described by Krasner and Rankow [8] in 2004 and are listed below. Described as 'laws', the guidance is applicable in most situations, but anatomical variation exists, and so judicious application is required in the clinical setting.
(c) 'Laws' for the identification of the pulp chamber floor:
    - **Law of centrality**: The floor of the pulp chamber is always located in the centre of the tooth at the level of the cementoenamel junction (CEJ).
    - **Law of concentricity**: The walls of the pulp chamber are always concentric to the external surface of the tooth at the level of the CEJ.
    - **Law of the CEJ**: The CEJ is the most consistent and repeatable landmark for locating the position of the pulp chamber. In cases of pulp canal obliteration, the use of this landmark to aid in the location of the pulp chamber floor

may be particularly helpful. The expected required depth of access cavity can be determined by measuring/comparing the distance between CEJ and an occlusal reference point using either a UNC-15 probe or the access bur itself

(d) Laws for the identification of root canal orifices:
   - **Law of symmetry 1**: Except for maxillary molars, the orifices of the canals are equidistant from a line drawn in a mesio-distal direction through the pulp chamber floor (Fig. 16.9).
   - **Law of symmetry 2**: Except for maxillary molars, the orifices of the canals lie on a perpendicular line drawn in a mesio-distal direction across the centre of the floor of the pulp chamber (Fig. 16.9)
   - **Law of colour change**: The colour of the pulp-chamber floor is always darker than the walls (Fig. 16.10).
   - **Law of orifice location 1**: Orifices of the root canals are always located at the junction of the walls and the floor (Fig. 16.10).
   - **Law of orifice location 2**: Orifices of the root canals are located at the angles in the floor-wall junction (Fig. 16.11).
   - **Law of orifice location 3**: Orifices of the root canals are located at the terminus of the root developmental fusion lines.

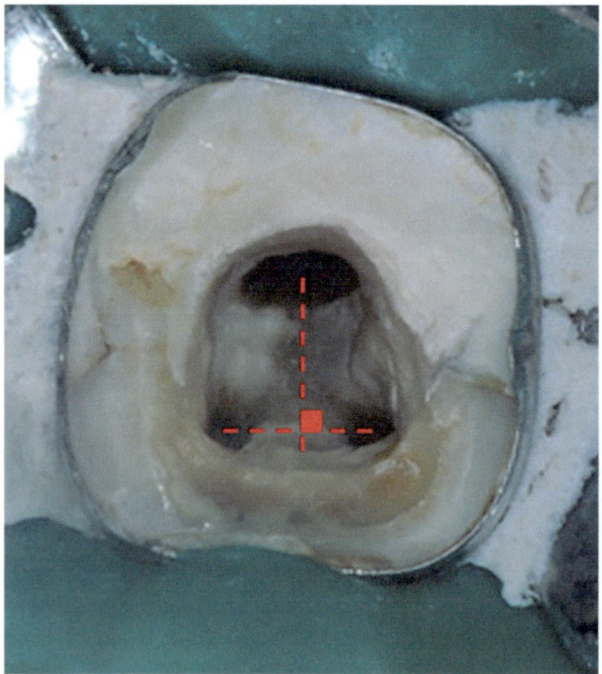

Fig. 16.9 Lines superimposed over the pulp chamber floor of a mandibular first molar to demonstrate adherence to the 'laws' of the symmetry

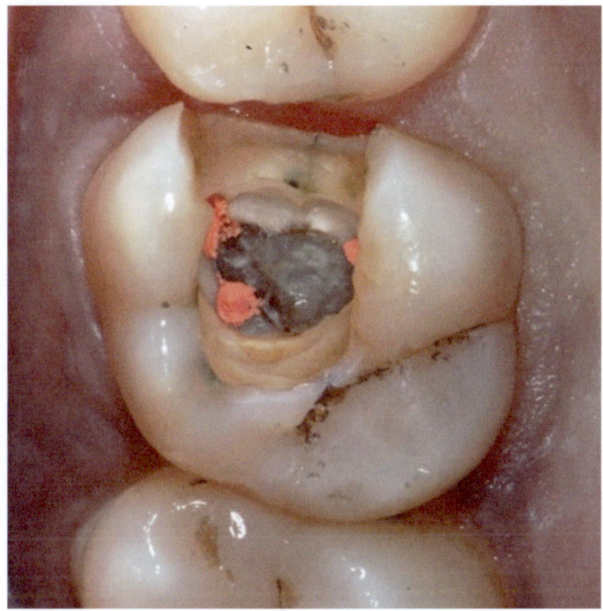

Fig. 16.10 Maxillary first molar with failed primary RCT in which MB2 had not been previously located

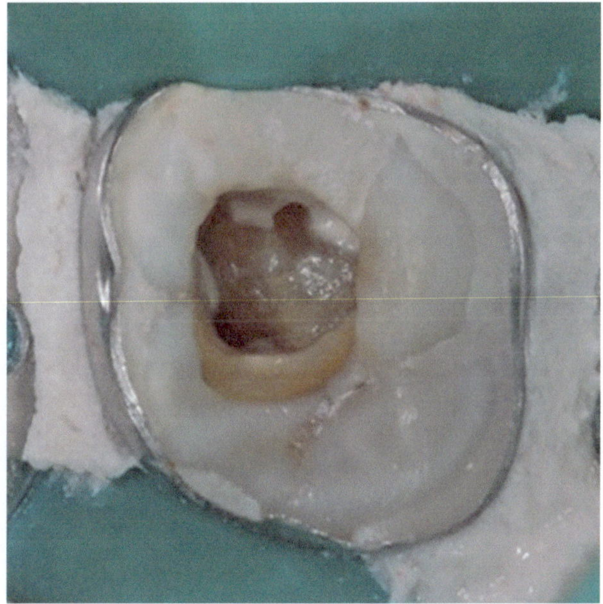

Fig. 16.11 Intra-operative view of the same tooth, after identification and shaping of MB2

(e) In vital teeth, a root canal orifice may be identified from a bleeding point in the floor of the pulp chamber.
(f) Where it is uncertain whether a bleeding point represents a root canal orifice or perforation, an apex locator connected to the end of a DG-16 probe or endodontic file (when rubber dam is in place) can be placed on the bleeding point. A perforation will register as a 'zero-reading'.
(g) The degradation of organic tissue by sodium hypochlorite produces gaseous products, which, within a pulp chamber filled with this irrigant, can sometimes be seen to bubble up from their point of origin—helping to identify the position of root canal orifices.
(h) Where a root has a single canal, the canal will be centred within the root. However, where a root has more than one root canal, the root canals will be 'off-centre'. Where one root canal has been identified, and a second suspected, but not yet found, an angled LCPA radiograph may be taken (with a file inserted inside the located canal) to determine whether this is centred or not.
(i) The closer the root canal orifices are to each other, the more likely they are to merge into a single canal within the root.
(j) Maxillary first molar teeth generally have four root canals: mesio-buccal (MB) 1, MB2, disto-buccal, and palatal. Untreated MB2 canals are a common cause of endodontic failure in these teeth [9], as the MB2 orifice can be challenging to locate, especially without the use of magnification. Görduysus et al. (2001) [10] reported that the MB2 orifice was often found on a line between the MB1 and palatal root canal, usually within 2 mm of the MB1 orifice (Fig. 16.11).

16.8 Optimisation of RCT/RCReTx

(a) Following restorability assessment, any missing axial walls should ideally be (temporarily) restored (Fig. 16.4) with a glass-ionomer cement +/– an orthodontic band (in posterior teeth) or composite resin (directly or via a temporary crown). This facilitates the creation of a four-walled access cavity, which provides the following advantages:
    - Alongside the use of rubber dam, contributes to effective intra-appointment isolation
    - Creates a reservoir for irrigants to pool and exchange
    - Ease of temporisation (if multi-visit treatment), allowing efficient and effective attainment of an inter-appointment coronal seal
    - Reduces the risk of coronal fracture
(b) The replacement of metallic restorations with non-metallic direct restorations reduces aberrant electronic apex locator readings via short-circuiting.

16.9 Protection of the Tooth and Temporisation

(a) The stiffness, and resistance to fracture, of teeth which are undergoing or which have undergone RCT/RCReTx, is significantly reduced, especially in posterior teeth, where one or more marginal ridges have been lost [11]. Ultimately, the predictability of survival posterior root filled teeth is enhanced by provision of a definitive cast cuspal-coverage restoration (ideally cast) [12]. However, prior to definitive restoration of posterior teeth, undergoing or which have undergone RCT/RCReTx, the following precautions can be taken to reduce the risk of fracture:
   - Placement of an orthodontic band (Fig. 16.11).
   - Reduction of cusps by 2 mm and provision of occlusal coverage with a 2 mm layer of either glass ionomer cement (GIC) or composite resin to contribute to a more uniform loading of the tooth tissue. Where there is already inter-occlusal space (e.g. posterior open bite, deficient opposing restoration, etc.), then occlusal reduction may not be necessary prior to provision of the build-up.
   - Provision of a temporary crown and (re)accessing through it.

(b) Where the RCT/RCReTx is being carried out over more than one session, inter-appointment temporisation can be achieved by dressing the root canal(s) with non-setting calcium hydroxide, placement of a piece of sponge into the access cavity (allowing room for a depth temporary restorative material coronally), and placement of a temporary restoration, such as GIC or Intermediate Restorative Material (IRM) (Dentsply Sirona, Charlotte, North Carolina, USA).

We hope that these top tips will provide a useful guide for achieving efficient and effective endodontic access. The advice given may require some adaptation to individual clinical circumstances.

16.10 Conclusion

Endodontic access is a fundamental stage in the provision of optimal root canal treatment. A good knowledge of endodontic anatomy to guide orientation and minimising tooth tissue removal is important to allow unimpeded access to the canal system during biomechanical preparation.

References

1. Abbott PV. Assessing restored teeth with pulp and periapical diseases for the presence of cracks, caries and marginal breakdown. Aust Dent J. 2004;49:33–9.
2. Smith RJR, McColl E, Bryce GE. Top tips for restoration of root-filled teeth: part 1 – minimally invasive techniques for anterior teeth. Br Dent J. 2022;233:592–4.
3. Smith RJR, McColl E, Bryce GE. Top tips for restoration of root-filled teeth: part 2 – management of broken-down anterior teeth. Br Dent J. 2022;233:704–7.

4. Smith RJR, McColl E, Bryce GE. Top tips for restoration of root-filled teeth: part 3 – posterior teeth. Br Dent J. 2022;233:830–2.
5. Patel S, Brown J, Semper M, Abella F, Mannocci F. European Society of Endodontology position statement: use of cone beam computed tomography in endodontics. Int Endod J. 2019;52:1675–8.
6. Kahler B. Present status and future directions – managing discoloured teeth. Int Endod J. 2022;55:922–50.
7. Tomson PL. A guide to good endodontic practice. British Endodontic Society; 2022. https://britishendodonticsociety.org.uk/_userfiles/pages/files/a4_bes_guidelines_2022_hyperlinked_final.pdf. Accessed November 2023.
8. Krasner P, Rankow H. Anatomy of the pulp chamber floor. J Endodont. 2004;30:516.
9. Wolcott J, Ishley D, Kennedy W, Johnson S, Minnich S, Meyers J. A 5 yr clinical investigation of second mesiobuccal canals in endodontically treated and retreated maxillary second maxillary molars. J Endodont. 2005;31:262–4.
10. Görduysus MO, Görduysus M, Friedman S. Operating microscope improves negotiation of second mesiobuccal canals in maxillary molars. J Endodont. 2001;27:683–6.
11. Reeh ES, Messer HH, Douglas WH. Reduction in tooth stiffness as a result of endodontic and restorative procedures. J Endodont. 1989;15:512–6.
12. Aquilino SA, Caplan DJ. Relationship between crown placement and the survival of endodontically treated teeth. J Prosthet Dent. 2002;87:256–63.

Minimally Invasive Techniques for Endodontically Treated Anterior Teeth

17

R. J. R. Smith, Ewen McColl, and G. Ewen Bryce

Learning Points

- Recall the various mechanisms that can result in tooth discolouration.
- Appreciate the non-vital bleaching technique and the various methods that can be provided.
- Recognise the technique to provide a restoration within the access cavity, which is important for coronal seal and minimising further discolouration.
- Understand when a porcelain laminate veneer can be provided for discoloured anterior units.

17.1 Introduction

Trauma to anterior teeth is a common cause of pulp necrosis and subsequent requirement for root canal treatment (RCT). Pulp pathosis in such teeth is usually mediated via bacterial ingress through cracks/fractures, +/− damage to the blood supply of the tooth. In such cases, the bulk of tooth tissue may be relatively intact (though often discoloured to some extent). In this paper, we offer advice for restorative management of such teeth, via minimally invasive techniques.

R. J. R. Smith
Defence Centre for Rehabilitative Dentistry, Aldershot, UK

E. McColl (✉)
Peninsula Dental School, Plymouth, UK
e-mail: ewen.mccoll@plymouth.ac.uk

G. E. Bryce
Restorative Dentistry, Defence Centre for Rehabilitative Dentistry, Aldershot, UK

E. McColl, A. Alani (eds.), *Practical Tips in Clinical Dentistry*, BDJ Clinician's Guides, https://doi.org/10.1007/978-3-031-90355-7_17

17.2 Assessment

(a) Prior to (re)restoration of a root-filled tooth, clinical and radiographic assessment should determine the following: the restorability of the tooth, nature of any discolouration, technical quality of the root-filling, periapical health, and presence of root fractures or resorption lesions. We advocate the removal of all restorative materials as part of the restorability assessment.

(b) When clinical or radiographic signs/symptoms of non-resolving endodontic pathology or the root-filling is technically sub-optimal (e.g. voids or does not extend to within 2 mm of the radiographic apex [1]), then root canal re-treatment +/− referral to a specialist endodontist is advised prior to bleaching (if required) and definitive restoration (Figs. 17.1 and 17.2).

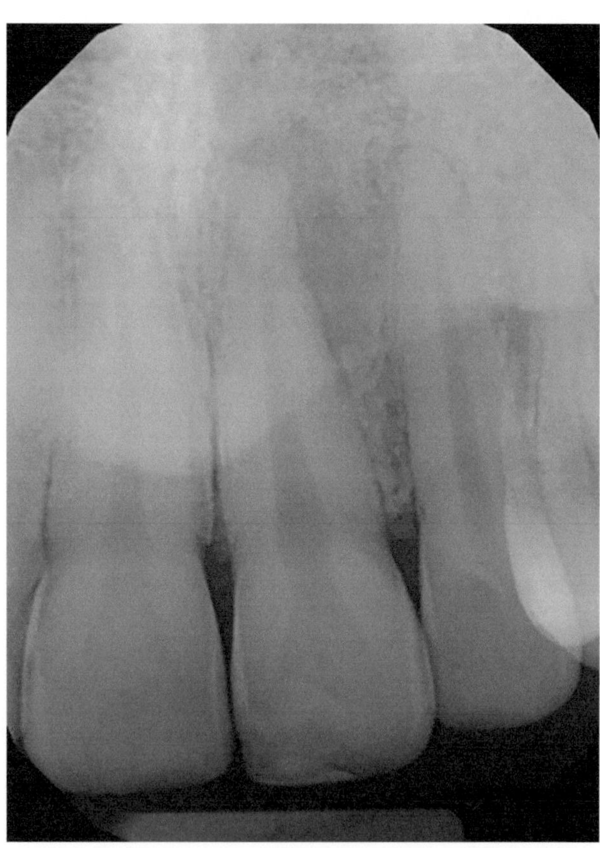

Fig. 17.1 Previously traumatised, non-vital, 21 tooth in a young adult. Wide root canal. Large eccentrically positioned periapical lesion

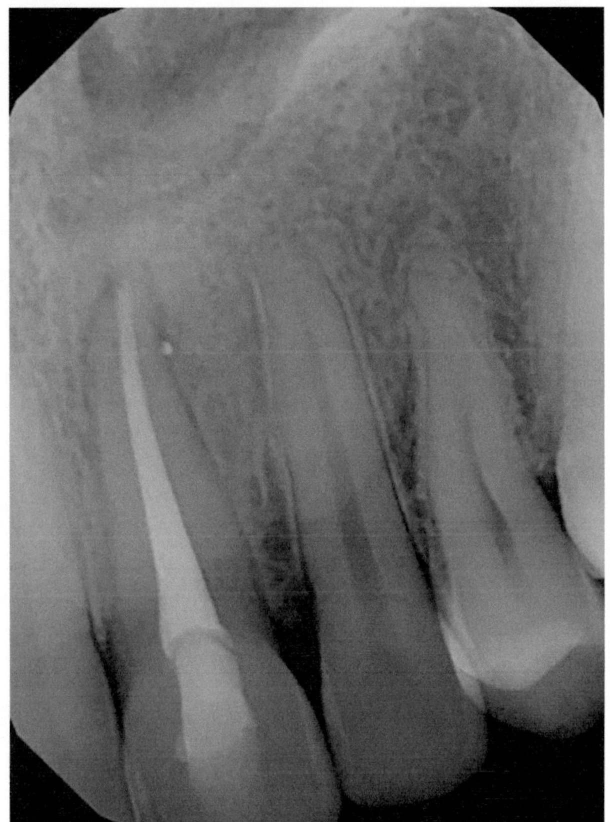

Fig. 17.2 Twelve-month follow-up radiograph. Unnecessary over-widening of the access cavity was avoided. Access cavity was restored using GIC (over the gutta-percha), flowable composite (over the GIC), and surfaced with a layer of nano-filled universal composite resin. Note filled lateral canal and healing of the periapical lesion

17.3 Discolouration

(a) Root-treated teeth can be discoloured due to one or more intrinsic or extrinsic mechanisms [2]; some of the most common ones are outlined in Table 17.1.

(b) Partial or complete calcification of the root canals (e.g. calcific metamorphosis) has a reported incidence of 4–24% following dental trauma [3]. The crowns of affected teeth classically have a yellow hue, and root canal calcification can be confirmed radiographically. Pulp testing in such teeth is unreliable [4], which can complicate decision-making. RCT is not indicated unless there are clear clinical or radiographic signs of pulpal pathosis, for instance, pain or periapical radiolucency. The appearance of both vital and non-vital teeth with calcific metamorphosis can generally be improved with bleaching, although the regime may need to be continued for up to 3 months to effect a discernible change. If vital bleaching is unsuccessful, then the aesthetics of the tooth can often be improved via minimal tooth preparation and provision of a low translucency opacious porcelain veneer (see Sect. 17.5).

Table 17.1 Intrinsic and extrinsic causes of discoloured root-treated teeth

	Mechanism	Appearance of crown	Management
Intrinsic	Leakage of haemolytic breakdown products into dentine, subsequently metabolised by bacteria	Uniform grey appearance	Bleaching
	Remnants of pulp tissue in pulp horn(s)	Localised grey/brown discolouration in coronal-third	Mechanical and chemical debridement of the pulp horns +/− bleaching
	Partial or complete calcification of root canal(s)	Uniform yellow appearance	Bleaching
	Gutta-percha or root canal sealer within pulp chamber	Localised band of discolouration, consistent with the coronal extent of material	Removal of materials from pulp chamber +/− bleaching as required
	Mineral trioxide aggregate (MTA) (via bismuth oxide component)	Dependent on the coronal extent of the MTA but often localised to the gingival-third	Opacious veneering material to disguise
Extrinsic	Dietary (e.g. tea, coffee, red wine, etc) or tobacco-related stain	May be adsorbed onto the surface of the tooth but may also leach into tooth tissue via craze and crack lines	Bleaching followed by surface sealing with resin bonded composite to prevent further ingress of stain

17.4 Non-vital Bleaching

(a) Root-filled teeth, discoloured via organic pigment staining, are amenable to non-vital bleaching. Prior to definitive restoration, bleaching can be delivered either via an internal ('walking-bleach') approach (e.g. sealing bleach into the pulp chamber) or a combined internal/external approach (e.g. bleach is placed into the pulp chamber, as well as a custom-made bleaching tray).

(b) Historically, 35% hydrogen peroxide was commonly used for bleaching non-vital teeth in conjunction with the walking-bleach technique. However, since 2012, the maximum allowable concentration of hydrogen peroxide in dental bleaching products within the EU/UK has been limited to 6% [5]. In the authors' experience, bleaching agents at this lower concentration are ineffective for use with the walking-bleach technique but are suitable for use with the combined internal/external bleaching technique. Whilst some relapse in discolouration may occur over time, due to the infiltration of pigments via craze and crack-lines, 85% colour stability for bleached teeth has been reported at 25 years [6]. The risks and benefits of bleaching should be weighed up and discussed with the patient as part of the consent process.

(c) The authors' protocol for internal/external bleaching includes the following steps:

- Pre-operative photographs of the tooth are taken alongside a representative shade tab to enable an objective assessment of the relative success of treatment.
- Impressions for study casts are taken, and a lab-made flexible or Essix-type bleaching tray is requested.
- Rubber dam isolation of the affected tooth (and adjacent teeth to facilitate orientation of the bur within the palatal access cavity). Under magnification (loupes or microscope if available), dental materials are then carefully removed from the pulp chamber in two stages: bulk removal and removal of remnants. Bulk removal of restorative materials is undertaken with a long-tapered course diamond bur in a high-speed handpiece, taking care to avoid the removal of tooth tissue. If a well colour-matched restorative material has been used previously, this can be difficult to visualise. Rubbing the tip of a metal probe over the walls of the access cavity will tend to leave a grey mark on composite/glass-ionomer cement (GIC) remnants but will not mark dentine/enamel and helps to avoid unnecessary removal of tooth tissue. Any small tags of restorative material can often be dislodged with a DG16 probe or ultrasonic scaler, whilst root canal sealer residue can be removed from the walls by scrubbing them with a Tepe brush (TePe, Malmö, Sweden) soaked in a suitable solvent (e.g. eucalyptus oil). The pulp horns are then explored with a DG16 probe. Where necessary, access to the pulp horns can be further developed with a suitably sized Meisinger pulp chamber bur prior to chemical debridement/disinfection with 1–5% sodium hypochlorite solution.
- The gutta-percha (GP) root-filling should then be trimmed back to a level 2 mm apical to the amelo-cemental junction (ACJ) using either a heated plugger, ultrasonic scaler, or Gates Glidden drill. The root-filling should then be sealed via careful placement of a 2 mm layer of GIC up to the level of the ACJ [7]. The seal protects the root-filling from bacterial ingress and potentially offers more protection to the ACJ zone to collateral damage from the bleaching agent: a potential risk factor for external cervical resorption. In placing the seal, care should be taken to avoid GIC getting onto the walls of the pulp chamber (above the level of the ACJ), as this will inhibit the permeation of bleach into dentine in that area. The authors find that by using an encapsulated GIC, a line of material can be piped across the back of a gloved hand and the setting carefully monitored until it starts to enter the rubbery phase, at which point a portion of the material is then carried over to the tooth and packed down with a Machtou plugger.
- Sometimes, removing the discoloured materials from the pulp chamber negates the need for bleaching, and once the pulp chamber has been cleared of debris, the (dis)colouration of the tooth and requirement for bleaching should be reassessed.
- Where progression to internal/external bleaching is indicated, several syringes of either 10% or 16% carbamide peroxide (respectively, releasing 3.6% or 5.7% hydrogen peroxide) should be issued to the patient and a

demonstration given as to how to place bleaching gel into both the access cavity and bleaching tray (at the position corresponding to the tooth to be bleached). We advise our patients to wear their bleaching tray for 2–4 h per day initially, and if no side effects are encountered after the first 2 days (e.g. troublesome chemical irritation of the gingivae or dentine sensitivity), then the frequency and duration of wear (up to overnight wear) can be increased by the patient. The patient is instructed on how to keep the access cavity clean at home using a suitably sized TePe brush +/– lavage with tap water via a syringe with a 23-gauge blunt-ended needle (Monoject, Kendall, Nashville, USA).

- The patient should attend for review at 1, 2, and 4 weeks to assess the progress of the treatment.
- If the pulp chamber has been prepared in accordance with this protocol and the patient is compliant with the bleaching regime, the majority of improvement tends to occur within the first week. However, where required, limited further whitening can often be achieved by extending the bleaching duration to 4 weeks. Following the completion of non-vital bleaching, the access cavity should be definitively restored as soon as possible. Where surface craze/crack-lines are present on the labial aspect, sealing of the surface layer with bonded composite resin can reduce the risk of rebound discolouration.

17.5 Restoration of the Access Cavity

(a) Following completion of RCT (or bleaching), the access cavity should be definitively restored as soon as possible to help support residual tooth structure and create an effective coronal seal. Meticulous technique is required to avoid the creation of air inclusions within the restoration.

(b) In the depths of the access cavity, where dentine bonding agent and composite resin cannot be predictably cured, GIC can be packed in place as a base using the methods previously discussed.

(c) At cavity depths of <5 mm, predictable light curing can be achieved. Light curing from the incisal aspect should be supplemented with additional light curing from the labial and palatal aspects (where a limited amount of light may penetrate the tooth tissue). Following acid etching and application/cure of a dentine bonding agent, the base may be (further) built up using a flowable composite resin such as smart dentine replacement (SDR) (Dentsply Caulk, Milford, USA). This material has excellent wettability and readily adapts to the cavity walls. To avoid air inclusions, the applicator tip of the flowable composite should be inserted into the cavity base before slowly injecting the material and simultaneously withdrawing the applicator from the cavity. The material will tend to slump due to gravity and, if required, can be quickly manipulated with a probe prior to curing.

(d) The final increment of composite should be a harder wearing universal-type composite such as Filtek Supreme XTE (3 M ESPE, Seefeld, Germany). The use of a composite modelling instrument, such as OptraSculpt (Ivoclar Vivadent, Amherst, USA), improves the efficiency and accuracy of composite placement prior to finishing with a composite polishing system (as required).

17.6 Definitive Direct Vs Indirect Restoration

(a) Composite resin provides an effective definitive direct restoration in a root-filled anterior tooth where >50% of coronal tooth tissue remains and there is sufficient pulp chamber to retain the core [8]; there is a ring of enamel for bonding; and tooth discolouration can be camouflaged by composite overlay. However, the clinician must consider that the dentine-resin bond strength may be reduced via:
   - The presence of restorative material residue on the dentine surface and within the medial end of the dentinal tubules.
   - Differences in the nature of the dentine substrate within the pulp chamber compared to that on the outer aspects of the tooth, namely: pre-dentine vs dentine, and wider diameter of dentinal tubules on the inner aspect of the tooth.

(b) Where a discoloured root-filled anterior tooth has not responded to bleaching and the patient is seeking a restoration to camouflage this, a porcelain laminate veneer restoration may be appropriate, where the tooth is largely unrestored (except for the access cavity), the enamel on the labial face of the tooth is intact and bruxing, or parafunctional forces can be controlled.

17.7 Porcelain Laminate Veneers

(a) The provision of a porcelain laminate veneer often requires tooth preparation, which is an irreversible process. To provide a sufficient thickness of opacious material, a veneer on a discoloured tooth will often need to be ≥0.7 mm (although this can be thinner in non-discoloured cases). Alternatively, a shallower tooth preparation can be undertaken, accepting that this will increase the mesial-distal thickness of the crown.

(b) The relative advantages of using an indirect restoration to mask out discoloured tooth tissue should be balanced against the disadvantages of reducing tooth structure, potentially increasing the risk of crown fracture, and should be fully discussed with the patient as part of the consent process.

(c) When specifying porcelain laminate veneers for discoloured teeth, the authors include the following aspects on the labwork prescription:
   - Material: e.g. lithium disilicate with opaquing layer.
   - Shade map of the tooth tissue.
   - Desired shade and characterisation of veneer.

17.8 Conclusions

In this chapter, we have explored the various ways in which a tooth can discolour and the methods and means to correct this from minimally invasive approaches to more invasive and the provision of indirect restorations. An important factor to consider is the relative reduction and removal of tooth tissue and the subsequent restorative burden this may create in the future for the patient.

References

1. Ng Y-L, Mann V, Rahbaran S, Lewsey J, Gulabivala K. Outcome of primary root canal treatment: systematic review of the literature—part 2. Influence of clinical factors. Int Endod J. 2008;41:1026–46.
2. Ahmed H, Abbot P. Discolouration potential of endodontic procedures and materials: a review. Int Endod J. 2012;45:883–97.
3. McCabe P, Dummer P. Pulp canal obliteration: an endodontic diagnosis and treatment challenge. Int Endod J. 2012;45:177–97.
4. Oginni A, Adekoya-Sofowara C, Kolawole K. Evaluation of radiographs, clinical signs, and symptoms associated with pulp canal obliteration: an aid to treatment decision. Dent Traumatol. 2009;25:620–5.
5. General Dental Council. Position statement on tooth whitening. 11 July 2016. https://www.gdc-uk.org/DownloadHelper.aspx?docID=79862d90-5a1e-437d-8bdd-d511ab64b8cb. Accessed 11 June 2022.
6. Amato A, Caggiano M, Pantaleo G, Amato M. In-office and walking bleach dental treatments on endodontically treated teeth: 25 years follow-up. Minerva Stomatol. 2018;67:225–30.
7. Rotstein I, Zyskind D, Lewinstein I, Bamberger N. Effect of different protective base materials on hydrogen peroxide leakage during intracoronal bleaching in vitro. J Endodont. 1992;18:114–7.
8. Zarow M, Ramírez-Sebastià A, Paolone G, et al. A new classification system for the restoration root filled teeth. Int Endod J. 2018;51:318–34.

Restoring Broken-Down Endodontically Treated Anterior Teeth

18

R. J. R. Smith, Ewen McColl, and G. E. Bryce

Learning Points

- Understand the indications for crowns in anterior units.
- Recall indications for posts in anterior teeth.
- Appreciate the different types and materials for posts and how this impacts the tooth tissue and the subsequent definitive restoration.
- Recall the process of post provision from impression-making to cementation.

18.1 Introduction

Root-filled anterior teeth have reduced tooth structure, associated with previous caries, fractures, restorative interventions, and access cavity preparation. In this paper, we offer advice for restorative management of 'broken-down' anterior teeth, characterised by loss of >50% coronal tooth tissue.

18.2 Assessment

(a) Initial clinical and radiographic examination, followed by restorability assessment (including removal of restorations from the tooth in question), should be undertaken prior to confirming whether a root-filled tooth is predictably restorable, and if so by what means.

R. J. R. Smith
Defence Centre for Rehabilitative Dentistry, Aldershot, UK

E. McColl (✉)
Peninsula Dental School, Plymouth, UK
e-mail: ewen.mccoll@plymouth.ac.uk

G. E. Bryce
Restorative Dentistry, Defence Centre for Rehabilitative Dentistry, Aldershot, UK

E. McColl, A. Alani (eds.), *Practical Tips in Clinical Dentistry*, BDJ Clinician's Guides, https://doi.org/10.1007/978-3-031-90355-7_18

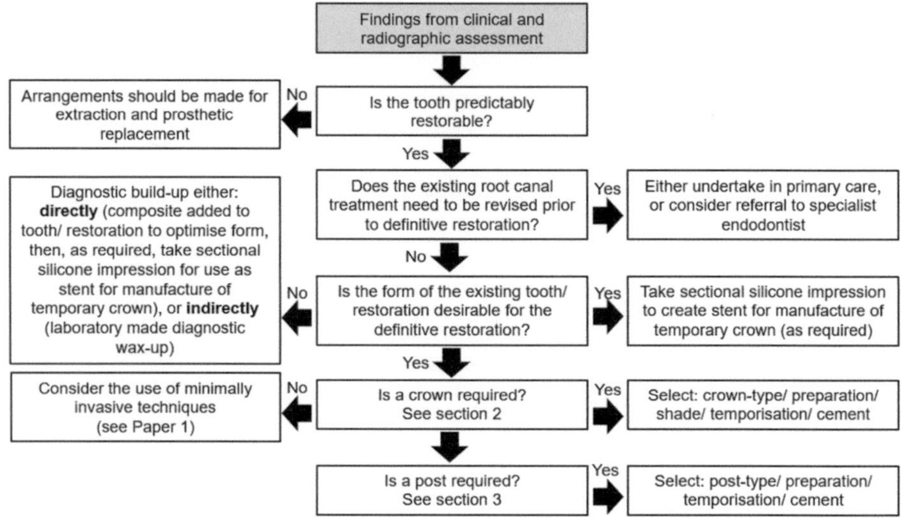

Fig. 18.1 The findings at assessment inform the treatment planning process

(b) The findings at assessment inform the treatment planning process, which are summarised in the flow chart (Fig. 18.1).

18.3 Crowns

(a) A crown is appropriate where <50% of the coronal tooth structure remains; tooth tissue is of poor quality (e.g. developmental disorders); insufficient enamel remains for predictable resin bonding; history of failed composite/porcelain veneers; and severe discolouration, which has not responded to bleaching, or the tooth is subject to heavy occlusal loading.
(b) If a crown for an anterior tooth is indicated, excellent aesthetics and functional outcomes can be achieved with lithium disilicate glass ceramic crowns, which can be bonded to tooth tissue. However, where there is heavy occlusal loading (e.g. in bruxist patients), a layered zirconia or porcelain-fused-to-metal crown may be more suitable.
(c) The overall shade/characterisation of the crown should be specified, along with the shade of the 'stump' (as the laboratory technician will need to take this into account when specifying the relative opacity of the substructure if a glass ceramic crown is prescribed).

18.4 Function of a Post

(a) Posts are indicated when there is insufficient coronal tooth tissue to retain a core.
(b) Posts do not improve the fracture resistance of teeth [1].

18.5 Types of Post

(a) Posts may be classified as either prefabricated (e.g. glass fibre, metal or ceramic) or custom-made (e.g. cast metal post/core). The authors use either glass fibre or cast metal post/cores, which are discussed below.

(b) Glass fibre posts. These are made from unidirectionally arranged glass fibres embedded within a resin matrix. They are cemented in place with a dentine-bonded resin cement prior to core build-up with a composite resin.
   - Advantages: Fibre posts can be placed at the same time as obturation, improving the immediate coronal seal; tapered designs conform better to the root canal anatomy than conventional parallel-sided cast post/core systems and may be more conservative of tooth tissue; fracture of fibre post-treated teeth is more likely to be retrievable compared to those treated with cast posts/cores [2].
   - Disadvantages: Mechanical preparation of the post space (if required) will weaken the tooth; debonding of fibre posts is a common cause of failure [3] and is a symptom of the challenges of dentine bonding within a sub-optimal intra-radicular environment (e.g. predentine vs dentine, smear layer, altered dentine due to endodontic irrigants, sealer residue); and, where post debond has occurred, this may precipitate fracture of the post/core, microleakage, and caries.

(c) Cast post/cores. These are integral precious metal cast post/core (example in Fig. 18.2), which are constructed in the laboratory from either a Duralay (Reliance Dental, Alsip, USA) direct post/core pick-up or impression.
   - Advantages: No interface between post and core—integral unit; can be used to retain a core when there is no ferrule (though not ideal) [4].
   - Disadvantages: Mechanical preparation of the post space is almost always required and will weaken the tooth; forces are transmitted to the thinner apical root structure and can precipitate root fracture; catastrophic fracture is more likely in teeth treated with cast post/cores versus teeth with a fibre post [5]; and, due to the requirement for post-preparation and post-fit on separate occasions, there is a risk of inter-appointment coronal leakage.

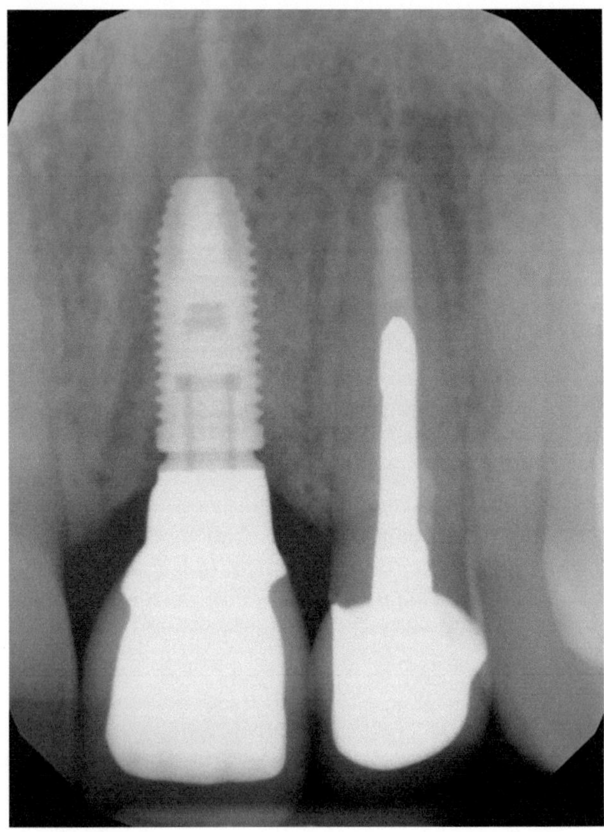

Fig. 18.2 Patient had experienced trauma to the 21 and 22 teeth. The 21 tooth was deemed non-restorable and replaced with an implant supported crown. The 22 tooth was extensively damaged, and following root canal treatment, a Type IV gold post/core was fabricated via the Duralay pick-up technique, and restored with a layered zirconia crown

18.6 Choosing a Post

(a) Decisions on whether a post is indicated, and if so which type, are principally guided by the amount of residual tooth structure.
(b) A useful classification to guide decision-making for post placement has been proposed by Zarow et al. (2018) [6]:
    - Class 0 (no post recommended): >50% of coronal structure, >2 walls intact, and sufficient pulp chamber to support core.
    - Class 1 (fibre post recommended): <50% coronal tooth structure, ≤2 walls, and > 2 mm ferrule.
    - Class 2 (crown lengthening or ortho extrusion recommended): absence of ferrule. Following crown lengthening or orthodontic extrusion, the type of post required will be guided by the height of tooth tissue available for the ferrule effect.
    - Class 3 (cast gold alloy post/core recommended): ≤2 walls, <2 mm ferrule.

18.7 Timing of Post Space Preparation

(a) Whenever possible, the post space should be prepared at the obturation visit because:
- Rubber dam isolation will already be in place, reducing the risk of contamination of the root canal.
- The clinician will be familiar with the anatomy of the root canal system, reducing the risk of iatrogenic damage.
- Preparation of the post space will disturb the apical root-filling. Where the root canal sealer has set, this disturbance could increase the risk of micro-leakage. However, if the post space preparation is finalised immediately following obturation, the sealer will not set by this point, and there is a chance that unset sealer could re-adapt to fill any gaps between the root-filling and root canal walls.

18.8 Recommendations for Determining Post Length

(a) The post should extend to two-thirds of the length of the root [7] or at least equal to the height of crown [8].
(b) To preserve the apical seal, the post space should not extend closure than 5 mm from the terminus of the root-filling [9].

18.9 Recommendations for Determining Post Width

(a) The volume of remaining tooth tissue, rather than the type of post, is the better predictor of tooth survival [10]. Therefore, post preparation should be conservative of both coronal and radicular dentine.
(b) The authors recommend that the minimum thickness of posts should be 1.5 mm.
(c) Whilst various approaches to post space preparation exist, the authors recommend a conservationist approach and that a minimum of 1 mm of circumferential root dentine thickness remains [11]. The following points should be considered when estimating the thickness of residual root dentine:
- Roots often have external concavities within their mesial/distal surfaces, especially where more than one root canal is present. Therefore, when assessing a long-cone periapical (LCPA) radiograph, it is easy to overestimate the amount of dentine thickness remaining due to superimposition phenomenon.
- Unless considerably angled in the horizontal plane, a LCPA radiograph will not provide information about dentine thickness in the labio-palatal/lingual dimension.

18.10 Undertaking Post Space Preparation

(a) Step 1: Removal of gutta percha (GP). Once the desired length of post is determined, GP is removed to that depth using a Gates Glidden bur or heated plugger. To assist in length control, a rubber bung can be placed onto a plugger and positioned at a pre-measured distance from the tip. Bungs placed on a Gates Glidden drill will tend to move along the shank during drill rotation, and it is useful to be aware that the position of the neck of the Gates Glidden drill relative to the incisal edge of the tooth can be referenced as 17 mm.

(b) Step 2: Post spaces can be prepared using either a parallel-sided twist drill or a tapered twist drill. A parallel-sided drill will cut a post space to a uniform width and generate a 90° floor-wall junction, which can precipitate areas of stress concentration in the apical area. In contrast, a tapered twist drill allows for greater conservation of dentine and a more rounded shape in the apical aspect of the preparation. Twist drills have a latch grip for use with a slow-speed handpiece but may also be operated using a latch-grip hand driver or even simply rotated between thumb and index finger (which allows for greater control in drilling). Post systems employ a series of twist drills of varying diameters. The narrowest drill to bind should be used first, sequentially followed by larger sizes as required. Finally, any remnants of gutta-percha and sealer on the walls of the post space can be removed with a Hedström file, kinked at the tip, to allow canal wall scraping, followed by scrubbing with a Tepe brush (TePe, Malmö, Sweden) soaked in a suitable solvent (e.g. eucalyptus oil).

(c) Step 3: Where an indirect post/core is prescribed and therefore risk of inter-appointment leakage exists, the root-filling should be sealed with a 1–2 mm barrier of Intermediate Restorative Material (IRM) (Dentsply Caulk, Milford, USA). The IRM should be allowed to start to set prior to packing a suitably sized ball of the material in place with a Machtou plugger. The coronal extension of this seal should be confirmed by re-measuring the depth of the post space. If excess material has been inadvertently placed, this can be quickly removed by the use of a pre-measured twist drill.

18.11 Clinical Records for Cast Metal Post/Cores

(a) Following preparation of the post space, an impression post should be selected, which corresponds to the width of the final twist drill to be taken to full-length. The walls of the post space are then coated with a thin layer of petroleum jelly using a thick paper point or TePe brush in order to help block out any undercuts and facilitate ease of retrieval of materials introduced to the post space during record taking.

(b) Records for the post/core labwork can be obtained via either:

- Taking an impression. A plastic impression post (e.g. ParaPost XP, Coltène/Whaledent AG, Altstätten, Switzerland) is positioned into the post space, and a working impression taken using either a single-phase polyether impression material (e.g. Impregum, 3 M ESPE, Seefeld, Germany) or a light-bodied/heavy-bodied silicone combination can be used.

- Duralay (Reliance Dental, Alsip, USA) direct post/core pick-up. The plastic impression post is adjusted to fit such that the head of the post nestles within the confines of the proposed core. The coronal third of the post is then built up using increments of Duralay applied with a composite manipulation brush. The post should be mobilised and re-seated prior to the full set to ensure that it can ultimately be removed from the post space. The tooth should then be prepared for a crown with the post/core in situ. If a lab-made temporary crown is required, an impression can be taken with the pattern in place (alginate may be accurate enough for this), prior to removing the pattern and temporising the tooth.

18.12 Cementation of Posts

(a) General advice:

- The post should be tried in to confirm it can be seated to the full depth of the preparation. If the post does not go to length, careful assessment should be undertaken to determine why and adjustments made as necessary:
  - To the casting itself in the case of a cast post/core.
  - To the post space preparation, not the post, in the case of a fibre post. Alternatively, a narrower fibre post may be used.
- Final cleaning of the post space should be completed by using an ultrasonic scaler (with fine long tip) on low-power +/− Tepe brush, rinsed with sterile water or normal saline via a syringe, and dried with paper points.
- A self-etching composite resin cement (e.g. RelyX Unciem, 3 M ESPE, Seefeld, Germany) is recommended for fibre posts, which can also be used for cast post/cores. However, cast post/cores may also be cemented with a suitable GIC (e.g. AquaCem, Dentsply Sirona, Charlotte, USA) or a resin-modified GIC (e.g. Fuji PLUS, GC Corporation, Tokyo, Japan).
- Where the cement product is presented with a fine-tipped applicator (e.g. RelyX Unicem), the incidence of voids within the cement layer can be minimised by priming the tip to expel any air bubbles, placing the application tip at the base of the post space prior to injection of the cement, and keeping the tip within the cement mass whilst simultaneously injecting and withdrawing the tip from the canal. The post is then slowly inserted to length, prior to removing the cement excess and light curing (as required).
- Where a fine application tip is not supplied with the chosen cementation product, the freshly mixed cement should be quickly loaded into the post space using a suitable instrument (e.g. DG16 probe) and used to liberally coat the post, prior to pump priming the post into position.
- In the case of fibre posts: Any excess length of the post (above the level of the desired core) should be removed with a high-speed handpiece, and following acid-etching and application of a dentine bonding agent, the core

should then be built up with composite resin and prepared to the required dimensions.

18.13 Provisionalisation

(a) It may be necessary to place a provisional (post-)crown in the following situations:
    - To assess the form and function of the restoration.
    - To assess the impact of significant changes to aesthetics.
    - To translate desirable changes to form, function, and aesthetics into the definitive restoration.
    - Inter-appointment stabilisation between post (or crown) preparation and fit.
    - To stabilise a particular tooth, which is involved in an overall comprehensive restorative plan, pending completion of other elements.
    - To stabilise a tooth whilst monitoring periapical healing.

(b) Temporary post-crowns have a propensity for marginal leakage [12], and further to adequate protection of the apical root filling (as previously discussed), should only be used a short-term measure.

(c) In situations where temporisation of a post space is required, but where a post-crown can be avoided (to minimise the risk of [re]contamination of the root canal system), this can be achieved by:
    - Placement of non-setting calcium hydroxide and a pellet of endodontic sponge (coronally) into the post space, followed by closure of the access cavity with IRM. At a subsequent appointment, the IRM can be readily removed with an ultrasonic scaler and the post space washed out.
    - Coordination of the direct sealing of the access cavity with provision of an Essix-type overdenture (which must be requested from the lab in advance).

(d) A chair-side provisional post-crown can be constructed where a suitable pre-operative silicone stent is available, by:
    - Customising a suitable temporary metal post (e.g. ParaPost) to the correct length.
    - Seating the temporary post to the full depth of the post space.
    - Syringing bis-acryl composite resin (e.g. ProTemp4, 3 M ESPE, Seefeld, Germany) around the post/prep and into the silicone stent prior to seating the stent.
    - After the bis-acryl composite resin has set, the post/crown can then be removed from the mouth, excess material removed, the crown polished, and cemented with a non-eugenol temporary cement (e.g. Fuji Temp LT, GC Corporation, Tokyo, Japan).

(e) Where a lab-made provisional crown has been requested, following cementation of the definitive post/core and refinement of the margins of the crown preparation, the temporary crown can be tried in. The temporary restoration can be relined as necessary using bis-acryl composite resin prior to cementation with a temporary cement.

18.14 Root-Filled Anterior Teeth in Heavily Loaded Situations

(a) The reduction in tooth structure associated with RCT and restorative procedures weakens teeth [13]. Additionally, de-innervation of teeth can predispose to occlusal overloading [14]. Where parafunction is suspected or confirmed and/or where a root filled-tooth is involved in dynamic occlusion, this further pre-disposes to over-loading and fracture. Where such situations are identified, consideration should be given to:
  - Design of the definitive restoration to reduce or relieve participation of the root-filled tooth in dynamic occlusion (e.g. by reducing the steepness of cuspal-inclines).
  - Use of cast post/cores where the effectiveness of the ferrule-effect is in doubt.
  - Provision of an occlusal splint for night-time wear.

(b) Root-filled teeth make sub-optimal bridge abutments and increase the risk of root fracture in abutment teeth. In clinical situations, where there are no alternatives to a root-filled tooth-supported bridge, the following should be considered:
  - The abutment tooth-type should be at least the same size (or ideally larger) than that of the pontic (e.g. maxillary central incisor acting as abutment for bridge replacing contralateral central incisor, or ipsilateral lateral incisor).
  - For a resin-bonded bridge, ideally, the labial aspect of the abutment tooth should be intact, and the palatal/lingual aspect should have >50% of enamel remaining. Any defective composite resin restorations should be replaced. The mechanical resistance form for the wing of the bridge can be enhanced by cutting a 1–1.5 mm box within the composite within the access cavity, ensuring that the walls of the box are in line with path of insertion of the bridge. To further enhance micro-mechanical retention prior to bonding, the palatal surface of the tooth should be air-abraded under rubber dam isolation with 50-micron alumina powder.
  - A fixed/fixed or fixed/moveable bridge design using either conventional or resin-bonded retainers can be employed where additional support is considered necessary over and above that which can be provided by a cantilever arrangement.

18.15 Conclusion

The restoration of anterior units with significantly reduced supragingival tooth volume requires a good awareness of occlusion whilst also ensuring optimal coronal seal to maintain endodontic health. Anatomical parameters such as root length and canal wall thickness play a role in post design. Maintenance of coronal seal during post-construction and delivery is an important aspect contributing to the final outcome. Where high occlusal loads are present, some precaution is required on units with reduced tooth volume.

References

1. Fokkinga W, Bell A-M, Kreulan C, Lassila L, Vallittu P, Creugars N. Ex vivo fracture resistance of direct resin composite complete crowns with and without posts on maxillary premolars. Int Endod J. 2005;38:230–7.
2. Zhou L, Wang Q. Comparison of fracture resistance between cast posts and fiber posts: a meta-analysis of literature. J Endodont. 2013;39:11–5.
3. Rasimick B, Wan J, Musikant B, Deutsch A. A review of failure modes in teeth restored with adhesively luted endodontic dowels. J Prosthodont. 2010;19:639–46.
4. Maroulakos G, Nagy W, Kontogiorgos E. Fracture resistance of compromised endodontically treated teeth restored with bonded post and cores: an in vitro study. J Prosthet Dent. 2015;114:390–7.
5. Franco E, Lins do Valle A, Pompeia Fraga de Almeida A, Rubo J, Pereira J. Fracture resistance of endodontically treated teeth restored with glass fiber posts of different lengths. J Prosthet Dent. 2014;111:30–4.
6. Zarow M, Ramírez-Sebastià A, Paolone G, et al. A new classification system for the restoration root filled teeth. Int Endod J. 2018;51:318–34.
7. Goodacre C, Spolnik K. The prosthodontic management of endodontically treated teeth: a literature review, II, maintaining the apical seal. J Prosthodont. 1995;4:51–3.
8. Sorensen J, Martinoff J. Clinically significant factors in dowel design. J Prosthet Dent. 1984;52:28–35.
9. Camp L, Todd M. The effect of dowel preparation on the apical seal of three common obturation techniques. J Prosthet Dent. 1983;50:664–6.
10. Naumann M, Schmitter M, Frankenberger R, Krastl G. 'Ferrule comes first. Post is second!' Fake news and alternative facts? A systematic review. J Endodont. 2018;44:212–9.
11. Lloyd P, Palik J. The philosophies of dowel diameter preparation: a literature review. J Prosthet Dent. 1993;69:32–6.
12. Fox K, Gutteridge D. An in vitro study of coronal microleakage in root-canal-treated teeth restored by the post and core technique. Int Endod J. 1997;30:361–8.
13. Reeh E, Messer H, Douglas W. Reduction in tooth stiffness as a result of endodontic and restorative procedures. J Endodont. 1989;15:512–6.
14. Randow K, Glantz K. On cantilever loading of vital and non-vital teeth. An experimental clinical study. Acta Odontol Scand. 1986;44:271–7.

Restoring Endodontically Treated Posterior Teeth

19

R. J. R. Smith, Ewen McColl, and G. E. Bryce

Learning Points

- Recall the biometric measurements required to assess tooth structure prior to treatment.
- Understand the need to restore teeth endodontically treated in a timely manner to avoid unnecessary coronal leakage or issues with structural integrity and potential breakdown.
- Recognise the need for core build-up and how this relates to the subsequent preparation and restoration.
- Appreciate the advantages and disadvantages of direct vs indirect restoration.
- Identify clinical factors that will influence material choice for the final restoration.

19.1 Introduction

A tooth requiring root canal treatment (RCT) has often previously experienced caries, trauma, or restoration. RCT further injures the tooth through multiple mediums, including quantitative removal of tooth structure for endodontic access, qualitative deterioration of tooth structure via root canal irrigants, and de-innervation leading to reduced neurosensory feedback to occlusal loading. Subsequently, the root-filled tooth is at significantly increased risk of (non-restorable) fracture and requires

R. J. R. Smith
Defence Centre for Rehabilitative Dentistry, Aldershot, UK

E. McColl (✉)
Peninsula Dental School, Plymouth, UK
e-mail: ewen.mccoll@plymouth.ac.uk

G. E. Bryce
Restorative Dentistry, Defence Centre for Rehabilitative Dentistry, Aldershot, UK

E. McColl, A. Alani (eds.), *Practical Tips in Clinical Dentistry*, BDJ Clinician's Guides, https://doi.org/10.1007/978-3-031-90355-7_19

careful restorative consideration. Part 3 of this series outlines key factors to consider when planning restoration of root-filled posterior teeth.

19.2 Saving or Replacing an Existing Restoration

(a) A restorability assessment should be undertaken before RCT and include the removal of all existing restorative materials in order to be able to identify caries, cracks, and marginal leakage [1]. However, exceptionally, when a tooth requires RCT treatment subsequent to recent placement of a restoration (within last 6 months) and the treating clinician is familiar with the amount, distribution, and quality of the tooth tissue that remained at the time of restoration, endodontic access can be prepared through an existing restoration. However, it should be borne in mind that creating an endodontic access cavity through an existing restoration (especially cast restorations) often hinders proper orientation, makes root canal identification more challenging, and increases the likelihood of excessive removal dentine as well as the risk of perforation. Where a restoration has been compromised via preparation of an endodontic access cavity, it should be replaced following completion of the RCT.
(b) Where a tooth has an existing prosthetic crown, taking a pre-operative sectional silicone impression prior to the restorability assessment facilitates the subsequent manufacture of an indirect temporary restoration using a bis-acryl composite resin (e.g. ProTemp4, 3 M ESPE, Seefeld, Germany).

19.3 Assessing Tooth Structure

(a) The margins of a cast restoration should ideally encircle the prepared tooth structure to create a ferrule. Desirable features of a ferrule have been reported to include the following: tooth tissue encircled by the ferrule should be >1 mm in height [2], >1.5 mm in thickness [3], and ideally extend circumferentially around the tooth [4]. As a diagnostic aid, to determine whether an adequate ferrule effect can be generated, a crown margin may be prepared at the time of restorability assessment to quantify how much dentine remains.
(b) Where inadequate supra-gingival coronal dentine remains, additional height for the preparation may be gained via subgingival margin placement. The supracrestal attachment of the periodontium comprises both connective tissue and junctional epithelium and has been reported to be 2.04 mm thick on average [5]. Encroachment of the restorative margin into the supracrestal attachment is associated with inflammation +/− loss of periodontal supporting tissue [6]. Therefore, the clinician should undertake six-point probing around the tooth to establish the profile of the periodontal pockets and avoid placement of the margin closer than 0.5 mm from the depth of the gingival sulcus [7]. Alternatively, surgical crown lengthening can be employed to increase the amount of available supra-gingival dentine available.

19.4 Timing

(a) It is the authors' opinion that the risk of fracture and possible subsequent need for extraction outweighs the risk of delaying definitive restoration to confirm apical healing. Indeed, it has been shown that delayed provision of a definitive restoration for root-filled teeth has been shown to be associated with increased risk of tooth loss [8]. Therefore, where possible, a definitive core with cuspal coverage should be placed at the obturation appointment or as soon as possible after this. However, provision of a definitive cast restoration should be delayed if the tooth remains symptomatic (e.g. tenderness, non-healing sinus, or suppuration) following RCT, pointing to failure of the endodontic treatment and need for root canal re-treatment +/− referral to a specialist endodontist.
(b) Where doubt exists as to whether the RCT has been successful, then a root-filled posterior tooth should be provisionally restored with either a definitive core incorporating cuspal coverage or a temporary crown, prior to definitive management.

19.5 Pulp Chamber Management

(a) Root-filling material, which extends into the pulp chamber, should be removed prior to the restoration of the tooth in order to maximise the available space for retention of the core. Gutta-percha can easily be easily removed with a heated plugger or ultrasonic scaler (used for up to 10 s at a time, without water coolant, in order to guard against the risk of thermal injury to the tooth and supporting tissues).
(b) Remnants of unset sealer on the floor and walls of the pulp chamber should be removed using a solvent such as pure eucalyptus oil or an ethanol-based cleaner (e.g. AH Plus Cleaner, Dentsply, Konstanz, Germany) in conjunction with a cotton wool pledget held by tweezers or a microbrush (e.g. Ultrabrush, Microbrush International, Grafton, USA).
(c) Where the root canals are not going to be used to contribute towards retention of the core (see next section), then root canal orifices should be sealed to reduce the risk of (re)contamination of the root canal system in the event of future marginal breakdown around the core material. The rubber dam should remain in place until the orifices are sealed and ideally until the completion of core placement. An orifice seal can be achieved by removing the coronal 2 mm of GP from the root canal orifice with a heated plugger, ultrasonic scaler, or (less ideally) a Gates Glidden drill. The coronal 2 mm of each root canal is then sealed with glass ionomer cement (GIC). The use of a resin modified GIC provides the clinician with a level of control over the setting of the material, which can be initially manipulated with a Machtou plugger under illumination incorporating a blue-light filter; curing can be carefully accelerated by reflecting the unfiltered operating light into the pulp chamber (via a dental mirror) prior to further manipulation of the material, before commencing to final curing with a

conventional light curing unit. Alternatively, if amalgam is to be used as the core material, then Intermediate Restorative Material (Dentsply Caulk, Milford, USA) can be placed, which makes use of the inherent antibacterial properties of this zinc-oxide eugenol-containing material.

19.6 Core Placement

(a) Cavity preparation prior to core placement in a posterior tooth includes: removal of any unsupported enamel, use of the pulp chamber to enhance retention and resistance form, reduction of guiding cusps by 2 mm, reduction of balancing cusps by 1.5 mm, rounded internal angles, and preparation of a 90° cavo-surface angle to create a 'butt finish'.

(b) Either amalgam or composite is advised as core material in posterior teeth. Amalgam is a tried and tested material, offers good longevity, is strong in compression, offers good contrast with tooth tissue allowing ease of preparation, and is less technique-sensitive than composite alternatives. The mechanical retention of an amalgam core can be enhanced via the extension of amalgam 2–4 mm into the orifice of each root canal. However, in a modified approach to that proposed by Nayyar [9], we advocate that to avoid further structural weakening of the tooth, root canals should not be further prepared to facilitate amalgam packing. Alternatively, retention may be enhanced via amalgam bonding [10].

(c) Composite resin provides a contemporary alternative to amalgam. However, the challenges of achieving predictable light-activated polymerisation of resin monomers at depths greater than 5 mm have been reported [11]. To benefit from the properties of a composite resin material whilst negating the risk of incomplete polymerisation, the authors advocate the use of dual-cured composite resin for core build-up (e.g. ParaCore, Coltène/Whaledent AG, Altstätten, Switzerland). This material also has the following additional advantages: dentine bonding; efficient bulk placement of material (as a monobloc), so saving time and increasing the likelihood that RCT and definitive core placement can be completed within a single visit; can be prepared for an indirect restoration within 4 min of placement; and the white colour contrasts with tooth tissue, which proves useful during tooth preparation procedures.

19.7 Definitive Direct Vs Indirect Restorations

(a) Cast restorations are recommended for the definitive restoration of root-filled molar teeth [12, 13] (Figs. 19.1, 19.2, 19.3, 19.4 show some of the stages in the restoration of a root-filled 37 tooth). However, compared to molars, premolars have relatively thinner axial walls. Therefore, the preparation of a premolar for a given type of indirect restoration will result in a proportionally greater loss of coronal tooth tissue compared to the same type of preparation in a molar tooth.

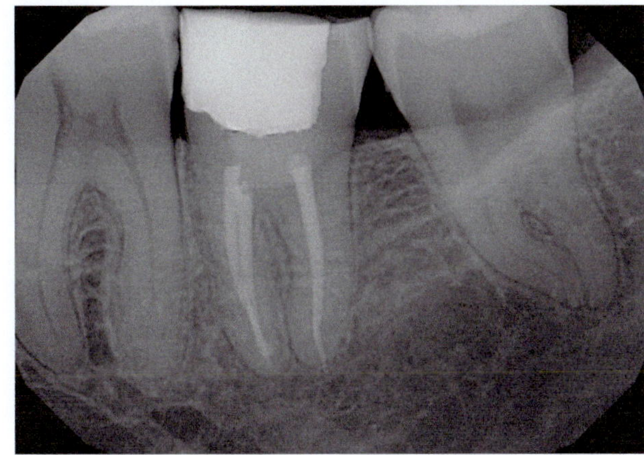

Fig. 19.1 Post-operative long-cone periapical radiograph of a 37 tooth following completion of root canal treatment and placement of a composite resin core

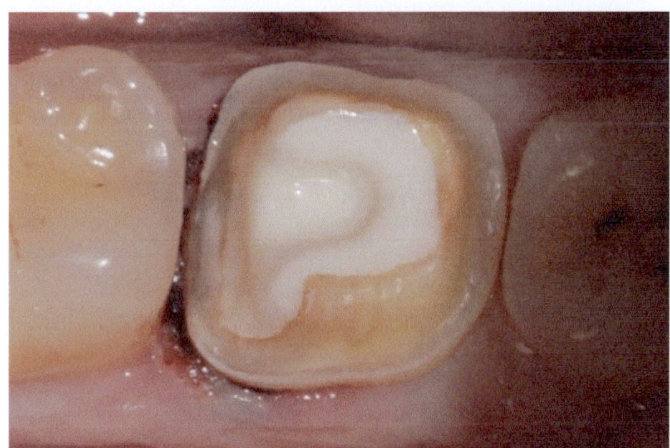

Fig. 19.2 Crown preparation 37 tooth. Box cut within the confines of the composite resin core to enhance retention and resistance form

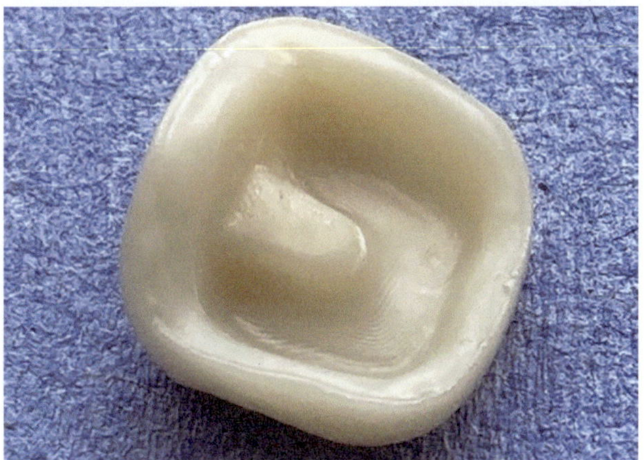

Fig. 19.3 Full-coverage, monolithic, zirconia crown for 37 tooth (detail of fitting surface)

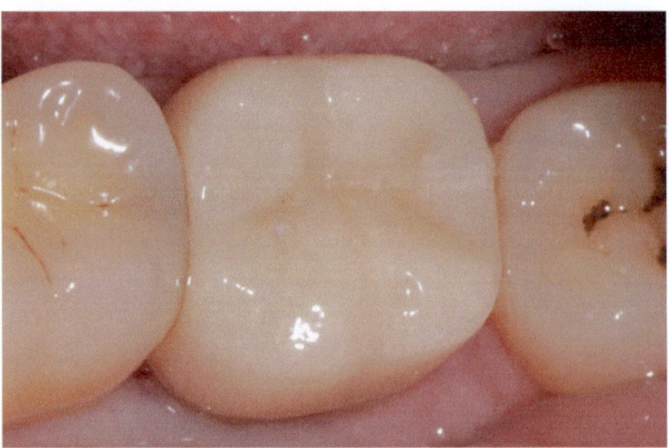

Fig. 19.4 Fitted zirconia crown

Where insufficient coronal tissue remains to retain a core in a premolar, a post will often be required.

(b) As an alternative to a cast restoration, where a circumferential ring of enamel remains, a definitive cuspal-coverage direct composite resin restoration may be placed. Alternatively, where insufficient enamel remains for predictable enamel bonding, amalgam may be used to provide a definitive cuspal-coverage restoration.

19.8 Use of Posts in Posterior Teeth

(a) Post placement to retain cores in molar teeth is not necessary [14] and should be avoided, as it can weaken teeth, predispose to root fracture, or result in perforation. Therefore, methods to enhance retention of the core in a molar should be limited to a modified Nayyar core or the use of a bonded amalgam or composite material, as previously outlined.

(b) In contrast, fibre posts in root-filled premolar teeth have been reported to be beneficial in aiding core retention where two or fewer axial walls remain [15]. However, there is a negative correlation between the amount of coronal tooth structure remaining and the likelihood of mechanical failure of a fibre post-treated tooth [16]. The inherent flexure of fibre posts can precipitate marginal leakage, caries, and, ultimately, fracture of the core. Where a ferrule is not achievable, or as an alternate to fibre posts, clinicians may opt to place a cast precious metal post and core prior to crowning the tooth [17]. The criteria for assessment and placement of posts was discussed in part 2 of this series.

19.9 Design Considerations for Indirect Restorations

(a) The preparation of posterior root-filled teeth for indirect restorations should be conservative whilst meeting the requirements for cuspal coverage and adequate retention/resistance form. For example, an onlay design should be chosen where the buccal and lingual/palatal walls are intact. However, where three walls are compromised, but one proximal wall remains, a three-quarter crown may be appropriate. Only where all four axial walls have been previously compromised is a full-veneer preparation recommended.

(b) Where a root-filled posterior tooth with a class-I access cavity has a circumferential band of enamel remaining, an 'endocrown' can provide a very conservative cast cuspal-coverage solution [18]. Endocrowns are monolithic porcelain (or gold) cast cuspal-coverage restorations, which utilise the pulp chamber for retention and have been reported to provide a high level of success at 10 years [19].

19.10 Material Choice for Indirect Restorations

(a) Gold alloys (type III or IV) are excellent for cuspal protection of root-filled teeth, owing to their strength in thin section (facilitating conservative tooth preparations) and capacity for bonding to tooth tissue. However, patients may not accept gold in the aesthetic zone.

(b) Lithium di-silicate glass ceramic restorations (e.g. eMax, Ivoclar Vivadent, Schaan, Lichtenstein) are not as strong as gold but have excellent aesthetic properties and can be bonded to tooth tissue, so facilitating a conservative tooth preparation.

(c) Monolithic yttrium-stabilised zirconia restorations (e.g. Procera, Nobel Biocare, Kloten, Switzerland) are stronger than lithium disilicate restorations, but when finished with an overlying layer of feldspathic porcelain, the fracture resistance of the restoration drops to that of the weaker material (e.g. the feldspathic porcelain). Zirconia cannot be predictably bonded to tooth tissue and so carries the disadvantage of requiring a conventional tooth preparation to derive the necessary retention and resistance form. Adjustment of the crown creates a roughened surface, which, if not adequately polished, can abrade the opposing tooth. If the patient is a bruxist and will not tolerate gold, monolithic zirconia would be an acceptable choice for a crown on a posterior tooth.

As stated previously, these top tips are based mainly from experience and may need some adaptation to an individual's circumstances and practice. We hope this series will be a useful reference for managing the restoration of root-filled teeth.

19.11 Conclusions

There are a plethora of options for restoring the root canal-treated posterior tooth on completion of endodontics. The restoration has a dual role of cuspal coverage, to prevent catastrophic fracture, and coronal seal, to prevent endodontic failure. Invariably, choice from the different materials available will have an aesthetic component despite superior functional and occlusal qualities of gold alloy.

References

1. Abbot P. Assessing restored teeth with pulp and periapical diseases for the presence of cracks, caries and marginal breakdown. Aust Dent J. 2004;49:33–9.
2. Sorensen J, Engleman M. Ferrule design and fracture resistance of endodontically treated teeth. J Prosthet Dent. 1990;63:529–36.
3. Haralur A, Al-Qahtani A, Al-Qarni M, Al-Homrany R, Aboalkhair A. Influence of remaining dentin wall thickness on the fracture strength of endodontically treated teeth. J Conserv Dent. 2016;19:63–7.
4. Arunpraditkul S, Saengsanson S, Pakviwat W. Fracture resistance of endodontically treated teeth: three walls versus four walls of remaining coronal structure. J Prosthodont. 2009;18:49–53.
5. Gargiulo A, Wentz F, Orban B. Dimensions and relations of the dentogingival junction in humans. J Periodontol. 1961;32:261–7.
6. Jepsen S, Caton J, Albandar J, et al. Periodontal manifestations of systemic diseases and developmental and acquired conditions: consensus report of workgroup 3 of the 2017 world workshop on the classification of periodontal and Peri-implant diseases and conditions. J Clin Periodontol. 2018;45:219–29.
7. Kois J. The restorative-periodontal interface: biological parameters. Periodontol. 2000;1996(11):29–38.
8. Lynch C, Burke F, Ríordáin R, Hannigan A. The influence of coronal restoration type on the survival of endodontically treated teeth. Eur J Prosthodont Restor Dent. 2004;12:171–6.
9. Nayyar A, Walton R, Leonard L. An amalgam coronal-radicular dowel and core technique for endodontically treated posterior teeth. J Prosthet Dent. 1980;43:511–5.
10. Sagsen B, Aslan B. Effect of bonded restorations on the fracture resistance of root filled teeth. Int Endod J. 2006;39:900–4.
11. Herrero A, Yaman P, Dennison J. Polymerization shrinkage and depth of cure of packable composites. Quintessence Int. 2005;36:25–31.
12. Aquilino S, Caplan D. Relationship between crown placement and the survival of endodontically treated teeth. J Prosthet Dent. 2002;87:256–63.
13. Ng Y-L, Mann V, Gulabivala K. A prospective study of the factors affecting outcomes of non-surgical root canal treatment: part 2: tooth survival. Int Endod J. 2011;44:610–25.
14. Sorensen J, Martinoff J. Intracoronal reinforcement and coronal coverage: a study of endodontically treated teeth. J Prosthet Dent. 1984;51:780–4.
15. Ferrari M, Vichi A, Fadda G, et al. A randomized controlled trial of endodontically treated and restored premolars. J Dent Res. 2012;9:72–8.
16. Ferrari M, Cagidiaco M, Goracci C, et al. Long-term retrospective study of the clinical performance of fibre posts. Am J Dent. 2007;20:287–91.
17. Sarkis-Onofre R, Fergusson D, Cenci M, Moher D, Pereira-Cenci T. Performance of post-retained single crowns: a systematic review of related risk factors. J Endodont. 2007;43:175–83.
18. Bindl A, Mörmann W. Clinical evaluation of adhesively placed Cerac endo-crowns after 2 years—preliminary results. J Adhes Dent. 1999;1:255–65.
19. Belleflamme M, Geerts S, Louwette M, Grenade C, Vanheusden A, Mainjot A. No post—no core approach to restore severely damaged posterior teeth: an up to 10-year retrospective study of documented endocrown cases. J Dent. 2017;63:1. https://doi.org/10.1016/j.jdent.2017.04.009.

Endodontic Prognosis 1

20

Prashanti Eachempati, Andrew Harris, Guy Lambourn,
Tony Francis, and Ewen McColl

Learning Points

- Appreciate the categorisation of prognostic factors into three phases.
- Recall the structural and pathological signs that reduce prognosis.
- Understand how the various stages of endodontic treatment modify the prognostic outcome.

20.1 Introduction

In this second part of our series on comprehensive dental treatment planning, we continue our exploration of the factors influencing the long-term prognosis of teeth. Building upon the foundation laid in previous chapters, which focused on restorative factors, we now shift our attention to endodontic considerations in tooth-by-tooth prognosis (Fig. 20.1).

P. Eachempati
Peninsula Dental School (University of Plymouth), Derriford Dental Education Facility, Plymouth Science Park, Plymouth, UK

Prosthodontics, Manipal University College Malaysia, Melaka, Malaysia

A. Harris · G. Lambourn
Peninsula Dental School (University of Plymouth), Derriford Dental Education Facility, Plymouth Science Park, Plymouth, UK

T. Francis
Department of Conservative and Endodontics, Manipal University College Malaysia, Melaka, Malaysia

E. McColl (✉)
Peninsula Dental School, Plymouth, UK
e-mail: ewen.mccoll@plymouth.ac.uk

E. McColl, A. Alani (eds.), *Practical Tips in Clinical Dentistry*, BDJ Clinician's Guides, https://doi.org/10.1007/978-3-031-90355-7_20

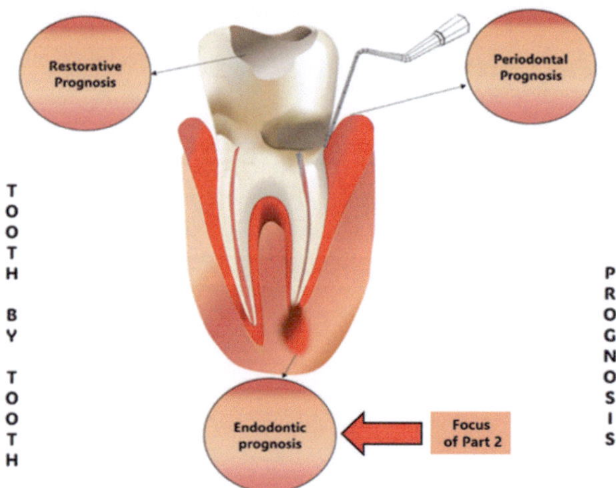

Fig. 20.1 Diagram representing the three critical areas for tooth-by-tooth prognosis

Endodontic factors play a crucial role in determining the success and longevity of dental treatments, alongside restorative and periodontal aspects. In this article, we discuss the complexities of endodontic prognosis, aiming to provide general practitioners with a structured framework for evaluating the prognosis of individual teeth.

Utilising established classification systems and terminology prevalent in dental literature, we aim to simplify the understanding of endodontic prognosis. By categorising prognoses as "good," "questionable," and "poor," we seek to enhance clarity and facilitate effective communication among dental professionals [1].

To differentiate between subcategories within the "good," "questionable," and "poor" prognosis classifications, in part 1 of this series, we specified whether a factor indicated as good or fair prognosis (both grouped under "good") or a compromised or non-salvageable prognosis (both grouped under "poor"). This approach allowed us to achieve a gradation of prognosis. For example, when we classify a tooth prognosis as "compromised", it suggests that treatment may be an option, though the prognosis is poor. This can be explained to the patient, allowing them to decide if they are willing to accept the potential risk of increased failure. In contrast, a "non-salvageable" prognosis indicates that attempting treatment is futile, and extraction is likely the best solution.

20.2 Endodontic Factors

We categorise factors influencing prognosis into three distinct phases [2]:

- Pre-operative.
- Intra-operative.
- Post-operative.

Each phase plays a crucial role in the overall success of endodontic treatment, from initial diagnosis to long-term outcomes.

20.2.1 Pre-Operative Factors

Pre-operative factors can be divided into two main categories: patient-related factors and tooth-related factors [2] (Table 20.1 and Fig. 20.2).

20.2.1.1 Pre-Operative Patient-Related Factors

Age and Gender [3]

While age and gender may not directly affect endodontic prognosis [4], it's important to recognise that certain medical conditions, which may be more prevalent in specific age groups or gender, can influence healing processes [3]. For instance, conditions like diabetes, which are more common in older individuals, can lead to delayed healing and heightened risk of complications [5]. Some studies have indicated that women are more susceptible to endodontic flare-ups than men [6]. However, other research has shown no correlation between gender and pain after endodontic treatment [6].

Systemic Conditions

Akin to the well-established association between periodontitis and other inflammatory conditions, there is a suggested link between compromised systemic health and the success or survival rate of root canal therapy [7]. Systemic conditions may exert a detrimental effect on the outcome of root canal therapy by perpetuating an inflammatory state and impairing the host's ability to undergo effective repair processes.

Tips

- Take a detailed medical history and review the patient's medications, for potential impacts on healing or complications to treatment delivery.
- Explain the potential impact of their systemic condition on dental treatment and healing. Emphasise the importance of managing their overall health to improve treatment outcomes.
- Suggest lifestyle modifications that can help manage systemic inflammation, such as quitting smoking, reducing sugar intake, and maintaining a balanced diet.
- Monitor the healing process, scheduling regular follow-ups to detect any signs of delayed healing or complications at an early stage.

20.2.1.2 Pre-Operative Tooth-Related Factors

- *Tooth type*: Although molars are often considered more complex due to their multi-rooted structure and intricate canal systems, with thorough assessment and meticulous treatment planning, their prognosis can be similar to that of anterior teeth [8].

Table 20.1 Prognosis based on various pre-operative factors

Stage	Category	Factor	Parameters to consider	Prognosis	
Pre-operative	Patient-related	Age/gender	Younger age group	Good	Good
			Older age group	Fair	
		Systemic condition	No medical conditions	Good	
			Conditions leading to delayed healing or immunocompromised	Fair	
	Tooth-related	Tooth type	Single rooted	Good	Good
			Multi-rooted with uncomplicated anatomy	Fair	
			Multi-rooted with complex root canal anatomy	Questionable	
			Retreatment	Compromised	Poor
		Tooth position in arch	Tooth with proximal contacts on both sides	Good	Good
			Terminal teeth or those without neighbouring adjacent contacts	Fair	
		Structural damage Coronal residual wall (CRW)	4 CRW (>2 mm thickness and height measured from the base of the cusp)	Good	Good
			3 CRW (>2 mm thickness and height measured from the base of the cusp)	Fair	
			2 CRW (>2 mm thickness and height measured from the base of the cusp)	Questionable	
			1 CRW remaining with adequate ferrule	Compromised	Poor
			1 CRW with no ferrule	Non salvageable	
		Presence of cracks	Sound intact teeth	Good	Good
			Cracks confined to the enamel or superficial dentine	Fair	
			Cracks extending into the pulp chamber	Fair	Good
			Cracks extending below the cemento-enamel junction	Compromised	Poor
			Vertical root fracture	Non-salvageable	
		Vitality of pulp and periapical lesions	Vital pulp	Good	Good
			Necrotic non-vital pulp	Fair	
			Necrotic non-vital pulp with a small periapical lesion	Fair	Good
			Necrotic non-vital pulp with a large periapical lesion	Fair	Good

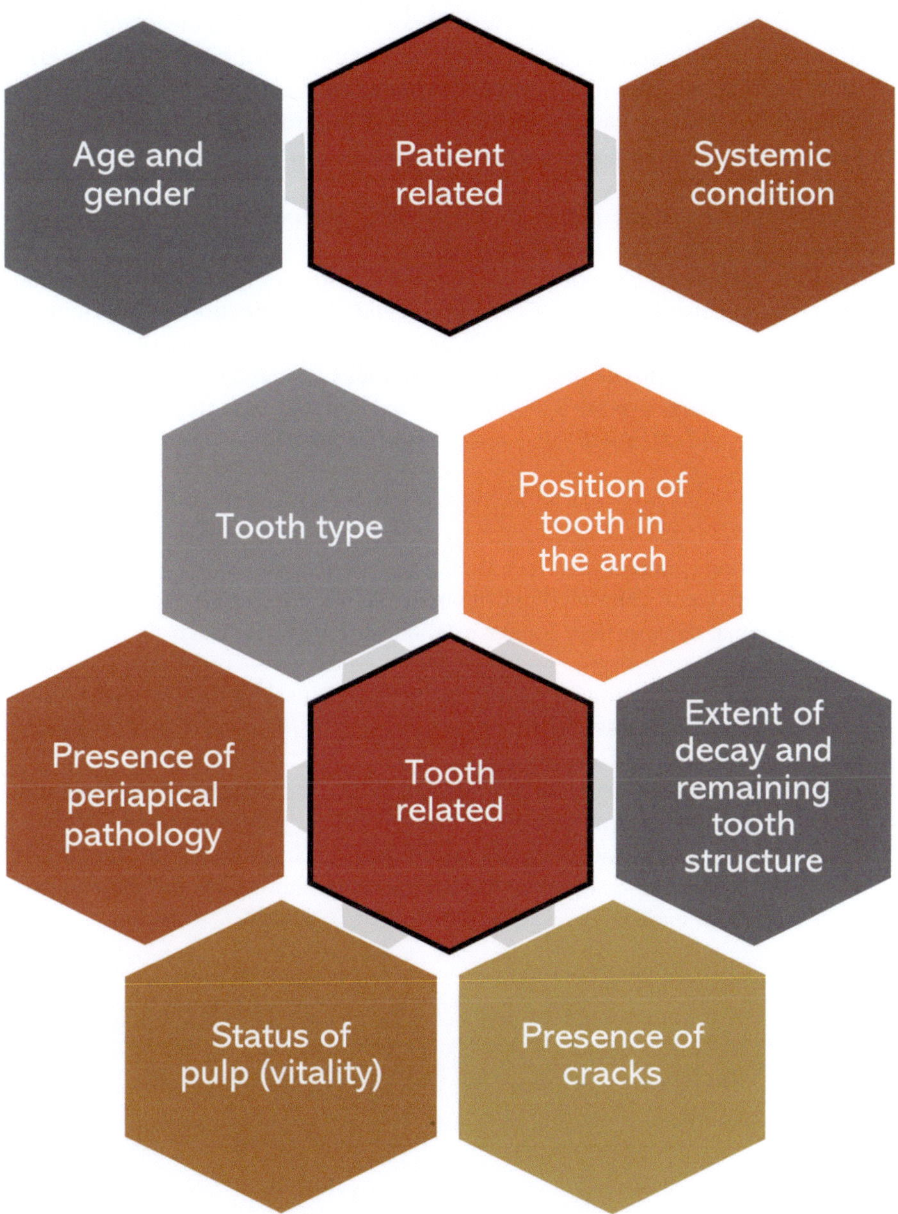

Fig. 20.2 Pre-operative factors influencing endodontic prognosis

- *Position of tooth in the arch*: The location of the tooth within the dental arch can influence its prognosis [2, 9]. Terminal teeth (those at the end of the arch) or those without neighbouring adjacent contacts may experience higher occlusal forces, leading to increased risk of fractures or failures [2].
- *Extent of decay or damage to remaining tooth structure*: The amount of decay or structural damage to the tooth can impact its prognosis. Evaluate the remaining tooth structure and the potential for restoring the tooth to function effectively [10–14] (Fig. 20.3).
- *Presence of Cracks:* Cracks in teeth can significantly compromise their structural integrity, increasing the risk of failure post-endodontic treatment. Determine the location and extent of the crack. Cracks confined to the enamel or superficial dentin may have a better prognosis, while cracks extending into the pulp chamber or root structure pose a higher risk. Vertical root fractures are particularly problematic and often indicate a poor prognosis [15].

Tips

- For evaluating complex root canal anatomy, utilisation of imaging techniques such as cone-beam computed tomography (CBCT) can provide greater detail of the root canal system than longer established techniques such as radiography (Fig. 20.4a, b).
- For teeth without proximal contacts, assess the occlusal load and consider occlusal adjustments if necessary.
- In case of insufficient tooth structure, consider pre-treatment measures such as building up the tooth structure or placing a temporary crown to protect the tooth during endodontic treatment.
- Use advanced diagnostic tools like magnification (loupes or microscopes) and illumination (fibre-optic lights or transillumination) during clinical examinations to detect cracks early.

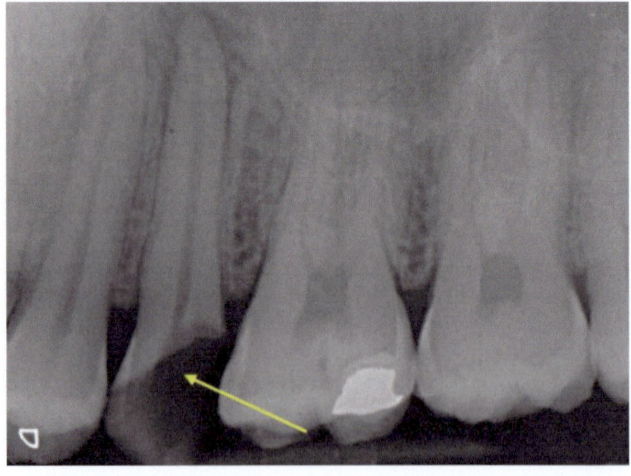

Fig. 20.3 Amount of decay or structural damage impact prognosis

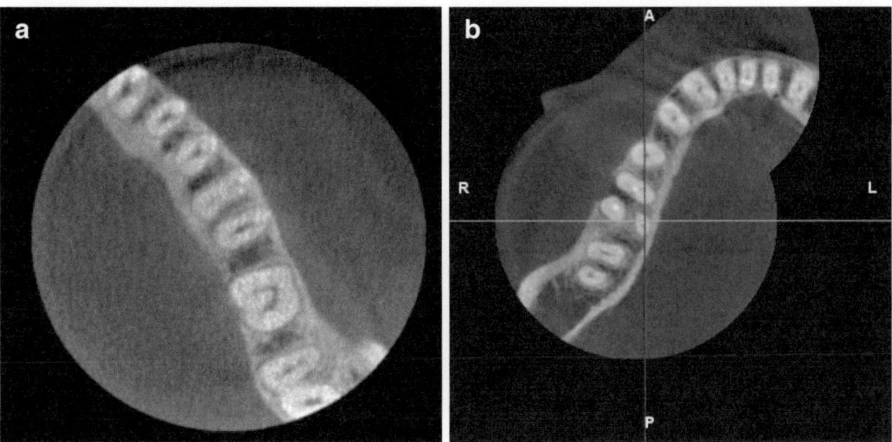

Fig. 20.4 (**a**) CBCT image showing a C-shaped canal in LL7. (**b**) CBCT image showing bifurcated distal root in LR6

- Ensure that the tooth can be adequately restored post-treatment to withstand functional demands (e.g. crowns).

It has been reported that in pre-operative lesions the odds of treatment success decrease by 14% for every increase of 1 mm in diameter [2]. Possible reasons for this include greater bacterial diversity, cystic change or extra-radicular infection, and deeper microbial penetration into areas of complex anatomy, rendering root canal systems more difficult to clean [16].

Status of Pulpal Tissue

Teeth with a vital pulp generally have a better prognosis than those with a necrotic pulp or associated chronic apical periodontitis. However, a recent review reported that there is no significant difference in outcomes between vital and non-vital pulps unless apical pathology is present [8] (Fig. 20.5). There is however unequivocal evidence that the presence of apical pathology significantly reduces prognosis, and it has been reported that roots with a periapical lesion (preoperatively) had 49% lower odds of success (as measured by absence of periapical pathology) than roots without them [2].

Presence of Periapical Pathology

Periapical pathology indicates an active infection, which may compromise treatment outcomes [2, 8, 16, 17]. Evaluate the size and extent of periapical lesions using radiographs (Fig. 20.6). Larger periapical lesions often indicate a more extensive infection and may have a lower prognosis. Treatment success rates decrease as lesion size increases due to higher microbial loads and greater difficulty in achieving complete disinfection. Other prognostic considerations are the presence of a preoperative sinus, which increased the likelihood of tooth loss by 120% [16].

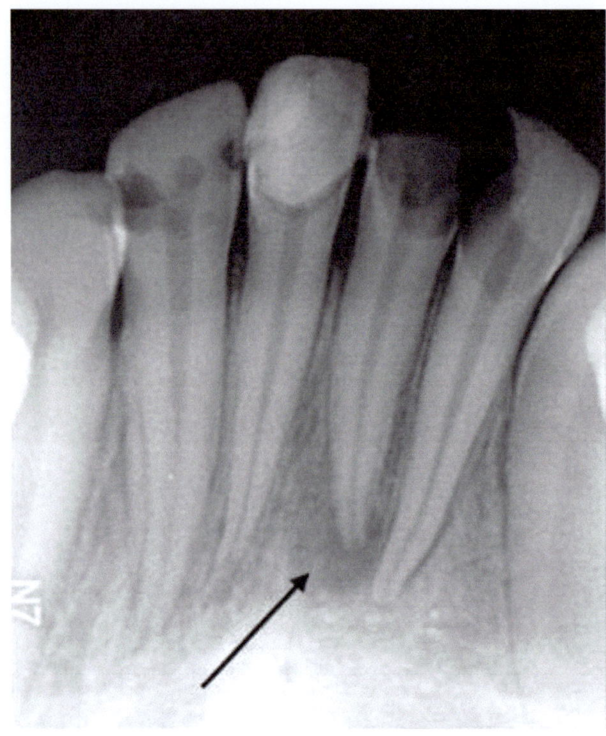

Fig. 20.5 Pre-operative pulpal and periapical tissue evaluation. Radiolucency indicated periapical pathology

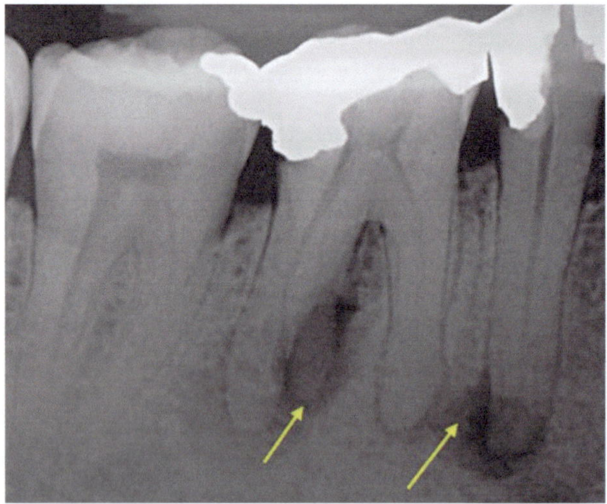

Fig. 20.6 Evaluate the size and extent of periapical lesions

Tips

- Utilise periapical radiographs and, if necessary, CBCT scans to evaluate the size [17], location, and extent of periapical lesions. Look for signs of bone loss, radiolucencies, and other indicators of apical pathology (Fig. 20.6).
- Assess clinical symptoms such as pain, swelling, tenderness to percussion, and the presence of a sinus tract [16]. These signs can provide insight into the severity of the infection and the body's response.
- For large or symptomatic lesions, consider creating an access point to allow for drainage of purulent material. This can help reduce infection load and alleviate symptoms.
- Manage infection and inflammation with appropriate medications. Use calcium hydroxide as an intracanal medicament to disinfect and promote healing [18].

Prognosis based on these various pre-operative factors is presented below (Table 20.1).

20.2.2 Intra-Operative Factors (Fig. 20.7)

20.2.2.1 Achieving Apical Patency

The most important factor when treating a tooth with apical periodontitis is the ability to negotiate the main root canal system in its entirety from the coronal entrance to the apical exit. The inability to achieve technical patency may be due to anatomical features, such as complex root system architecture, or iatrogenic errors, such as debris build-up or fractured instruments [8]. A previous prospective study indicated that roots with apical periodontitis that achieved apical patency were twice as likely to heal [2]. Additionally, for every 1 mm short from the apical terminus, there was a corresponding 12% reduction in the odds of resolution [2].

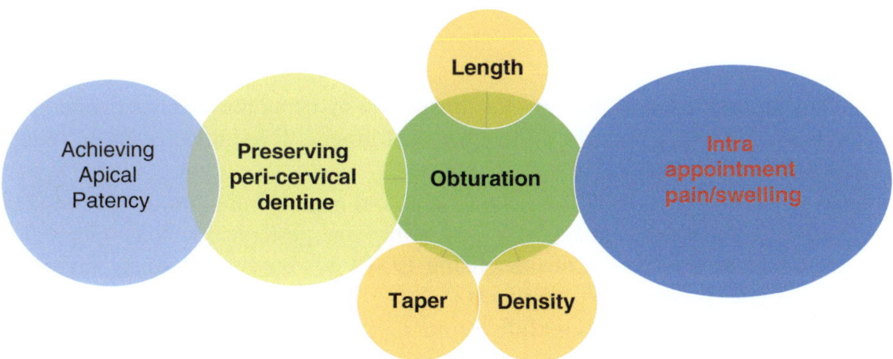

Fig. 20.7 Intra-operative factors influencing endodontic prognosis

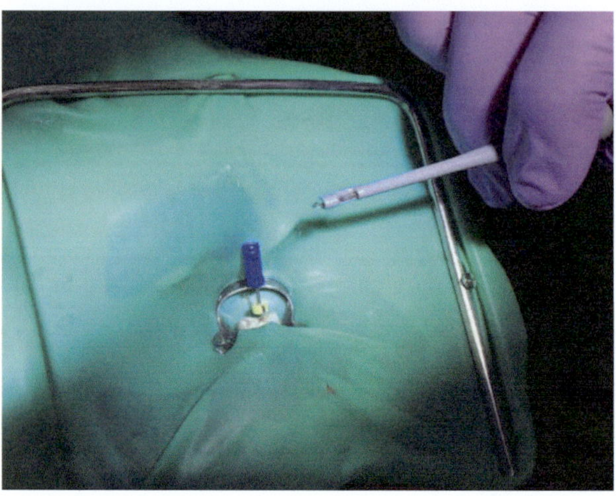

Fig. 20.8 Accurately determine the working length using electronic apex locators

Tips

- Accurately determine the working length using electronic apex locators (Fig. 20.8) and radiographic confirmation. This ensures thorough cleaning and shaping up to the apical terminus.
- Use small, flexible hand files or the newer glide path rotary files to gently negotiate the canal to its full length [19]. Establish patency and a smooth glide path for further instrumentation.
- Advanced rotary and reciprocating instruments [20] can aid in preservation of the apical patency throughout instrumentation. These instruments are designed to navigate complex canal systems with reduced risk of procedural errors.
- Be aware of anatomical variations such as curved or narrow canals. Use pre-curved files that can navigate complex root canal anatomies.
- Meticulously irrigate with 1% sodium hypochlorite to remove debris and prevent blockages. Employ irrigant activation techniques such as a simple manual dynamic agitation or passive ultrasonic activation to enhance irrigation effectiveness.
- Avoid excessive forces during instrumentation by using torque control endodontic handpieces and periodically inspect instruments for signs of wear to reduce the risk of fracture.
- Advanced irrigation techniques, such as apical negative pressure irrigation [21], could be considered especially in teeth with large periapical lesions for predictable canal disinfection. Consider using EDTA to remove the smear layer and allow deeper penetration of irrigants.
- For re-treated tooth, focus on fully removing or significantly reducing the filling material within the root canals during retreatment to ensure thorough cleaning and disinfection [22].

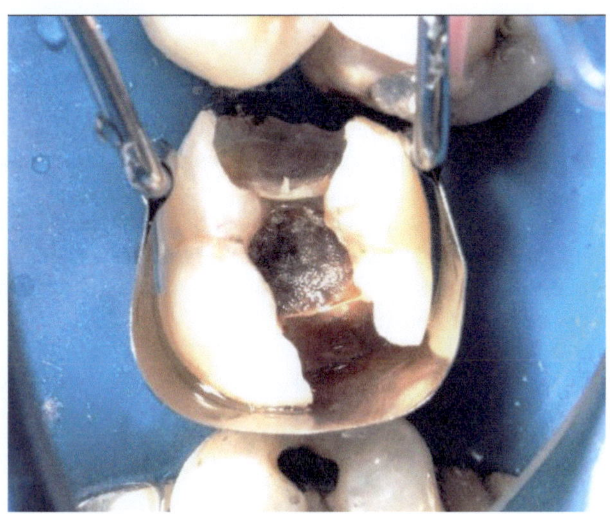

Fig. 20.9 Reduction in the number of residual coronal walls can compromise prognosis

20.2.2.2 Preservation of Peri-Cervical Dentine

Peri-cervical dentine (PCD) is crucial for transmitting and dissipating masticatory forces, residing approximately 4 mm above and below the crestal bone. Loss of PCD during root canal access preparation can weaken the tooth, making it more susceptible to fractures, compromising prognosis. This coupled with reduction in the number of residual coronal walls can further compromise prognosis (Fig. 20.9).

The production of large cavity preparations during root canal therapy can undermine and reduce PCD. This has led to a shift towards more conservative access cavities (CAC) with the aim of retaining more tooth structure [23, 24]. Conservative access cavities (CAC) aim to retain more tooth structure compared to traditional access cavities (TAC), enhancing structural support. Ultra-conservative access cavity design [25] (UCAC) further minimises tooth structure removal by creating separate cavities for different canal systems in molars [2, 8, 23, 24].

Tips

- PCD serves as an important foundation for restorations such as crowns or onlays, which are often placed after root canal therapy to protect the tooth. Utilise techniques like CAC and UCAC to preserve PCD and maintain the structural integrity of the tooth for better prognosis [23, 24].
- Although UCAC [25] preserves more tooth structure and provides improved support, it can limit access for complete debridement and visualisation, potentially impacting disinfection and obturation. Hence, its use should be guided by clinical judgment to balance structural preservation with optimal chemo-mechanical debridement.

20.3 Conclusion

In conclusion, we have discussed the importance of pre-operative factors and highlighted two critical intra-operative factors: achieving apical patency and preserving peri-cervical dentine. These elements play a significant role in the long-term prognosis of teeth from an endodontic perspective. To aid clinicians in making informed decisions, we have provided a prognostic table to facilitate easier clinical decision-making. In Part 2b, we will continue our discussion by exploring additional intra-operative factors such as obturation and intra-operative flare-ups, as well as post-operative considerations.

Acknowledgement We would like to acknowledge the figure contributions from the Department of Oral Medicine and Radiology and the Department of Conservative and Endodontics at Manipal University College Malaysia, Melaka, Malaysia (Figs. 20.4a, b, 20.8, and 20.9), and the Department of Oral Medicine and Radiology at Bapuji Dental College and Hospital, Davangere, Karnataka, India (Figs. 20.3, 20.5, and 20.6).

References

1. Eachempati P, Lambourn G, Harris A, McColl E. Top tips for treatment planning: tooth-by-tooth prognosis—part 1: restorative prognosis. Br Dent J. 2024;236:738–41.
2. Ng YL, Mann V, Gulabivala K. A prospective study of the factors affecting outcomes of non-surgical root canal treatment: part 1: periapical health. Int Endod J. 2011;44:583–609.
3. Kwak Y, Choi J, Kim K, Shin SJ, Kim S, Kim E. The 5-year survival rate of nonsurgical endodontic treatment: a population-based cohort study in Korea. J Endod. 2019;45:1192–9.
4. Shakiba B, Hamedy R, Pak JG, Barbizam JV, Ogawa R, White SN. Influence of increased patient age on longitudinal outcomes of root canal treatment: a systematic review. Gerodontology. 2017;34:101–9.
5. Segura-Egea JJ, Martín-González J, Cabanillas-Balsera D, Fouad AF, Velasco-Ortega E, López-López J. Association between diabetes and the prevalence of radiolucent periapical lesions in root-filled teeth: systematic review and meta-analysis. Clin Oral Investig. 2016;20:1133–41.
6. Bassam S, El-Ahmar R, Salloum S, Ayoub S. Endodontic postoperative flare-up: an update. Saudi Dent J. 2021;33:386–94.
7. Niazi SA, Bakhsh A. Association between endodontic infection, its treatment and systemic health: a narrative review. Medicina (Kaunas). 2022;58:931.
8. Gulabivala K, Ng YL. Factors that affect the outcomes of root canal treatment and retreatment-a reframing of the principles. Int Endod J. 2023;56:82–115.
9. Aquilino SA, Caplan DJ. Relationship between crown placement and the survival of endodontically treated teeth. J Prosthet Dent. 2002;87:256–63.
10. Cloet E, Debels E, Naert I. Controlled clinical trial on the outcome of glass fiber composite cores versus wrought posts and cast cores for the restoration of endodontically treated teeth: a 5-year follow-up study. Int J Prosthodont. 2017;30:71–9.
11. Juloski J, Radovic I, Goracci C, Vulicevic Z, Ferrari M. Ferrule effect: a literature review. J Endod. 2012;38:11–9.
12. Nagasiri R, Chitmongkolsuk S. Long-term survival of endodontically treated molars without crown coverage: a retrospective cohort study. J Prosthet Dent. 2005;93:164–70.
13. Cagidiaco MC, García-Godoy F, Vichi A, Grandini S, Goracci C, Ferrari M. Placement of fiber prefabricated or custom made posts affects the 3-year survival of endodontically treated premolars. Am J Dent. 2008;21:179–84.

14. Ferrari M, Vichi A, Fadda GM, Cagidiaco MC, Tay FR, Breschi L, Polimeni A, Goracci C. A randomized controlled trial of endodontically treated and restored premolars. J Dent Res. 2012;91:72S–8S.
15. Leong DJX, de Souza NN, Sultana R, Yap AU. Outcomes of endodontically treated cracked teeth: a systematic review and meta-analysis. Clin Oral Investig. 2020;24:465–73.
16. Ng YL, Mann V, Gulabivala K. A prospective study of the factors affecting outcomes of non-surgical root canal treatment: part 2: tooth survival. Int Endod J. 2011;44:610–25.
17. Karamifar K, Tondari A, Saghiri MA. Endodontic periapical lesion: an overview on the etiology, diagnosis and current treatment modalities. Eur Endod J. 2020;5:54–67.
18. Kumar NK, Brigit B, Annapoorna BS, Naik SB, Merwade S, Rashmi K. Effect of triple antibiotic paste and calcium hydroxide on the rate of healing of periapical lesions: a systematic review. J Conserv Dent. 2021;24:307–13.
19. Aminsobhani M, Hamidzadeh F, Rezaei Avval A, Merrikhi F, Sadri E. Evaluation of the canal transportation following glide path preparation with different rotary systems: a comparative study. ScientificWorldJournal. 2022;2022:8087378.
20. Nouri H, Amini K, Jahromi MZ. Comparison of full rotation and reciprocating movements in regaining apical patency during endodontic retreatment. Dent Res J. 2021;18:85.
21. Konstantinidi E, Psimma Z, Chávez de Paz LE, Boutsioukis C. Apical negative pressure irrigation versus syringe irrigation: a systematic review of cleaning and disinfection of the root canal system. Int Endod J. 2017;50:1034–54.
22. Trierveiler Paiva RC, Solda C, Vendramini F, Vanni JR, Baldissarelli Marcon F, João Fornari V, Martins Hartmann MS. Regaining apical patency with manual and reciprocating instrumentation during retreatment. Iran Endod J. 2018;13:351–5.
23. Sabeti M, Kazem M, Dianat O, Bahrololumi N, Beglou A, Rahimipour K, et al. Impact of access cavity design and root canal taper on fracture resistance of endodontically treated teeth: an ex vivo investigation. J Endod. 2018;44:1402–6.
24. Jurado CA, Amarillas-Gastelum C, Tonin BSH, Nielson G, Afrashtehfar KI, Fischer NG. Traditional versus conservative endodontic access impact on fracture resistance of chairside CAD-CAM lithium disilicate anterior crowns: an in vitro study. J Prosthodont. 2023;32:728–34.
25. Abou-Elnaga MY, Alkhawas MBAM, Kim HC, Refai AS. Effect of truss access and artificial truss restoration on the fracture resistance of endodontically treated mandibular first molars. J Endod. 2019;45:813–7.

Endodontic Prognosis 2

21

Prashanti Eachempati, Andrew Harris, Guy Lambourn, Tony Francis, and Ewen McColl

Learning Points

- Recall how the various different features of the final obturation can affect prognosis.
- Understand the significance of pain and swelling as an indicator for future treatment.
- Appreciate the importance of cuspal coverage in the longevity of the root canal treated unit.

21.1 Introduction

In this chapter, we continue our discussion by exploring additional intra-operative factors and post-operative considerations. To recap, Fig. 21.1 illustrates the intra-operative factors we have covered thus far: achieving apical patency and preserving peri-cervical dentine. In this part, we will further discuss intra-operative factors,

P. Eachempati
Peninsula Dental School (University of Plymouth), Derriford Dental Education Facility, Plymouth Science Park, Plymouth, UK

Prosthodontics, Manipal University College Malaysia, Melaka, Malaysia

A. Harris · G. Lambourn
Peninsula Dental School (University of Plymouth), Derriford Dental Education Facility, Plymouth Science Park, Plymouth, UK

T. Francis
Department of Conservative and Endodontics, Manipal University College Malaysia, Melaka, Malaysia

E. McColl (✉)
Peninsula Dental School, Plymouth, UK
e-mail: ewen.mccoll@plymouth.ac.uk

E. McColl, A. Alani (eds.), *Practical Tips in Clinical Dentistry*, BDJ Clinician's Guides, https://doi.org/10.1007/978-3-031-90355-7_21

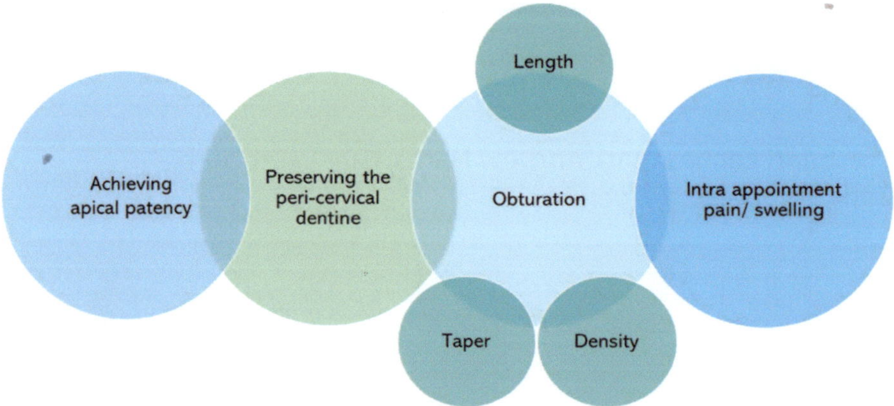

Fig. 21.1 Intra-operative factors influencing endodontic prognosis

such as the length, density, and taper related to obturation, as well as managing intra-operative flare-ups. Additionally, we will address post-operative considerations that influence the overall success and longevity of endodontic treatments. Our aim is to provide comprehensive prognostic guides for clinicians, ensuring well-informed decision-making throughout the treatment process.

21.2 Intra-Operative Factors

21.2.1 Obturation

21.2.1.1 Length of the Root Canal Filling

Numerous studies have investigated various aspects of filling length, including short, flush, and long fillings, as well as comparisons between overfilled and overextended fillings and studies on leakage. However, only a few studies have examined the impact of leaving a chemo-mechanically debrided root canal unfilled on treatment outcomes. These studies attributed about 40% to 60% of endodontic treatment failures to inadequate obturation of the root canal system [1]. Traditionally, these failures were believed to arise from issues such as overfilling, underfilling, and the overall poor quality of root fillings.

Initially, it was believed that an unfilled root canal would cause stagnation of tissue fluids within the "hollow tube", leading to sustained periapical inflammation. Later studies refuted this, finding no significant differences in periapical healing between teeth with and without obturation [2]. The quality of the coronal restoration was found to be more crucial for periapical health than the root filling [3].

Given the current evidence, it is premature to disregard the obturation step. Root canal filling should still be performed to address any lingering infection after cleaning and shaping. Additionally, it may help prevent microbial leakage to the periapex if the coronal seal is compromised, though evidence for this is limited. Clinical decision-making should prioritise the patient's specific needs rather than rigidly adhering to a single method.

Root fillings extending to within 2 mm of the apex have been associated with success rates of 81%. [2] This could be attributed to the effective disinfection of the canals, particularly at the apical portion, achieved through thorough instrumentation and irrigant penetration, which allowed the root fillings to extend similarly [1, 4].

Tips

- Use electronic apex locators, as suggested previously, to determine the precise working length [5]. This helps in avoiding over- or under-preparation of the canals and placement of the final root filling at the desired length.
- If you are uncertain, always double-check the working length (WL). A cone-fit radiograph with the master gutta-percha (GP) point in place can be extremely helpful if the WL is in question or if a WL radiograph was not been previously taken. Ensure that the filling material is within the optimal range of 0–2 mm from the apex.
- Obturation techniques such as warm vertical compaction or continuous wave condensation can help achieve optimal fill even in complex canal anatomies.

21.2.1.2 Density of Root Canal Obturation

Obturation aims to provide a satisfactory apical seal and three-dimensional filling of the canals. Although the concept of a "hermetic seal" has been questioned by recent studies, achieving a good three-dimensional fill can mitigate residual infection after chemo-mechanical debridement [4, 6]. While assessing three-dimensional obturation with two-dimensional imaging is challenging, technically "satisfactory" obturations (absence of voids) are associated with significantly improved success rates [1, 4]. A radiographically dense root filling has been considered to additionally aid in preventing microbial seepage for a short while, in the event the coronal seal is compromised [7].

Tips

- In addition to the tips provided above for achieving good obturation, integrating strategies, such as utilising magnification and illumination, employing specific obturation techniques like lateral condensation or warm vertical compaction to achieve a uniform and void-free obturation, and confirming void absence with radiographs, further enhances the quality of obturation and contributes to improved prognosis.
- Sealers fill the vacant space between the prepared dentinal wall and the core filling material, establishing a good seal in the root canal system.

When using traditional sealers like resin-based and calcium hydroxide-based sealers, ensure that the core filling material occupies most of the canal space, minimising the amount of sealer used. This helps prevent sealer-related problems such as disintegration, dissolution, or shrinkage. Newer calcium silicate-based sealers, with their superior biomechanical properties, can simplify this process and reduce the time needed for obturation [8].

21.2.1.3 Taper of Root Canal Obturation

Preparing and creating a taper in the root canals enhances irrigation dynamics and effective chemo-mechanical debridement [9, 10]. This tapering also reduces the risk of extruding irrigants and obturating materials. While over-tapering can lead to weakening of roots by compromising the PCD, under-shaping can result in compromising the prognosis.

21.2.2 Intra-Appointment Pain and Swelling

The presence of pain and swelling between operative appointments, often termed as inter-appointment flare-ups, has been associated with poorer treatment outcomes deteriorating endodontic prognosis [11]. These flare-ups are considered as exacerbations of periapical inflammation or infections and can occur due to various reasons, such as inadequate asepsis, disinfection, improper irrigation, or material extrusion during the root canal procedure.

Extensive inter-appointment swelling can impair mouth opening, compromising the quality of subsequent treatments. Additionally, damage to the provisional restoration during a prolonged inter-appointment period for pain and swelling to subside can lead to coronal microbial leakage, further affecting the tooth's prognosis.

Current evidence suggests that inter-appointment flare-ups may indicate a more aggressive host-microbial interaction at the periapical region [4]. This interaction involves the persistence or proliferation of microorganisms within the periapical tissues despite initial treatment attempts. These microorganisms can provoke an inflammatory response, leading to symptoms such as pain and swelling. These errors can cause tissue irritation and exacerbate periapical inflammation [4, 11].

Tips

- To avoid the complication of intraoperative pain and swelling and improve prognosis, we can follow these additional tips:
- Utilise rubber dam isolation for an aseptic operating field, which helps prevent contamination of the root canal system and reduces the risk of postoperative complications (Fig. 21.2).

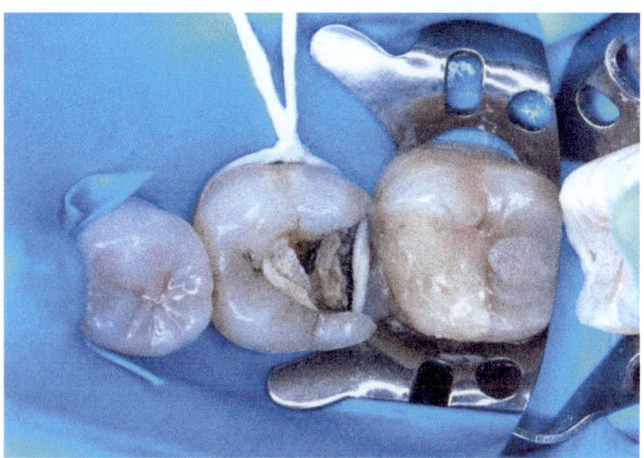

Fig. 21.2 Utilise rubber dam isolation for an aseptic operating field

- Adopt a conservative and gentle approach during canal instrumentation to avoid excessive pressure or trauma to periapical tissues. This helps minimise tissue irritation and reduces the likelihood of postoperative pain and swelling.
- Employ intermittent irrigation techniques using side-vented needles to flush debris and disinfect the root canal system effectively. This reduces the risk of extrusion of irrigants beyond the apex while enhancing irrigation efficacy without causing irritation to the periapical tissues.
- Provide clear postoperative instructions to patients, including guidance on managing discomfort, swelling, and any potential complications following the procedure. Prescribe appropriate analgesics and recommend adjunctive measures such as cold compresses or anti-inflammatory medications to alleviate postoperative symptoms (Fig. 21.3).

Stage	Category	Factor	Parameters to consider	Prognosis	
Intra-operative	Apical patency	Previously untreated/ Primary RCT	Negotiable	Good	
			Inability to achieve technical patency (debris/ complex anatomy)	Questionable(For every 1mm short from the apical terminus-prognosis changes from questionable to poor)	
		Retreatment	Able to remove a significant amount of the existing root filling material	Questionable	
			Inability to remove filling material	Non-Salvageable	Poor
	Peri-cervical dentine (PCD)	Access cavity preparation and remaining coronal walls	Adequate preservation of PCD with UCAC or CAC forms	Good	Good
			CAC preparations needing some removal of tooth structure, adequate coronal residual walls	Fair	
			TAC needing greater removal of tooth structure, adequate coronal residual walls	Questionable	
			TAC needing greater removal of tooth structure, compromised coronal residual walls	Comprom-ised	Poor
	Obturation	Length of root canal obturation	Root filling extending 0 - <1mm short of radiographic apex	Good	Good
			Root fillings ending at the radiographic apex (or 1-2mm short)	Fair	
			Root fillings with biomimetic sealers ending beyond the radiographic apex (overfilling)	Fair	Good
			Root fillings with traditional sealers ending beyond the radiographic apex (overfilling)	Questionable	
			Root filling ending >2mm short of radiographic apex (underfilling)	Comprom-ised	Poor
		Density of root canal obturation	No void present in the root canal obturation	Good	Good
			Void(s) limited to coronal third	Fair	
			With void(s) within the mid/apical third	Comprom-ised	Poor
		Taper of root canal obturation	Consistently tapered from coronal part to apex	Good	Good
			Inadequate taper	Fair	
			Inconsistent or irregular taper (over or under shaped)	Compromised	Poor
	Intra-appointment pain and swelling		Asymptomatic between appointments (no flare ups)	Good	Good
			Symptomatic between appointments (flare ups)	Fair	

Fig. 21.3 Prognosis based on these various intra-operative factors is presented

21.3 Post-Operative Factors

Coronal leakage is a major cause of endodontic failure in a tooth with thoroughly disinfected root canals [3]. Even a well-obturated canal does not provide an enduring barrier to bacterial penetration for extended durations; thus, we rely on the restoration for the long-term integrity of the coronal seal. Inadequate quality of the coronal restoration contributes to unsuccessful outcomes.

After access cavity restoration, endodontically treated teeth are often restored with full-coverage crowns to ensure optimal structural support and protection [12]. Restorations should serve primarily three functions: the protection of the root canal treatment from microleakage and subsequent failure, fracture protection from occlusal forces, and providing the contacts and contours to support a healthy attachment apparatus around the treated tooth.

The necessity for cuspal coverage should be assessed on a tooth-by-tooth basis, considering factors such as remaining tooth structure, presence of cracks, and opposing dentition. According to the latest recommendations from the European Society of Endodontology [13], most posterior teeth with at least one missing proximal wall require cuspal coverage restorations.

Recent advancements in adhesive dentistry and biomimetic principles are challenging the routine use of full-coverage crowns for endodontically treated teeth [14]. Biomimetic dentistry focuses on preserving as much tooth structure as possible and replicating natural biomechanics through minimally invasive preparations and selective caries removal (Figs. 21.4 and 21.5).

The biomimetic restoration protocol emphasises modern adhesion techniques and stress-reduced cavity preparation to minimise the configuration factor (C-factor) and reduce stress in dental composite restorations [15].

Tips

- Familiarise yourself with biomimetic dentistry principles aimed at preserving natural tooth structure and biomechanics. Incorporate minimally invasive techniques and selective caries removal to enhance long-term outcomes of restorative procedures.
- Recognise that the approach to restorative treatment for endodontically treated teeth may vary depending on factors such as remaining wall volume and type of

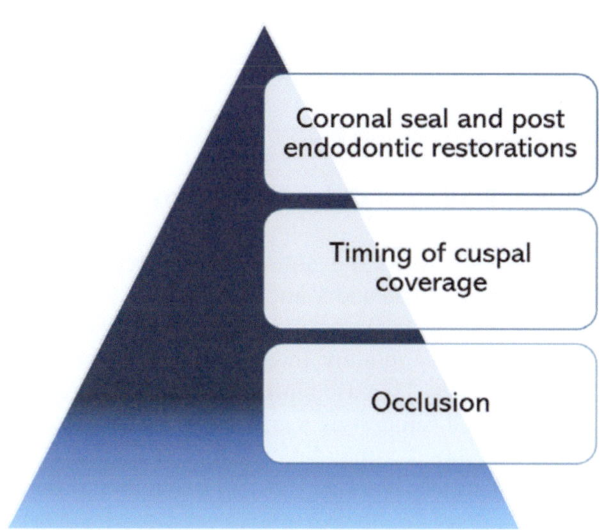

Fig. 21.4 Post-operative factors for endodontic prognosis

Stage	Category	Parameters to consider	Prognosis	
Post-operative	Coronal seal & post endodontic restoration	Adequate coronal restoration: A well bonded coronally sealing restoration which appears intact radiographically	Good	
		Inadequate coronal restoration: Final restoration appears sub-optimal radiographically with open margins or positive margins	Questionable	
		Inadequate coronal restoration: recurrent caries, partial temporary fillings or no filling.	Compromised	Poor
	Timing of cuspal coverage	Restored with direct or indirect definitive restoration with no or minimal delay	Good	Good
		Restored with direct or indirect definitive restoration with delay of less than four months	Fair	
		Restored with direct or indirect definitive restoration with delay of greater than four months	Questionable	
		Teeth receiving no definitive cuspal coverage restoration	Compromised	Poor
	Occlusion	Canine guidance with no lateral excursive contacts on the tooth	Good	Good
		Group function with smooth lateral excursive contacts distributed on all teeth	Fair	
		Any occlusal scheme with eccentric contacts / heavy lateral loading on the tooth	Compromised	Poor

Fig. 21.5 Prognosis based on these various post-operative factors is presented

access cavity preparation. Customise treatment plans to suit each patient's unique needs and circumstances.

- For anterior teeth, consider direct composite restoration for intact marginal ridges, while previously heavily restored teeth may require either direct composite or indirect restoration.
- In posterior teeth, direct composite restoration is suitable for those with intact marginal ridges, while previously heavily restored teeth may benefit from direct composite with reinforced ultrahigh-molecular-weight polyethylene fibre (UHMWPEF), possibly leading to indirect restoration or crown placement [13].
- Previously crowned posterior teeth with lost marginal ridges may require a reinforced core with either a conventional post, a UHMWPEF fibre post, or an endo crown.

21.3.1 Timing of Cuspal Coverage

Pratt et al. (2016) [15] examined the impact of the timing of cuspal coverage after root canal treatment and found that teeth receiving crowns more than 4 months after the procedure were almost three times more likely to be extracted compared to those restored within 4 months. Interestingly, after the 4-month mark, the failure rate did not significantly increase until 18 months post-treatment, at which point the rate of failure surged, suggesting a critical period for fracture development [15].

Teeth restored with indirect restorations within 6 months of root canal treatment had a higher survival rate (93.1%) compared to those with direct fillings (89.8%)

[15]. It was also noted that teeth with a more favourable prognosis might have been preferentially restored with indirect restorations.

The survival rate of root-filled teeth without crowns was satisfactory up to 3 years (84% ± 9%) but declined thereafter. Outcomes after 5 years between teeth restored with direct and indirect restorations showed no difference. However, at the 10-year mark, teeth with indirect restorations had superior outcomes [16].

Tips
- Periodically assess the need for cuspal coverage restoration during follow-up appointments, especially for teeth with delayed restoration, to prevent complications and ensure optimal prognosis.
- Educate patients about the importance of timely restoration after root canal treatment and encourage compliance with recommended treatment timelines to improve treatment outcomes and long-term tooth survival.

21.3.2 Occlusion

Occlusion plays a significant role in the prognosis of endodontically treated teeth, although conclusive evidence is lacking [17]. Proper occlusion ensures that forces are distributed evenly across the dental arch, reducing the risk of excessive stress on individual teeth, including those that have undergone endodontic treatment. Occlusal forces can impact the longevity of restorations placed on endodontically treated teeth. Proper occlusion ensures the stability and durability of restorations, reducing the risk of failure.

Tips
- When considering occlusal guidance, it's important to note that, in cases where it is desirable to avoid lateral forces on compromised posterior teeth, canine guidance is preferred as it redirects forces away from these teeth. Alternatively, group function is ideal when the goal is to distribute these forces across multiple teeth.

21.4 Conclusion

In conclusion, the comprehensive evaluation of endodontic prognosis involves a meticulous consideration of pre-operative, intra-operative, and post-operative factors. Each phase contributes uniquely to the long-term success of root canal therapy, emphasising the importance of patient-specific assessments and tailored treatment plans. By integrating advanced diagnostic tools and adhering to evidence-based practices, dental practitioners can enhance treatment outcomes and patient satisfaction. Effective communication with patients regarding prognosis classifications—whether "good", "questionable", or "poor"—is essential in fostering informed decision-making and achieving optimal oral health outcomes.

Acknowledgement We would like to acknowledge the figure contributions from the Department of Conservative and Endodontics at Manipal University College Malaysia, Melaka, Malaysia.

References

1. Ng YL, Mann V, Gulabivala K. A prospective study of the factors affecting outcomes of non-surgical root canal treatment: part 1: periapical health. Int Endod J. 2011;44:583–609.
2. Sabeti MA, Nekofar M, Motahhary P, Ghandi M, Simon JH. Healing of apical periodontitis after endodontic treatment with and without obturation in dogs. J Endod. 2006;32:628–33.
3. Pirani C, Camilleri J. Effectiveness of root canal filling materials and techniques for treatment of apical periodontitis: a systematic review. Int Endod J. 2023;56:436–54.
4. Gulabivala K, Ng YL. Factors that affect the outcomes of root canal treatment and retreatment—a reframing of the principles. Int Endod J. 2023;56:82–115.
5. Nasiri K, Wrbas KT. Accuracy of different generations of apex locators in determining working length; a systematic review and meta-analysis. Saudi Dent J. 2022;34:11–20.
6. Somani R, Jaidka S, Singh DJ, Kaur N. Hermetic seal in Obturation: an achievable goal with recently introduced Cpoint. Int J Clin Pediatr Dent. 2019;12:410–3.
7. Ng YL, Mann V, Rahbaran S, Lewsey J, Gulabivala K. Outcome of primary root canal treatment: systematic review of the literature—Part 2. Influence of clinical factors. Int Endod J. 2008;41:6–31.
8. Lim M, Jung C, Shin DH, Cho YB, Song M. Calcium silicate-based root canal sealers: a literature review. Restor Dent Endod. 2020;45:e35.
9. Gomes BPFA, Aveiro E, Kishen A. Irrigants and irrigation activation systems in endodontics. Braz Dent J. 2023;34:1–33.
10. Buchanan LS. The standardized-taper root canal preparation—Part 1. Concepts for variably tapered shaping instruments. Int Endod J. 2000;33:516–29.
11. Bassam S, El-Ahmar R, Salloum S, Ayoub S. Endodontic postoperative flare-up: an update. Saudi Dent J. 2021;33:1056–62.
12. Fedorowicz Z, van Zuuren EJ, Schoones J. Antibiotic use for irreversible pulpitis. Cochrane Database Syst Rev. 2021;5:CD004969.
13. Mannocci F, Bhuva B, Roig M, Zarow M, Bitter K. European Society of Endodontology position statement: the restoration of root filled teeth. Int Endod J. 2021;54:1974–81.
14. Kimble P, Corso AM, Beattie M, Campos MS, Cavalcanti B. Biomimetics and the restoration of the endodontically treated tooth. Braz Dent Sci. 2023;26:e3668.
15. Pratt I, Aminoshariae A, Montagnese TA, Williams KA, Khalighinejad N, Mickel A. Eight-year retrospective study of the critical time lapse between root canal completion and crown placement: its influence on the survival of endodontically treated teeth. J Endod. 2016;42:1598–603.
16. Ferrari M, Ferrari Cagidiaco E, Pontoriero DIK, Ercoli C, Chochlidakis K. Survival rates of endodontically treated posterior teeth restored with all-ceramic partial-coverage crowns: when systematic review fails. Int J Environ Res Public Health. 2022;19:1971.
17. Abduo J, Bennamoun M, Tennant M, McGeachie J. Effect of prosthodontic planning on lateral occlusion scheme: a comparison between conventional and digital planning. J Appl Oral Sci. 2015;23:196–205.

Part III

Dental Trauma

Immediate Management of Dental Trauma

22

Clement Seeballuck, Sean Dolan, and Julie K. Kilgariff

Learning Points

- Recognise different sources of information on the management of acute dental trauma.
- Appreciate the need to screen for general injuries that may not involve the mouth and dental tissues.
- Understand the principles involved in stabilising and preserving injured tissues.
- Recall the need for ongoing monitoring and review.

22.1 Introduction

Traumatic dental injuries to the permanent dentition are estimated to have a global prevalence of 15.2% [1]. This equates to potentially over one billion people living today having experienced dental trauma.

The immediate management of dental trauma impacts the prognosis of the affected structures and therefore the outcome. This is of particular note when the periodontal ligament and pulp sustain severe injuries, more likely to have long-term sequelae and complicating management.

Given the unplanned nature associated with immediate trauma management, it is crucial that clinicians are well versed in appropriate management strategies and/or can quickly access current best practice guidance.

C. Seeballuck
Paediatric Dentistry, Dundee Dental Hospital and Research School, Dundee, UK

S. Dolan
Ninewells Hospital, Dundee, UK

J. K. Kilgariff (✉)
Endodontics, Dundee Dental Hospital and School, Dundee, UK
e-mail: julie.kilgariff@nhs.scot

E. McColl, A. Alani (eds.), *Practical Tips in Clinical Dentistry*, BDJ Clinician's Guides, https://doi.org/10.1007/978-3-031-90355-7_22

This article aims to provide key tips for the successful management of trauma affecting permanent teeth.

22.1.1 Be Informed

There are several relevant resources for trauma management, and up-to-date best practice guidance is free to access in the public domain. Online resources are frequently updated, and it is recommended clinicians likely to manage dental trauma consider incorporating regular guidance review into personal development plans.

The Dental Trauma Guide website [2] contains links to the 2020 International Association of Dental Traumatology Guidelines (IADT) [3] and detailed management steps for all types of dental trauma [4–6]. ToothSOS [7] is a mobile application, and Dental Trauma UK [8] is another site providing guidance for both clinicians and patients.

As the pulp is often affected in dental trauma, it is recommended that clinicians be familiar with both the American Association of Endodontists' consensus statement from 2008 (regarding diagnostic terms used in endodontics) [9] and the 2021 European Society of Endodontology position statement on the endodontic management of traumatised teeth [10].

Traumatic injuries can result in teeth remaining in aberrant positions. For example, an intruded tooth may fail to re-erupt spontaneously, or a displaced tooth may cause an occlusal interference. Orthodontic colleagues may be called upon to reposition and realign traumatised teeth, in which case, the 2020 'Guidelines for the Orthodontic Management of the Traumatised Tooth' [11] are of value.

Not only is information available, but online videos, such as those provided by the Dundee School YouTube page [12], guide clinicians on practical skills, e.g. placing a dental splint.

For gathering the key information needed during emergency trauma management, developing and using a pro forma has been shown to aid in data capture when used for referrals [13]. The use of pro formas can enhance the reliability and standardisation of dental trauma patient assessment. In designing a pro forma, it is important that the General Dental Council [14] and medicolegal requirements are met.

22.1.2 Screen for Medical Injuries and Safeguarding Concerns

If medical injuries are suspected, an urgent referral to Accident and Emergency (A + E) or oral and maxillofacial surgeons (OMFS) is recommended. It is advisable to have awareness of the local A + E department location, contact details, and urgent referral pathways.

Injuries, which are not life-threatening/severe, can potentially wait until initial dental trauma has been stabilised as this is likely to enhance the treatment outcome. Stabilisation is often best done by the patient's registered dentist in accordance with

IADT guidelines, prior to referring for a second opinion and/or management in a specialist dental centre (to a paediatric, restorative, or endodontic specialist), if this is needed. Severe dental trauma may require referral; less serious injuries rarely do.

In screening for urgent medical injuries, the 'ABCDE approach' as per resuscitation guidelines [15] can be used. Key injuries to screen for and rationalisation are summarised in Table 22.1.

Unfortunately, some dental trauma injuries are associated with non-accidental injury (NAI) and/or intimate partner violence (IPV), defined as 'any behaviour

Table 22.1 Relevant non-dental injuries

Injury	Reason for concern	Signs/symptoms
Head injury	Can be life threatening and neurologically disabling [16]	Assess for: – Altered mental state/confusion – Ask if patient has vomited and/or loss of consciousness – Clear fluid from the nose or bleeding from the ear A positive response to any of the above indicates a possible head injury, and urgent referral to A + E is indicated
Overdose	Trauma injuries are often painful, and the maximum analgesic dose may have been exceeded, which can be life threatening	An accurate analgesia history, regarding the type, timing, and dose, along with a full medical history, should be taken If overdose is suspected or known, contact the local A + E department for advice. Whilst awaiting medical advice, stabilise the dental injury
Facial fractures	Diagnosis allows timely referral to OMFS and appropriate management	Mid-face: Screen for visual disturbances and changes to face shape. Asymmetries may not be obvious due to swelling; however, if a patient has a significant mid-face swelling, OMFS assessment is recommended Ask the patient regarding visual changes, particularly double vision, restricted eye movement, or pain on upward gaze. If a fracture is suspected, contact OMFS Mandible: Malocclusion and step deformities can indicate a compound fracture of the mandible requiring prompt surgical management. Liaise with OMFS urgently Distinct mandibular fractures and le Fort fractures have been reported as having a greater association with dental injury than zygomatic arch or complex fractures [17]
Facial lacerations	May require closure	If a laceration is not actively bleeding, initial dental first aid to stabilise the dental injury can be carried out, particularly if the dental injury is time sensitive, e.g. replanting an avulsed tooth Lacerations with profuse bleeding, altered sensation, or vast amounts debris in the wound are best referred to A + E

within an intimate relationship that causes physical, psychological, or sexual harm to those in the relationship'. [18] A recent review of IPV found twice as many women were identified as victims when healthcare professionals inquired regarding abuse [19]. Figures from England and Wales estimate two million adults aged between 16 and 59 experienced domestic abuse in the year ending March 2018 [20].

Be aware of injuries, which appear suspicious, for example, perhaps the injury history and the injury itself do not sensibly align; the person or their accompanying persons behave out of the norm, e.g. a particularly overbearing partner. It can be helpful to see the patient unaccompanied, which is sometimes difficult to achieve; however, when taking radiographs, accompanying persons must leave the room, and this opportunity may be used to ask safeguarding questions.

The National Institute for Health and Care Excellence recommends that frontline staff know the signs to look for and are prepared to have a brief intervention with patients if there are fears abuse may have occurred. A helpful tool to use is 'Ask Validate Document Refer' [21] as summarised below.

- **Ask**: If concerning signs are noted or suspicion raised, **ask** the patient. This opens up the floor, inviting the patient to talk.
- **Validate:** If patients reveal abuse, **acknowledge** the wrong that has been done to them, and let them know it is not their fault.
- **Document:** Records must be **complete and contemporaneous** and may be used later in court. If consented to, **photographs** can be useful.
- **Refer**: Referral to local social services, appropriate shelters, or police, if necessary, may be required.

Abuse and IPV are very serious concern. This article cannot cover it in its entirety; seeking relevant safeguarding CPD for the benefit and welfare of all patients, and colleagues, is recommended.

If there are immediate concerns regarding the patient's safety, police may need to be involved. If there is reason to believe a person is in immediate danger, or that person is a danger to the public, it is recommended the police be called, dialling 999, if necessary. The General Dental Council Standard 4.3.1 acknowledges this [14].

22.1.3 Be Prepared Clinically: Consider a 'Trauma Toolkit'

For clinicians likely to manage immediate trauma cases, it can be helpful to have a 'trauma toolkit', enabling appropriate equipment to be quickly available chair side. Such toolkits can be developed with reference to guidelines.

As dental trauma cases can involve prosecution, taking photographic records is advised and many patients can supply pre-injury and injury photographs from their mobile phones, if the dental clinic does not have photographic facilities.

22.1.4 Aim to Stabilise, Preserve and Protect Tissues

Stabilising injured tissues involves prioritising the health and healing of the pulp and periodontal supporting apparatus. Favourable outcomes are when repair (i.e. scar tissue) or regeneration of tissues occurs, ideally the latter.

If the pulp is exposed, encourage healing by placing a material likely to stimulate this. Today, calcium silicate cements (CSC) are recommended and available in pre-mixed formulations such as Biodentine. The use of biocompatible and bioactive CSCs and the prevention of microbial contamination increase the likelihood of successful pulpal recovery. The use of a dental dam (if the pulp is exposed) is important to reduce the risk of microbial ingress and facilitate the use of sodium hypochlorite irrigation. Following placement of a CSC, an adhesive restoration should be placed. In some cases of pulpal exposure, partial pulpotomies are indicated (detailed in IADT guidelines) and are associated with high success rates.

Teeth, which have been moved into position, need the periodontal supporting apparatus stabilised. This will involve repositioning and retaining the tooth or teeth in their pre-injury position with a splint. Stabilisation in a harmonious static and functional occlusal relationship is key.

Root fractures must also be stabilised in this way, via splinting, to encourage the fracture site to heal. Splints should be placed so as not to interfere with periodontal tissue healing, the occlusion, or oral hygiene practices.

In considering protection, it is of note that the use of custom-made mouth guards for contact sports appear to significantly decrease the risk of orofacial trauma, as does early orthodontic correction of overjets of >6 mm in 6–13-year-old children [22]. Each of these prevention strategies is recommended for routine use, where appropriate.

22.1.5 Splinting and Maintaining Aesthetics

Splinting aims to stabilise the tooth in the pre-injury position and be easy to place and remove [23]. In some cases, ascertaining the pre-injury tooth position is challenging; radiographs and recent 'selfies' may be of help. Mixed dentition cases can be more complex to splint, and if needed, advice can be sought from specialist centres; however, teeth sufficiently loose to be an aspiration risk must be managed as a matter of urgency.

Once in place, a splint must reliably stay in situ, avoiding undue stress on the tooth or periodontal ligament and allowing for functional tooth movement. To achieve this, evidence supports the use of flexible composite and wire splints (wire diameter less than 0.4 mm) [24, 25].

Where teeth have been avulsed and lost, it is important to maintain aesthetics and the edentulous area (preventing drifting and tilting of neighbouring teeth), until definitive restoration. A 'Flipper' (partial denture replacing one or more teeth and clasping molars) or Essix retainer with pontic can be quickly made and effectively maintain the space and aesthetics.

22.1.6 Recognise More Serious Dental Trauma Injuries

Those injuries most damaging to the pulp and periodontal tissues are luxations, particularly lateral and intrusion, and avulsions. These injuries are most likely to develop challenging long-term sequelae, which must be monitored for (discussed later).

Those teeth that have been avulsed or intruded and have complications and teeth with cervical or crown root fractures are those most likely to be lost.

22.1.7 Follow-Up and Further Planning

Having dealt with immediate trauma stabilisation, longer-term planning must take a more holistic approach, including discussing patient expectations. The IADT guidelines provide follow-up schedule advice and possible complications arising from the trauma itself.

In the longer term, the general oral condition must be considered and, in particular, the aesthetics, function, and prognosis of traumatised teeth. If teeth have a guarded or poor outlook, whether from trauma, caries, or periodontal disease, factors in relation to tooth replacement must be assessed. This will include consideration of patient age, caries and periodontal status and risk, smile line, gingival phenotype, occlusal factors, the chances of further trauma, and the position and number of teeth likely to be lost. Specialist input may be of help if the loss of several teeth is anticipated.

22.1.8 Shared Decision-Making and Consent

To maximise the trauma outcome, accurate diagnoses, effective management, and prediction of prognosis are needed. These must be discussed with the patient in an understandable manner. Any treatment must be with the informed consent of the patient or, where necessary, the patient's advocate. Medicolegally, advice on the diagnosis, reasonable treatment options, and associated risks/benefits must be discussed and documented, along with referral arrangements, if relevant.

The Scottish initiative Realistic Medicine [26] is a useful resource regarding shared decision-making. This aims to help clinicians and patients communicate effectively about options. Patients may find the simple questions about treatment options particularly useful.

Following healthcare consultations, patients' retention of information is known to be low [27, 28]; this, coupled with a stressful trauma event, means that patients may not be receptive to information. It is therefore sensible to reiterate prognosis and long-term sequelae advice at follow-up appointments and consider sending summary letters or producing relevant patient information leaflets.

22.1.9 Sequelae

Ongoing clinical and radiographic monitoring is advisable because complications can arise more than 10 years after injury. Teeth with closed apices are more likely to have complications (Tables 22.2 and 22.3).

Table 22.2 Sequalae of traumatic dental injuries

Tooth colour changes	Rationale	Previous injury	Management
Yellow/ brown clinical crown	Usually associated with pulpal obliteration	Luxations	Sensibility test. If pulp is vital, monitor only +/− improve aesthetics If pulp is non-vital, endodontic treatment is more complex. Magnification required Consider specialist referral
Grey clinical crown	Blood products from pulpal haemorrhage	Luxations Avulsions Complicated crown fracture	Confirm loss of vitality, endodontically treat and improve aesthetics Alternatively, extract
Pink area in clinical crown	Shine through of invading tissue, usually from external cervical root resorption (ECRR)	Aetiology unclear but associations with previous trauma reported [29]	If very soon after trauma, may indicate tooth revascularisation. Monitor, frequently review, should reverse within days or weeks If several months/years after trauma and accompanied by subgingival cavity/defect, suspect ECRR. Refer urgently to specialist centre (endodontic, restorative or paediatric dentistry)

(continued)

Table 22.2 (continued)

Tooth colour changes	Rationale	Previous injury	Management
Loss of pulp vitality	**Rationale**	**Previous injury**	**Management**
More likely to arise in closed apex cases	Healing (repair/ regeneration) capacity of closed apex teeth is less than that of open apex, younger teeth Injuries which stretch (displacements) or sever the neurovascular bundle at the root end predispose to loss of vitality in closed apex cases Even in less severe injuries, traumatised teeth, which remain intact, may have unseen cracks present, which admit biofilm and can lead to the deterioration of pulp In fractured traumatised teeth, exposed dentine tubules and pulp can suffer microbial invasion Root fractures, where the segment coronal to the fracture has been displaced, are more likely to lose vitality	Luxations Avulsions Complicated crown fractures can challenge pulp survival	Identify loss of vitality as soon as possible and endodontically treat If a complex case (e.g. horizontal root fracture and coronal portion is non-vital), consider specialist referral for coronal segment to be managed as though an open apex is present

Table 22.3 Radiographically identified complications

Pulpal obliteration	Rationale	Previous injury	Management
Pulpal narrowing/ obliteration +/– yellow/ brown clinical crown	In more severe injuries, odontoblasts die, and differentiation of new odontoblast cells occurs Secretion of reparative dentine (bone-like tissue) commences in pulp chamber and along root canal system (RCS) walls, obliterating RCS	Mostly luxations	Sensibility test. If pulp is vital, monitor only +/– improve aesthetics If pulp is non-vital, endodontic treatment is more complex. Magnification required Consider specialist referral
Infection-related root resorption	**Rationale**	**Previous injury**	**Management**
External infection related root resorption (ERR)	Two situations are needed for ERR to arise: The root canal system must have microbial infection and in addition, damage or loss of cementum has occurred, and dentinal tubules are exposed to the PDL and bone [30]	Luxation Avulsion (with increased extra-oral dry time or non-physiologic storage medium)	Manage as per IADT guidelines Aim to extirpate pulp and prepare root canal system under dental dam and using sodium hypochlorite. Removal of necrotic canal contents aims to halt/ stabilise resorption Evidence of ERR at a horizontal root fracture site suggests the coronal fragment has become necrotic. Refer for endodontic management
Internal root resorption	Rare Destruction is seen within the root canal system and histologically metaplastic bone, or cementum-like tissue is seen adjacent to resorption	Aetiology unclear [31]	Refer urgently for specialist input because prognosis decreases if resorption perforates through radicular wall
External cervical root resorption (ECRR)	Thought to derive from inflammation following disruption of the PDL [32]	Aetiology unclear may report previous trauma	Refer urgently to specialist Centre (endodontic, restorative or paediatric dentistry)

(continued)

Table 22.3 (continued)

Pulpal obliteration	Rationale	Previous injury	Management
Replacement resorption (RR)	**Rationale**	**Previous injury**	**Management**
Replacement resorption leads to ankylosis	Compression of periodontal ligament (PDL) leads to macrophage and osteoclasts removing necrotic PDL fragments and infection related, or RR resorption may be seen	Intrusive luxation Avulsion (as extra-oral dry time increases, risk of RR increases)	Loss of tooth inevitable. Plan for future replacement If patient <18 years of age, consider disguising infra-occlusion using composite or decoronation until growth ceased alternatively, orthodontic space closure If patient >18 years of age, consider a fixed solution where possible: A resin-bonded bridge or dental implant. Removable options can be useful short term
Gingival recession or severe clinical attachment loss	**Rationale**	**Previous injury**	**Management**
Most likely in closed apex teeth which have been displaced	Maxillary cortical plate thinner and can fracture on lateral luxation If displaced teeth are not optimally repositioned, marginal bone loss is more likely	Lateral luxation Intrusive luxation Replanted avulsed teeth	Encourage excellent oral hygiene Consider referral to a specialist clinic. May need multidisciplinary input (restorative, orthodontic, paediatric dentistry)

22.2 Summary

Many clinicians work in dental settings, where patients sustaining trauma can present; however, this may be infrequent, heightening stress when dealing with trauma.

To support trauma management, consider displaying trauma management pathways in the clinic, for example, a flowchart with web links to best practice guidance, warning signs indicative of more serious medical injuries, contact numbers for local A + E, OMFS, and other dental specialist services.

The use of a pro forma can encourage robust and thorough trauma assessment, as well as be an educational tool. Having a 'trauma toolkit' either physically set up or as a laminated *aide memoire* list can facilitate speedy management when unscheduled, emergency trauma patients attend. To support good-quality patient communication, summary letters or information leaflets highlighting the timescales for follow-up, possible sequelae, and prognosis are helpful.

Trauma cases can highlight interesting clinical conundrums in their immediate and longer-term management. Peer discussion activities and sharing learning from cases are valuable, along with CPD activities. Many specialist societies have annual conferences of relevance to trauma management, which together with the points raised in this article, aim to equip clinicians with the knowledge and skills of ways in which to provide high-quality care when trauma is sustained to permanent teeth.

22.3 Conclusion

Traumatic dental injuries require rapid diagnosis and treatment; invariably, this is dependent on good clinical knowledge based on guidance to provide treatment efficiently and quickly to aid healing of teeth, soft tissues, and alveolus.

References

1. Petti S, Glendor U, Andersson L. World traumatic dental injury prevalence and incidence, a meta-analysis—one billion living people have had traumatic dental injuries. Dent Traumatol. 2018;34:71–86.
2. The Dental Trauma Guide. 2022. https://dentaltraumaguide.org/. Accessed Apr 2022.
3. International Association of Dental Traumatology. 2022. https://www.iadt-dentaltrauma.org/. Accessed Apr 2022.
4. Levin L, Day PF, Hicks L, et al. International Association of Dental Traumatology guidelines for the management of traumatic dental injuries: General introduction. Dent Traumatol. 2020;36:309–13.
5. Bourguignon C, Cohenca N, Lauridsen E, et al. International Association of Dental Traumatology guidelines for the management of traumatic dental injuries: 1. Fractures and luxations. Dent Traumatol. 2020;36:314–30.
6. Fouad AF, Abbott PV, Tsilingaridis G, et al. International Association of Dental Traumatology guidelines for the management of traumatic dental injuries: 2. Avulsion of permanent teeth. Dent Traumatol. 2020;36:331–42.
7. Khehra A, Cohenca N, Cehreli ZC, Levin L. The International Association of Dental Traumatology ToothSOS mobile app: a 2-year report. Dent Traumatol. 2021;37:145–50.
8. Dental Trauma UK. 2022. Available at: https://www.dentaltrauma.co.uk/. Accessed Apr 2022.
9. American Association of Endodontists. 2022. https://www.aae.org/specialty/wp-content/uploads/sites/2/2017/07/endodonticdiagnosisfall2013.pdf. Accessed 22 Feb 2022.
10. Krastl G, Weiger R, Filippi A, et al. European Society of Endodontology position statement: endodontic management of traumatized permanent teeth. Int Endod J. 2021;54:1473–81.
11. Sandler C, Al-Musfir T, Barry S, et al. Guidelines for the orthodontic management of the traumatised tooth. J Orthod. 2021;48:74–81.
12. Dundee Dental School. Dental trauma: management playlist. 2018. https://www.youtube.com/playlist?list=PLQ8ay5GGizJUCFHnULLw3HeLYVW6oPSgA. Accessed Apr 2022.
13. Djemal S, Chia M, Ubaya-Narayange T. Quality improvement of referrals to a department of restorative dentistry following the use of a referral proforma by referring dental practitioners. Br Dent J. 2004;197:85–8.
14. General Dental Council. Standards for the dental team. London: General Dental Council; 2013. www.gdc-uk.org. Accessed Apr 2022.
15. Resuscitation Council UK. 2021 Resuscitation guidelines. https://www.resus.org.uk/library/2021-resuscitation-guidelines. Accessed Apr 2022.
16. Teasdale GM. Head injury. J Neurol Neurosurg Psychiatry. 1995;58:526–39.
17. Ruslin M, Wolff J, Boffano P, Brand HS, Forouzanfar T. Dental trauma in association with maxillofacial fractures: an epidemiological study. Dental Traumatol. 2015;31:318–23.

18. World Health Organization. Global and regional estimates of violence against women. Prevalence and health effects of intimate partner violence and non-partner sexual violence. 2013. https://www.who.int/publications/i/item/9789241564625. Accessed Apr 2022.
19. O'Doherty L, Hegarty K, Ramsay J, Davidson LL, Feder G, Taft A. Screening women for intimate partner violence in healthcare settings. Cochrane Database Syst Rev. 2015;2015:CD007007. https://doi.org/10.1002/14651858.CD007007.pub3.
20. Office for National Statistics. Domestic abuse in England and Wales: year ending March 2018. https://www.ons.gov.uk/peoplepopulationandcommunity/crimeandjustice/bulletins/domesticabuseinenglandandwales/yearendingmarch2018. Accessed Jan 2022.
21. Gerbert B, Moe J, Caspers N, et al. Simplifying physicians' response to domestic violence. West J Med. 2000;172:329–31.
22. Schatz J-P, Ostini E, Hakeberg M, Kiliaridis S. Large overjet as a risk factor of traumatic dental injuries: a prospective longitudinal study. Prog Orthod. 2020;21:41. https://doi.org/10.1186/s40510-020-00341-5.
23. Sobczak-Zagalska H, Emerich K. Best splinting methods in case of dental injury—a literature review. J Clin Pediatr Dent. 2020;44:71–8.
24. Kahler B, Hu J-Y, Marriott-Smith CS. Splinting of teeth following trauma: a review and a new splinting recommendation. Aust Dent J. 2016;61:59–73.
25. Kwan SC, Johnson JD, Cohenca N. The effect of splint material and thickness on tooth mobility after extraction and replantation using a human cadaveric model. Dent Traumatol. 2012;28:277–81.
26. Realistic Medicine. 2022. https://www.realisticmedicine.scot/. Accessed Apr 2022.
27. Laws MB, Lee Y, Taubin T, Rogers WH, Wilson IB. Factors associated with patient recall of key information in ambulatory specialty care visits: results of an innovative methodology. PLoS One. 2018;13:e0191940. https://doi.org/10.1371/journal.pone.0191940.
28. Godwin Y. Do they listen? A review of information retained by patients following consent for reduction mammoplasty. Br J Plast Surg. 2000;53:121–5.
29. Irinakis E, Aleksejuniene J, Shen Y, Haapasalo M. External cervical resorption: a retrospective case-control study. J Endod. 2020;46:1420–7.
30. Abbott PV. Prevention and management of external inflammatory resorption following trauma to teeth. Aust Dent J. 2016;61(Suppl 1):82–94.
31. Patel S, Ricucci D, Durak C, Tay F. Internal root resorption: a review. J Endod. 2010;36:1107–21.
32. Chen Y, Huang Y, Deng X. External cervical resorption-a review of pathogenesis and potential predisposing factors. Int J Oral Sci. 2021;13:19. https://doi.org/10.1038/s41368-021-00121-9.

Traumatic Dental Injury Review: Part 1

23

Clement Seeballuck, Sean Dolan, and Julie K. Kilgariff

Learning Points

- Appreciate the need to revisit and confirm previous diagnoses at review.
- Understand that patients will require more information on their condition at review.
- Recall that long-term sequelae can develop and that a systematic schedule of review contributes to the early diagnosis of future conditions.

23.1 Introduction

Following initial stabilisation of traumatic dental injuries (TDIs) to permanent teeth, follow-up is likely to be required. This is often best carried out in general dental practice, easing barriers to accessing dental care, particularly in rural and isolated communities, and potentially enhancing the cost-effectiveness and sustainability of dental care. It is important that general dental practitioners (GDPs) are aware of which TDI injuries are the more serious and most likely to develop problematic consequences, requiring follow-up and potentially further dental intervention.

In a previous article, the immediate management of TDIs was discussed [1]. An accurate diagnosis will inform initial management, treatment required, and the follow-up regime. For follow-up to be effective, it is helpful if the clinician is aware of the original trauma diagnosis and the follow-up is in accordance with recognised

C. Seeballuck
Paediatric Dentistry, Dundee Dental Hospital and Research School, Dundee, UK

S. Dolan
Restorative Dentistry, Glasgow Dental Hospital and School, Glasgow, UK

J. K. Kilgariff (✉)
Endodontics, Dundee Dental Hospital and Research School, Dundee, UK
e-mail: julie.kilgariff@nhs.scot

E. McColl, A. Alani (eds.), *Practical Tips in Clinical Dentistry*, BDJ Clinician's Guides, https://doi.org/10.1007/978-3-031-90355-7_23

guidelines [2, 3]. Follow-up aims to facilitate early diagnosis, treatment, and/or referral of deleterious problems occurring as a result of the trauma, particularly because many problematic sequelae are asymptomatic and develop many months, or years, after the TDI [4–6].

This article and the second part guide and inform TDI follow-up, the investigations and special tests recommended, the reliability of these, and TDI sequelae to monitor for.

23.1.1 Confirm TDI Diagnosis

Trauma is seldom an anticipated or predictable event, with a range of case severity occurring, often with concurrent medical injuries, and potentially out-of-hours. This can lead to challenging circumstances in identifying, diagnosing, and stabilising TDIs, particularly when patient cooperation may be limited due to patient age and/or distress. In medical A&E services, access to take periapical and other intra-oral radiographs can be limited and impact the accurate diagnoses of injuries. For example, without a periapical, root fractures may not be identified and the injury insufficiently stabilised [7].

It is therefore important when examining a historical trauma case for the first time that the history and examination be carried out thoroughly and an open mind kept until the diagnosis is clarified. Be aware of potential misdiagnoses when initial management has been undertaken by a different clinician. If correspondence and/or dental records are available, reviewing these together with previous and current radiographs is sensible. Once the diagnosis is confirmed or an informed best guess made, the International Association of Dental Traumatology (IADT) [2] guidance should be referred to for recommended follow-up regimes and likely complications. The various relevant current guidelines in relation to TDIs have previously been discussed and readers are directed to this [1]. Pre-existing guidelines [8] have recently been reviewed and changes to recommended dental materials, follow-up timings, and diagnostic imaging regimes made.

23.1.2 Patient Education

Patients and, in the case of minors, their advocates must be made aware of potential TDI sequelae, the need for follow-up, and problematic signs/symptoms to look out for. Figure 23.1 illustrates a case example where the patient failed to return for review and at 4 months post injury, a hopeless outlook for the previously traumatised tooth evident. Although earlier attendance may not have changed the outlook in this case, it is essential that patients understand the importance of TDI follow-up, as early intervention can improve some outcomes.

Providing patients with the right information is therefore crucial and integral to shared decision-making and informed, valid consent [9–11]. Highlighting what patients should self-monitor for can be incorporated into a wider discussion

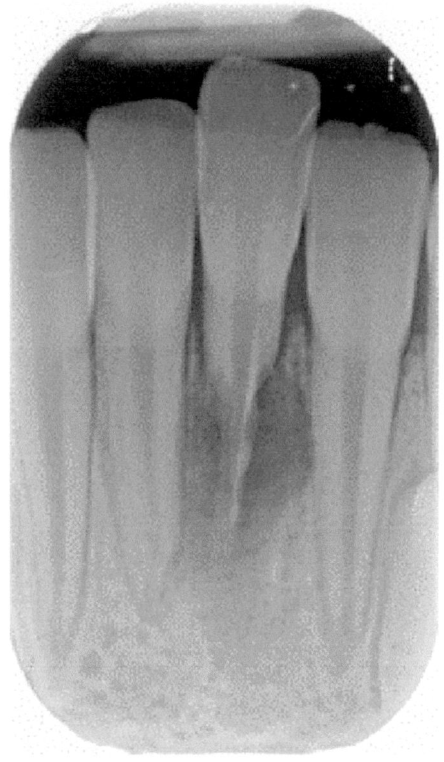

Fig. 23.1 Tooth 31 was replanted following avulsion. The patient re-attended some 4 months later, having missed intervening appointments. Replacement resorption is seen, and the outlook for 31 hopeless

regarding prognosis, expected outcome(s), and long-term treatment planning. There are evidence-based resources developed specifically for the public to refer to [12–15]. Patient information leaflets can be useful [16, 17], provided they are appropriately designed [18, 19]. Today, patients have unlimited access to online resources, of which content may not be quality assured. Therefore, providing accurate, comprehensive information directly to patients during dental visits may better guide realistic expectations and inform a self-monitoring toolkit of what to look out for and act on. Asking patients to make a dental appointment should they notice signs or symptoms such as pain, swelling, sinus tract, and tooth discolouration may enhance outcomes.

23.1.3 Be Aware of Potential TDI Sequelae

Table 23.1 summarises potential dental sequelae commonly encountered following a traumatic dental injury. The pulpal and periradicular diagnosis referred to are those used in the American Association of Endodontists 2008 Diagnostic Guidelines [20]. The impact of these injuries on tooth survival has been colour coded: green indicates sequelae unlikely to reduce tooth survival, amber highlights those which may reduce tooth survival, and red are sequelae likely to reduce tooth survival.

Table 23.1 TDI sequelae, significance, and management

TDI Sequelae Identified at follow-up	Signs	Symptoms	Significance & impact on tooth survival	Management
Change in tooth structure due to damage or subsequent loss of a coronal tooth fragment.*	Fractured tooth, Cracks, crazing/infractions within tooth structure	Patient may complain of sharp edges and/or aesthetic changes. Depending on extent of crack/fracture signs, and symptoms of reversible or irreversible pulpitis may be present.	Unlikely to reduce tooth survival. Impacts quality of life mainly, aesthetically, and potential functional implications (speech/ mastication). Pain may be present, due to dentine or pulp exposure and microbial ingress either directly (if the pulp is exposed) or indirectly via exposed dentinal tubules.	Evaluate extent of fracture to inform management. Cracks or crazes in the tooth can allow a portal of entry for infection, resin sealing of the crack may prevent this, decreasing permeability.[21] Pulpal exposure: A pulpotomy is carried out under aseptic conditions. Thereafter, the tooth fragment (if present) can be rehydrated (in saline) and reattached adhesively.[22] Reattachment can be done regardless of whether there is a pulpal exposure.
Pulp canal obliteration due to deposition of reactionary dentine.*	Yellow darkening of the tooth crown when viewed directly or via transillumination. Reduced or reducing response to sensibility testing because of reactionary dentine deposition (ie, vital pulp) Radiographic signs of a narrowing root canal system.	Nil, unless pulpal necrosis has occurred, but this is rare.	Unlikely to reduce tooth survival. Adversely affects aesthetics.	Unless overt signs or symptoms of pulpal necrosis are identified, management of the patient's aesthetic requirements only are required, along with clinical and radiographic monitoring in accordance with the TDI injury type. Previous luxation injuries are most associated with pulpal obliteration. Only 1% of such cases subsequently undergo pulpal necrosis.[23]
Pulpal necrosis.†	Greyish darkening of the tooth crown. Negative response to sensibility testing. In immature teeth with open apices, radiographic signs of arrested tooth development will be seen (cession of root development, no closure of root end). Compare it to contralateral tooth, in relation to the patient's age.	May have associated symptoms of pulpal necrosis and periradicular changes, such as intra or extra-oral swelling or a sinus tract, etc. Patient may complain regarding tooth discolouration.	May reduce tooth survival. Endodontic treatment is indicated. Highest success rates occur in the absence of periradicular radiographic changes. Diagnostic delay makes periradicular changes more likely. External inflammatory root resorption (EIRR) in acute or chronic periradicular inflammation can arise. This is due to microbial products from the necrotic pulp diffusing through dentinal tubules and stimulating osteoclastic resorption on the external root face.	Confirm pulpal necrosis using two or more investigations and/or tests and complete non-surgical endodontic treatment (in accordance with ESE guidelines,[22] prior to addressing any aesthetic concerns. Internal or external tooth whitening may be indicated. Products containing or releasing between 0.1 and 6% hydrogen peroxide cannot be used on under 18-year-olds unless used for treating or preventing disease.[24]
Periapical or periradicular periodontitis.†	Radiographically, widening of the periodontal ligament space (PDL), loss of lamina dura, and/or a frank radiolucency may be present.	Cases may be symptomatic (for example, affected teeth display tenderness to percussion), or asymptomatic.	May reduce tooth survival because presence of periradicular radiolucencies decrease endodontic treatment success.	In the absence of clinical signs or symptoms, seek further information to confirm pulpal necrosis (such as sensibility testing) prior to embarking on endodontic management. This is because widening of the PDL or a radiolucency can indicate microbes are present within the root canal system or can be due to the TDI severing of the neurovascular bundle causing localised inflammation.[25]
Acute apical abscess.§	Swelling of adjacent tissues	Spontaneous pain. Tooth tender to percussion and sulcular palpation	Potential for systemic involvement such as fever and lymphadenopathy. Indicative of pulpal necrosis and microbial colonisation of the root canal system.	Drainage is indicated, through the root canal system, removal of the tooth or incision into swollen soft tissue. Systemic involvement indicates antimicrobials may be required and readers are directed to relevant guidance.[26]
Chronic apical abscess.§	Sinus present on soft tissue that may be discharging or suppurating. A radiograph using a gutta percha point to trace the sinus can identify the causative tooth.[26]	Patient may present with little to no complaint	May revert to an acute apical abscess if drainage is halted. Can progress to a cystic lesion.[24]	The cause of the sinus is the tooth. Plan for tooth extraction or root canal treatment.
Tooth discolouration following endodontic management and access cavity restoration.*	Intrinsic discolouration of the clinical crown can arise as a result of dental materials used.	Patient may complain regarding tooth discolouration.	Unlikely to reduce tooth survival. Adversely affects aesthetic outcome	In recent years, modern endodontic materials, such as Mineral Trioxide Aggregate (MTA) (a calcium silicate-based cement, CSC) have been associated with tooth discolouration because of bismuth oxide contents, although contamination of endodontic materials with blood may be a factor also. Historically, amalgam used in access cavities can leach and affecting the crown colour. Other factors include secondary caries surrounding a leaking restoration. No significant discolouration has been found with modern generation CSCs which do not contain bismuth oxide.[27]
Internal inflammatory root resorption.†	Initially none, may be incidental radiographic finding. To occur, pulp must have some vitality, although can become necrotic eventually.	Often whilst pulp vital. Potentially irreversible pulpitis symptoms ensue. If necrosis occurs, signs and symptoms commensurate with this may occur.	May reduce tooth survival if resorption perforates tooth root. Early identification and management key. Coronal portion of pulp is often necrotic, apically it may be vital.[28]	Root canal treatment is indicated +/- antibiotic- corticosteroid pastes.[28] To obturate the tooth effectively, the extent of resorption requires to be known and heated obturation techniques needed. Referral to a specialist may be required.
External invasive root resorption (cervical root resorption).§	The pulp is most often vital. Patient may present noting a pink spot from the shine through of granulation tissue invading the tooth crown. The resorbed cervical area contains inflamed tissue that bleeds profusely on periodontal probing.[29] The aetiology is unclear, and trauma is but one implicating factor. A cause-and-effect relationship has not been established.[30]	Patients may report a change in aesthetics, bleeding on brushing from gingival inflammation in the resorbed area or pulpitis symptoms. Asymptomatic cases are also seen.	May reduce tooth survival. The extent of lesion must be considered when assessing the restorability.[30] Cases that have remained more coronal and have not entered the pulp have a better prognosis.[30]	Referral to a Restorative or Endodontic specialist is recommended as soon as possible to explore management options before the lesion potentially becomes too extensive to predictably treat.
External inflammatory root resorption (EIRR).§	Occurs as a result of pulpal necrosis. Radiographically lamina dura is no longer evident at the site of the resorption.	As per pulpal necrosis and the associated periradicular diagnosis.	May reduce tooth survival. Root canal system is infected.[28] *See 'Significance & impact' section of pulpal necrosis above.*	Confirm pulpal necrosis (eg, sensibility testing), extirpate as soon as possible to halt resorption. EIRR generally has a predictable outcome.[28] If diagnosed late, or if the crown: root ratio is less than 1:1, the outlook for the tooth may be reduced.
External Replacement resorption and ankylosis.§	Ankylosis may be determined by a high percussive note, loss of PDL space radiographically and absence of physiologic mobility. This may be accompanied by external replacement resorption.[31]	If the patient is younger and growing, a step in the occlusal level is likely to arise. Changes in gingival margin height can also occur and be noticeable.	Likely to reduce tooth survival. Progressive. Bone replaces entire tooth, leading to eventual tooth loss.	Monitor and plan for tooth loss and replacement. Focus on maintaining aesthetics as best possible.

Row colour: *green; †yellow; §red. Red rows are the most urgent to address; yellow have medium urgency; green are the least urgent.

A consequence of TDI can be the premature loss of a tooth, such as an avulsed tooth not recovered at the time of injury, or a tooth subsequently becoming unrestorable, such as that seen in Fig. 23.1. Premature tooth loss must be factored into treatment planning. The patient's age, tooth eruption stage, and occlusion will require consideration, along with potential specialist referral. In most cases, retaining teeth or a poor outlook and maintaining the space of teeth already lost due to TDI is recommended whilst treatment planning takes place.

23.1.4 Review and Document TDI Follow-Up Systematically

At each follow-up appointment, the aim is to identify if there has been a deterioration of the injured tooth or teeth and whether aesthetics and function are satisfactory. A patient history should be gathered, and clinical examination of the TDI-affected teeth (including neighbouring and opposing teeth), surrounding tissues, and a check of static and functional occlusion of TDI-affected teeth should be made. IADT guidelines [2] signpost review periods and when to sensibility test and radiograph TDI-affected teeth, depending on the injury previously sustained.

Comprehensive documentation is crucial for clinical notes [32]. A standardised method of recording a trauma review, such as using a pro forma, may help to mitigate human factors regarding information collection and enhance information gain [33, 34]. These can be designed to include information signposting appropriate review intervals in relation to the injury sustained.

At the TDI review appointment, ensuring a clear, accurate trauma diagnosis has previously been established and recorded. Enquiries should be made as to the development of signs or symptoms of pulpal, periodontal, or periradicular disease. Using a pain-recognised pain scale or pain assessment tool [35] can aid in capturing a pain history if problems are reported. The patient's view on the aesthetics of the TDI-affected teeth should be explored, together with asking about changes in tooth position and/or occlusion.

Sensibility tests are an important element of trauma review, but these do always reveal true pulpal status [36, 37]. Combining several tests and correlating these with signs and symptoms to determine pulpal diagnosis is the most robust approach, although still not 100% accurate [38]. Pulse oximetry is reportedly the most diagnostically accurate test; [39] however, this, together with laser Doppler flowmetry, is not commonly available or undertaken in dental clinics.

Figure 23.2 summarises the clinical examination, investigations, and special tests frequently undertaken at TDI follow-up. Videos demonstrating how to undertake these tests are available on the Dundee School of Dentistry YouTube Channel [40].

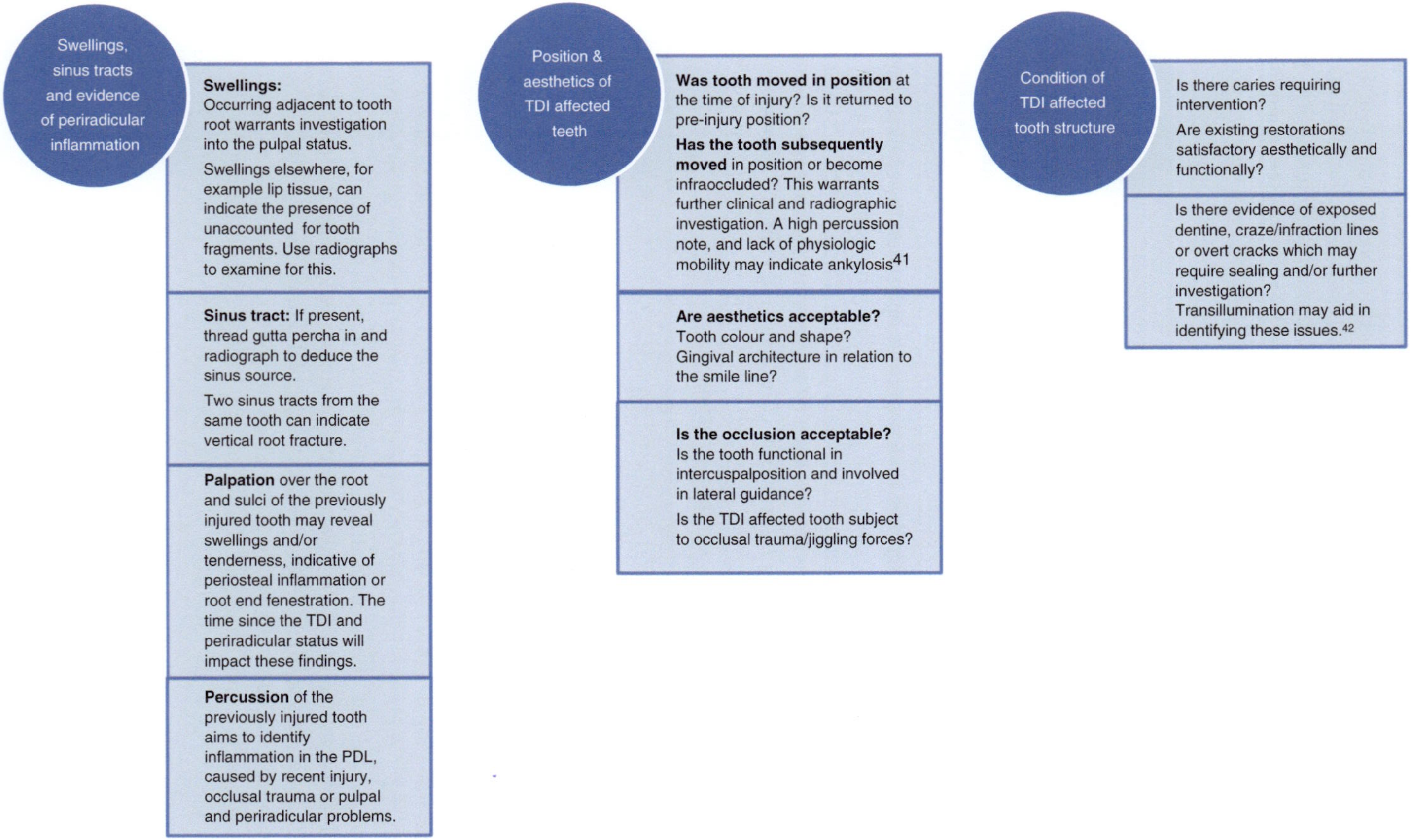

Swellings, sinus tracts and evidence of periradicular inflammation

Swellings:
Occurring adjacent to tooth root warrants investigation into the pulpal status.
Swellings elsewhere, for example lip tissue, can indicate the presence of unaccounted for tooth fragments. Use radiographs to examine for this.

Sinus tract: If present, thread gutta percha in and radiograph to deduce the sinus source.
Two sinus tracts from the same tooth can indicate vertical root fracture.

Palpation over the root and sulci of the previously injured tooth may reveal swellings and/or tenderness, indicative of periosteal inflammation or root end fenestration. The time since the TDI and periradicular status will impact these findings.

Percussion of the previously injured tooth aims to identify inflammation in the PDL, caused by recent injury, occlusal trauma or pulpal and periradicular problems.

Position & aesthetics of TDI affected teeth

Was tooth moved in position at the time of injury? Is it returned to pre-injury position?
Has the tooth subsequently moved in position or become infraoccluded? This warrants further clinical and radiographic investigation. A high percussion note, and lack of physiologic mobility may indicate ankylosis[41]

Are aesthetics acceptable?
Tooth colour and shape?
Gingival architecture in relation to the smile line?

Is the occlusion acceptable?
Is the tooth functional in intercuspalposition and involved in lateral guidance?
Is the TDI affected tooth subject to occlusal trauma/jiggling forces?

Condition of TDI affected tooth structure

Is there caries requiring intervention?
Are existing restorations satisfactory aesthetically and functionally?

Is there evidence of exposed dentine, craze/infraction lines or overt cracks which may require sealing and/or further investigation?
Transillumination may aid in identifying these issues.[42]

Fig. 23.2 (**a**) A summary of clinical follow-up of signs and symptoms. (**b**) A summary of utilising special tests and investigations at follow-up

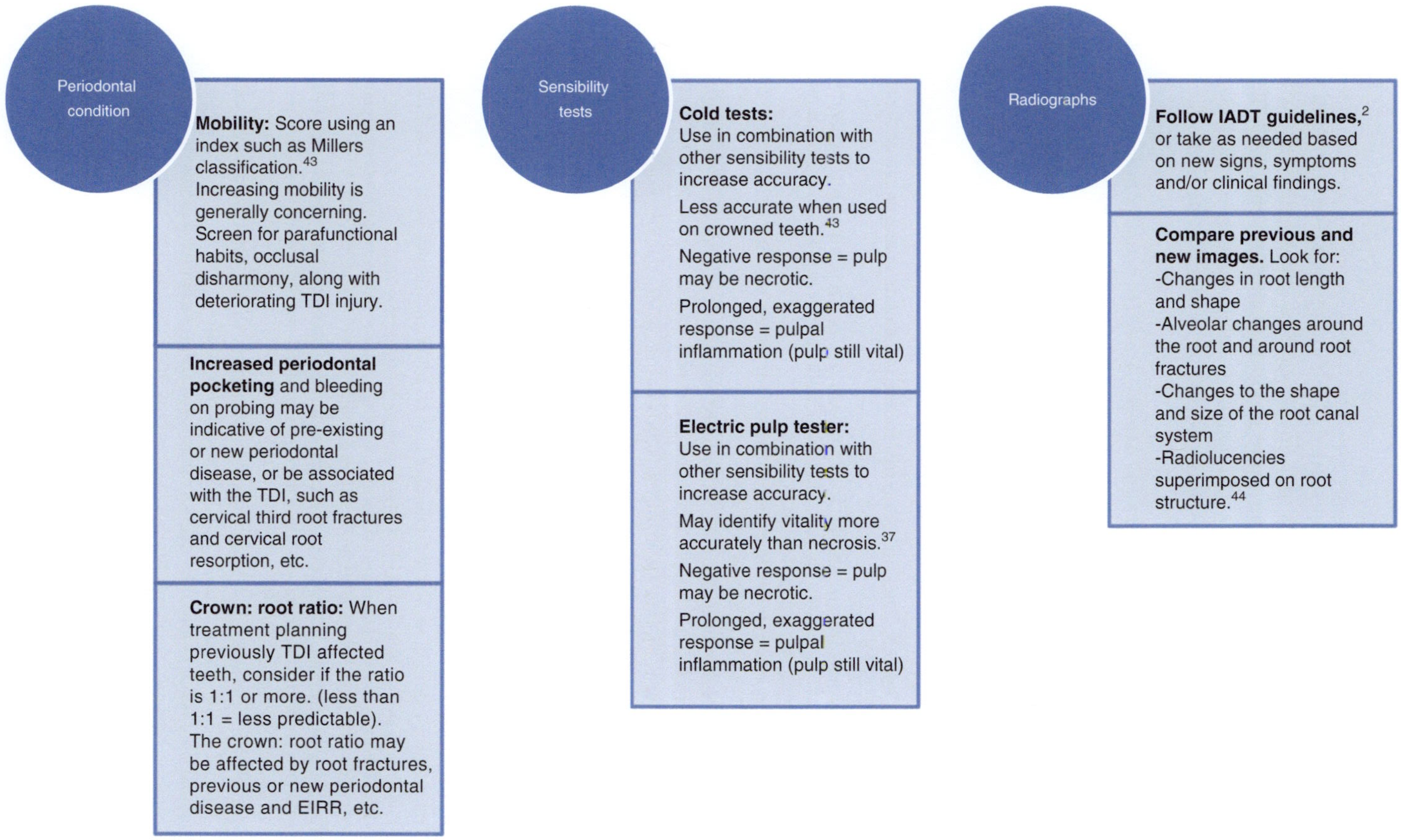

Periodontal condition

Mobility: Score using an index such as Millers classification.[43] Increasing mobility is generally concerning. Screen for parafunctional habits, occlusal disharmony, along with deteriorating TDI injury.

Increased periodontal pocketing and bleeding on probing may be indicative of pre-existing or new periodontal disease, or be associated with the TDI, such as cervical third root fractures and cervical root resorption, etc.

Crown: root ratio: When treatment planning previously TDI affected teeth, consider if the ratio is 1:1 or more. (less than 1:1 = less predictable). The crown: root ratio may be affected by root fractures, previous or new periodontal disease and EIRR, etc.

Sensibility tests

Cold tests:
Use in combination with other sensibility tests to increase accuracy.

Less accurate when used on crowned teeth.[43]

Negative response = pulp may be necrotic.

Prolonged, exaggerated response = pulpal inflammation (pulp still vital)

Electric pulp tester:
Use in combination with other sensibility tests to increase accuracy.

May identify vitality more accurately than necrosis.[37]

Negative response = pulp may be necrotic.

Prolonged, exaggerated response = pulpal inflammation (pulp still vital)

Radiographs

Follow IADT guidelines,[2] or take as needed based on new signs, symptoms and/or clinical findings.

Compare previous and new images. Look for:
-Changes in root length and shape
-Alveolar changes around the root and around root fractures
-Changes to the shape and size of the root canal system
-Radiolucencies superimposed on root structure.[44]

Fig. 23.2 (continued)

23.2 Conclusion

This chapter has discussed the importance of TDI diagnosis; the communication of TDI injury sequelae with patients and, in the case of minors, their guardians; the potential sequelae of TDIs and how these might impact tooth survival. The second part of this article expands on this and considers late trauma presentation, when to retain or extract teeth, and the role of dental implants in TDI-affected individuals.

All images, figures, and tables produced by the Dundee Dental Hospital and Research School with full permissions given for publication.

Conflict of Interest The authors have no conflicts of interest to declare.

References

1. Seeballuck C, Dolan S, Kilgariff J. Top tips for the immediate management of dental trauma. Br Dent J. 2022;233:8–12.
2. International Association of Dental Traumatology. IADT Guidelines for the evaluation and management of traumatic dental injuries. 2020. https://www.iadt-dentaltrauma.org/for-professionals.html. Accessed Nov 2023.
3. Sandler C, Al-Musfir T, Barry S, et al. Guidelines for the orthodontic management of the traumatised tooth. J Orthod. 2021;48:74–81.
4. Lin S, Pilosof N, Karawani M, et al. Occurrence and timing of complications following traumatic dental injuries: a retrospective study in a dental trauma department. J Clin Exp Dent. 2016;8:e429. https://doi.org/10.4317/jced.53022.
5. Dental Trauma Guide. Evidence based dental trauma treatment. https://dentaltraumaguide.org/evidence-based-dental-trauma-treatment/. Accessed Nov 2023.
6. Jackson NG, Waterhouse PJ, Maguire A. Factors affecting treatment outcomes following complicated crown fractures managed in primary and secondary care. Dent Traumatol. 2006;22:179–85.
7. Cohenca N, Silberman A. Contemporary imaging for the diagnosis and treatment of traumatic dental injuries: a review. Dent Traumatol. 2017;33:321–8.
8. Di Angelis AJ, Andreasen JO, Ebeleseder KA, et al. International Association of Dental Traumatology guidelines for the management of traumatic dental injuries: 1. Fractures and luxations of permanent teeth. Dent Traumatol. 2012;28:2–12.
9. NHS England. Shared Decision-Making: Summary Guide. 2019. https://www.england.nhs.uk/publication/shared-decision-making-summary-guide/. Accessed Nov 2023.
10. Scottish Government. Shared decision making in realistic medicine: what works. 2019. https://www.gov.scot/publications/works-support-promote-shared-decision-making-synthesis-recent-evidence/pages/3/. Accessed Nov 2023.
11. Scottish Government. Oral health improvement plan. 2018. https://www.gov.scot/publications/oral-health-improvement-plan/. Accessed Nov 2023.
12. International Association of Dental Traumatology. Information for patients. https://www.iadt-dentaltrauma.org/for-patients.html. Accessed Nov 2023.
13. Dental Trauma UK. Save a knocked out tooth. Information. https://www.dentaltrauma.co.uk/Index.aspx. Accessed Nov 2023.
14. Mobile application by the International Association of Dental Traumatology. ToothSOS. https://play.google.com/store/apps/details?id=com.iadtapp.toothsos&hl=en&gl=US&pli=1. Accessed Nov 2023.

15. Mobile application by the International Association of Dental Traumatology. ToothSOS. https://apps.apple.com/us/app/toothsos/id1368359249. Accessed Nov 2023.
16. Sustersic M, Gauchet A, Foote A, Bosson JL. How best to use and evaluate patient information leaflets given during a consultation: a systematic review of literature reviews. Health Expect. 2017;20:531–42.
17. Sustersic M, Tissot M, Tyrant J, et al. Impact of patient information leaflets on doctor–patient communication in the context of acute conditions: a prospective, controlled, before–after study in two French emergency departments. BMJ Open. 2019;9:e024184. https://doi.org/10.1136/bmjopen-2018-024184.
18. Herber OR, Gies V, Schwappach D, Thürmann P, Wilm S. Patient information leaflets: informing or frightening? A focus group study exploring patients' emotional reactions and subsequent behavior towards package leaflets of commonly prescribed medications in family practices. BMC Fam Pract. 2014;15:163. https://doi.org/10.1186/1471-2296-15-163.
19. Medina-Córdoba M, Cadavid S, Pérez-Acosta A, Amaya-Giraldo V. Factors that facilitate and hinder the comprehension of patient information leaflets (PILs): a brief scoping review. Front Pharmacol. 2021;12:740334. https://doi.org/10.3389/fphar.2021.740334.
20. Glickman GN. AAE consensus conference on diagnostic terminology: background and perspectives. J Endod. 2009;35:1619–20.
21. de Sousa APBR, França K, de Lucas RLVM, et al. In vitro tooth reattachment techniques: a systematic review. Dent Traumatol. 2018;34:297–310.
22. Krastl G, Weiger R, Filippi A, et al. European Society of Endodontology position statement: endodontic management of traumatized permanent teeth. Int Endod J. 2021;54:1473–81.
23. Robertson A, Andreasen FM, Bergenholtz G, Andreasen JO, Noren JG. Incidence of pulp necrosis subsequent to pulp canal obliteration from trauma of permanent incisors. J Endod. 1996;22:557–60.
24. General Dental Council. Tooth whitening position statement. 2016. https://www.gdc-uk.org/docs/default-source/what-is-the-legal-position/tooth-whitening-position-statementf08f3f9796b446d88663d00f035d4c13.pdf?sfvrsn=16f71e9_7. Accessed Nov 2023.
25. Abbott PV. Classification, diagnosis, and clinical manifestations of apical periodontitis. Endod Topics. 2004;8:36–54.
26. Scottish Dental Clinical Effectiveness Programme. Drug prescribing for dentistry. 3rd ed; 2016. https://www.sdcep.org.uk/published-guidance/drug-prescribing/. Accessed Jan 2024.
27. Torabinejad M, Parirokh M, Dummer PMH. Mineral trioxide aggregate and other bioactive endodontic cements: an updated overview—part II: other clinical applications and complications. Int Endod J. 2018;51:284–317.
28. Abbott PV, Lin S. Tooth resorption—part 2: a clinical classification. Dent Traumatol. 2022;38:267–85.
29. Heithersay GS. Clinical, radiologic, and histopathologic features of invasive cervical resorption. Quintessence Int. 1999;30:27–37.
30. Patel S, Saberi N, Pimental T, Teng P-H. Present status and future directions: root resorption. Int Endod J. 2022;55(Suppl 4):892–921.
31. Laddha A, Lau T, Wong Z, et al. Capturing the sound of ankylosis. Br Dent J. 2022;234:792–3.
32. GDC. Focus on Standards. Principle Four. https://standards.gdc-uk.org/pages/principle4/principle4.aspx. Accessed Nov 2023.
33. Djemal S, Chia M, Ubaya-Narayange T. Quality improvement of referrals to a department of restorative dentistry following the use of a referral proforma by referring dental practitioners. Br Dent J. 2004;197:85–8.
34. Smallwood N, Russell J, Forbes-Pyman R, Coates A. Do medical admission pro formas–improve the completeness of documentation? A multisite observational study. Fut Healthc J. 2018;5:121–5.
35. Gregory J. Use of pain scales and observational pain assessment tools in hospital settings. Nurs Stand. 2019;34:70. https://doi.org/10.7748/ns.2019.e11308.
36. Mejàre IA, Axelsson S, Davidson T, et al. Diagnosis of the condition of the dental pulp: a systematic review. Int Endod J. 2012;45:597–613.

37. Mainkar A, Kim S. Diagnostic accuracy of 5 dental pulp tests: a systematic review and meta-analysis. J Endod. 2018;44:694. https://doi.org/10.3390/ijerph19159599.
38. Donnermeyer D, Dammaschke T, Lipski M, Schäfer E. Effectiveness of diagnosing pulpitis: a systematic review. Int Endod J. 2022;56 Suppl 3:296. https://doi.org/10.1111/iej.13762.
39. Patro S, Meto A, Mohanty A, et al. Diagnostic accuracy of pulp vitality tests and pulp sensibility tests for assessing pulpal health in permanent teeth: a systematic review and meta-analysis. Int J Environ Res Public Health. 2022;19 https://doi.org/10.3390/ijerph19159599.
40. Dundee School of Dentistry YouTube Channel. https://www.youtube.com/@DundeeDentalSchool/about. Accessed Oct 2023.

Traumatic Dental Injury Review: Part 2 24

Clement Seeballuck, Sean Dolan, and Julie K. Kilgariff

Learning Points

- Recognise the challenges of managing previous dental trauma that presents delayed and without any previous treatment.
- Appreciate the need to recognise situations of safeguarding and how to act upon them in the correct manner.
- Understand the need for foresight in managing the traumatised dentition to recognise issues of space maintenance and the need for tooth replacement therapy into adulthood.

24.1 Introduction

This chapter follows on from the previous chapter [1] that discussed the importance of traumatic dental injury (TDI) follow-up and potential sequelae.

24.2 Stabilising Delayed Presentation TDIs

Immediate TDI management has previously been discussed [2]. Follow-up of TDIs allows the opportunity to ensure that injuries have been appropriately stabilised at, or close to, the time of injury and that the tissues affected are not deteriorating. However, patients may present sometime after initial injury, without

C. Seeballuck
Paediatric Dentistry, Dundee Dental Hospital and Research School, Dundee, UK

S. Dolan
Restorative Dentistry, Glasgow Dental Hospital and School, Glasgow, UK

J. K. Kilgariff (✉)
Endodontics, Dundee Dental Hospital and Research School, Dundee, UK
e-mail: julie.kilgariff@nhs.scot

E. McColl, A. Alani (eds.), *Practical Tips in Clinical Dentistry*, BDJ Clinician's Guides, https://doi.org/10.1007/978-3-031-90355-7_24

stabilisation having been achieved. Although it is not clear from current evidence how best to manage such situations, it seems appropriate to continue to apply the International Association of Dental Traumatology (IADT) guidelines as best as possible [3]. There are limitations however to accomplishing this when, for example, a tooth has moved in position because of a TDI and no attempt has been made to reposition it.

24.2.1 Delayed Presentation of Extruded or Laterally Luxated Teeth

Clinical decision-making and treatment provided will be impacted by the time lapse since injury. After 48 h post-injury, repositioning is more challenging because of inflammation and blood clot formation around displaced teeth, and treatment outcomes for delayed repositioning are unclear. Repositioning should still be attempted using careful 'watch-winding' type movements of the tooth, gripped using fingers or forceps positioned on the tooth crown only. This avoids damage to the periodontal ligament and cementum because damage may result in progressive resorption.

When a tooth has been repositioned, a periapical radiograph helps ascertain the accuracy of repositioning. Healing is better (outcomes enhanced) when teeth are returned to original positions. Articulating paper use is helpful to confirm that there is an intercuspal position contact (for functional teeth), but no excursive contacts, unless the tooth is involved in guidance. IADT guidelines should be consulted for splinting type and duration [3]. Typically a flexible splint using composite and wire is recommended and the traumatised tooth plus a tooth on either side included in the splint using 0.016″ (0.4 mm) stainless steel wire [3]. Oral hygiene instruction in relation to the splint and injury is recommended and may include short-term use of antimicrobial mouthwashes and softer toothbrushes whilst acute inflammation and pain subsides. Excellent personal care and regular follow-ups improve TDI healing [3].

Patients who sustain trauma with heavily restored dentition, including indirect restorations, can pose challenges for splinting. If teeth involved in the splint have ceramic restorations in situ, the ceramic will likely need to be etched using appropriate methods, such as hydrofluoric acid, to facilitate bonding [4]. Today, splints used should be passive, flexible (ensuring biological mobility) and cleansable and should stabilise the tooth into the appropriate position [5, 6].

Prior to splint removal, it is sensible to check that the splint has remained intact; if not, further splinting may be needed. Removal of composite affixed splints can be challenging as there is potential to damage the tooth surface when removing residual composite. Using an atraumatic technique, such as orthodontic bracket removers, ultrasonic scalers, or orthodontic tungsten carbide debonding burs and Soflex discs, can reduce potential enamel damage [7, 8].

24.2.2 Delayed Presentation of Intruded Teeth

Intrusions are the only displacement injuries in which immediate repositioning is not always advocated. Intruded teeth with open apices should be monitored only, regardless of the degree of intrusion for 4 weeks before considering intervention [3]. The 4-week clock starts from the date of injury. If, after 4 weeks, there is no improvement, input from orthodontic colleagues should be sought regarding extruding affected teeth.

Similarly, for teeth with a closed apex intruded less than 3 mm, monitoring for 8 weeks to allow for potential re-eruption is recommended [3]. A putty index, model, or photograph of the injury with a scale (e.g. using a periodontal probe) can aid review of whether there has been re-eruption. If the tooth is intruded beyond 3 mm, orthodontic extrusion or surgical repositioning is likely to be required. Alternatively, although not particularly reported in the literature, an aesthetic 'disguise' using composite buildups can be carried out in adults rather than repositioning, however, closed apex teeth are likely to require root canal treatment, and a composite tip will lengthen the endodontic working length, potentially complicating endodontic preparation and obturation (unless carried out prior to composite work). It is also crucial to consider any impact this may have on the gingival margin aesthetics. Careful, often multi-disciplinary treatment planning is warranted.

24.2.3 Delayed Presentation of Avulsed Teeth

Damage and drying of the periodontal ligament cells after a tooth has been avulsed for 30 min greatly reduces the outlook for the tooth. The best outcomes are seen when a tooth is replanted within 15 min [7]. For patients presenting within 48 h of injury, it may still be possible to replant the tooth. Step-by-step instructions and photographs for how to do this have recently been reported [9].

If the time-lag since injury does not preclude replanting, i.e. there is an open socket to reposition the tooth into, replanting is recommended because although the outlook for the tooth will be very poor, it may preserve hard and soft tissue whilst plans can be made for how to best replace the tooth aesthetically and functionally. Furthermore, replanting the tooth may prevent space closure and drifting of teeth prior to definitive treatment planning, and this may keep more options available as well as contributing to a more favourable outcome. Depending on the specific case, referral for specialist input may be useful, particularly in a growing patient who may benefit from multi-disciplinary treatment planning.

If replanting the tooth is not possible, alternative strategies to temporise and maintain space can be considered. These are discussed later.

To conclude, the initial TDI follow-up appointment may have additional elements to consider such as further radiographs, the removal of sutures, splints and the adjustment of occlusion and restoration placement or adjustment. Providing timely intervention to stabilise injuries potentially reduces the number of appointments needed later, reducing the burden of care goals set by local government [10] and may greatly enhance prognosis and improve patient outcomes.

24.3 Consider Safeguarding

Be aware of late presenting injuries that may be non-accidental. Up to 60% of child abuse cases have associated head and neck injuries, and 30% of these are intra-oral injuries [11, 12]. As previously discussed, clinicians have a responsibility to raise concerns if such injuries (particularly when repeated TDIs present) are potentially identified, particularly for vulnerable adults and children [2, 13]. Minors, repeatedly not being brought to follow-up TDI appointments, may be indicative of neglect and warrant investigation [14–17], although there may be valid reasons for non-attendance [18]. Sporadic attendance of minors, when symptoms have developed, may indicate neglect and in such cases other untreated disease, such as caries, erosion or periodontal disease may be present. The British Dental Association has published recommended actions for the dental team [19].

24.4 Know Where and When to Refer, If Needed

Serious TDIs, or those recognised as more challenging to manage, are summarised in Fig. 24.1. Studies show an increased likelihood of complications for luxation injuries and fractures with concomitant injuries have poor outlooks [20]. The injuries listed in Fig. 24.1 may be prudent to refer for specialist input.

Deleterious sequelae of TDIs seen at review may require onward referral or specialist advice. This is particularly for cases that appear to show evidence of certain resorption processes, such as replacement, internal and some cases of external inflammatory root resorption (depending on extent).

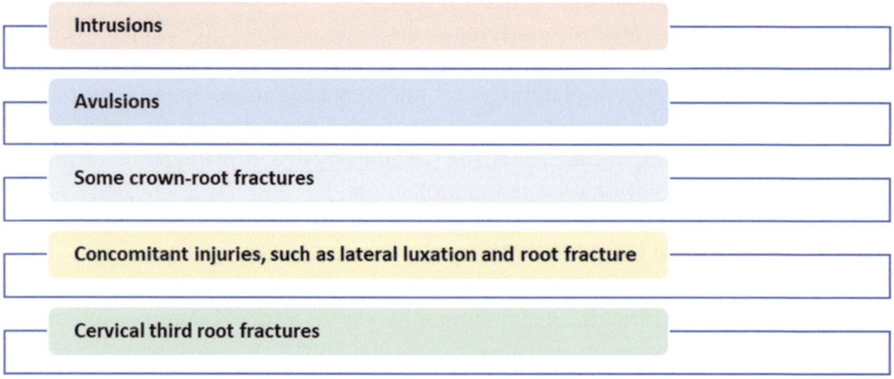

- Intrusions
- Avulsions
- Some crown-root fractures
- Concomitant injuries, such as lateral luxation and root fracture
- Cervical third root fractures

Fig. 24.1 TDIs which may warrant referral for specialist input

Both external inflammatory and internal root resorptions are halted by pulpal extirpation. Therefore, if the diagnosis is clear, extirpating and dressing the root canal system prior to referral is likely to halt the resorptive process. However, as Fig. 24.2a–c illustrate, the diagnosis may not be clear.

Unfortunately, replacement root resorption cannot be halted by pulpal extirpation but may progress slowly, especially in adult patients. In growing patients, replacement root resorption is particularly challenging because it impacts soft tissues and alveolar bone growth. Clinically, this manifests as alteration to gingival architecture and tooth infrapositioning, as shown in Fig. 24.3.

If tooth repositioning or space maintenance for TDI lost teeth has not been provided soon after injury, follow-up appointments can reveal occlusal interferences or space loss problems, as discussed later. Figure 24.4 illustrates a case where poor compliance wearing a removable partial denture following TDI injury has resulted in space loss.

Onward referrals to dental colleagues may include details of patient co-operation levels if this is likely to impact treatment planning and provision. This can be communicated by including a Modified Dental Anxiety Scale for adults [21] or Modified Child Dental Anxiety Scale for children [22].

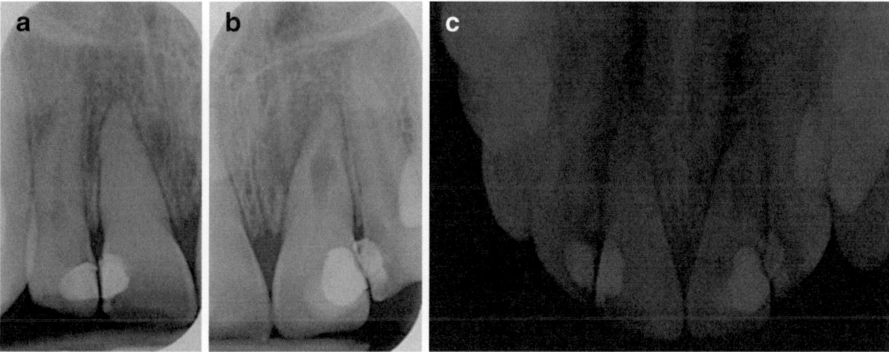

Fig. 24.2 A dentally anxious 16-year-old patient presented to their general dental practitioner some years following TDI. (**a**) Tooth 11 shows pulpal obliteration in the coronal portion of the root and an apical third root fracture. Clinically, 11 has no signs or symptoms. The radiographic appearance of 11 suggests stability because there are no alveolar changes or areas of resorption affecting the root end or horizontal root fracture area. Clinically, tooth 21 has a discharging sinus. Radiographically, there is a radiolucent lesion on the mid-third region of the root (**b** and **c**). From these images, it is difficult to ascertain whether the resorption is internal (and contained within the confines of the root canal system) and has perforated out with the root or is external. Further imaging is needed for planning the appropriate treatment in this case. In this situation, because the diagnosis of 21 is unclear, it is prudent to consider onward referral prior to extirpating the pulp

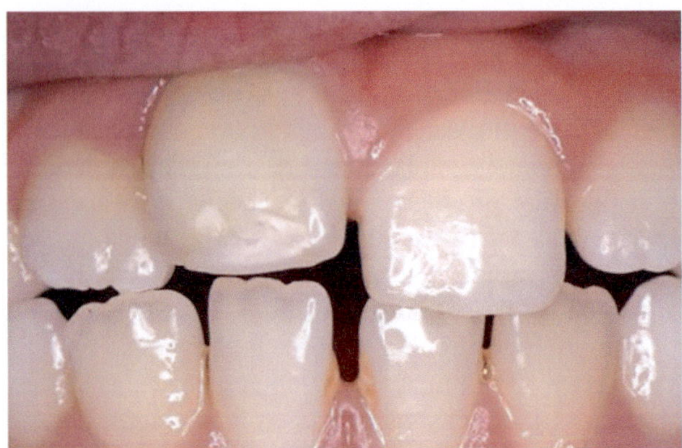

Fig. 24.3 Note the infra-occlusion and change in gingival margin level of tooth 11, which has become ankylosed following trauma in a paediatric patient

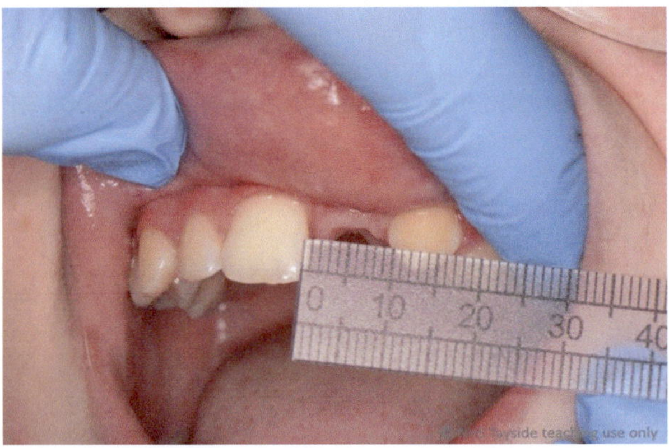

Fig. 24.4 This adolescent patient previously avulsed and lost 21 and 22. A partial denture was provided but not worn. Consequently, tooth 23 has erupted into the space of 22 and drifted mesially. The space available for restoration is significantly narrower mesio-distally than the width of the contralateral 12 and 11. This case requires multi-disciplinary input for an aesthetically and functionally satisfactory long-term outcome

However, onward referral to general medical practitioners may also be required for the patient and parent/guardians in relation to the psychological impact of TDIs, depending on the aetiology of the injury [23–25]. Children receiving sub-optimal TDI management may have reduced self-esteem [26]. Figure 24.5 illustrates a case where a patient raised concerns to a dentist about a TDI-related facial scar.

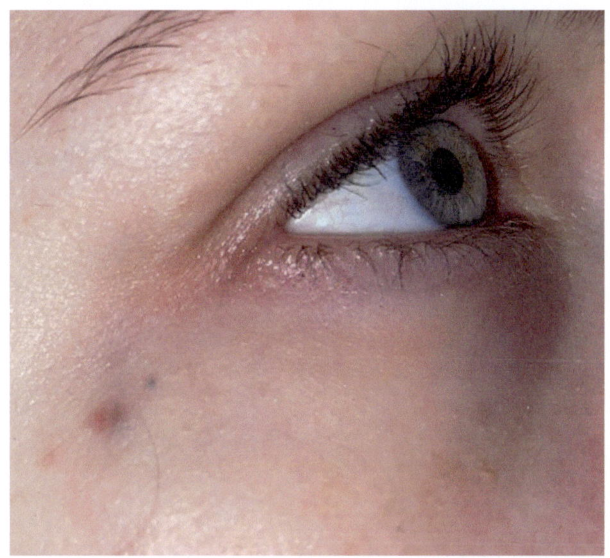

Fig. 24.5 This patient raised concern with a dentist about a facial scar post-TDI. Onward referral was sent, and a plastic surgery team addressed the facial skin discolouration arising from residual gravel in the scar

24.5 Maintaining Space in Growing Patients and Young Adults

When a TDI occurs, teeth may remain in the mouth, displaced, undisplaced or be avulsed. The most severe TDI injuries are generally accepted as intrusive luxations, lateral luxations with a concomitant root fracture and avulsions. Although not as severe an injury, cervical third root fractures are particularly challenging to stabilise because of the limited alveolar bone supporting the area and the potential ingress of microbes from the oral cavity to the fracture site. Likewise, some crown-root fractures result in significantly subgingival fractures, complicating tooth restoration. Teeth sustaining these injuries are vulnerable to being consigned for extraction by a clinician assessing the TDI; however, it is preferable to make every effort to retain teeth affected by all TDIs, even if this is short-term retention only. This is because retaining the TDI-affected tooth or teeth will help preserve hard (bone) and soft tissues and maintain space.

Following avulsions, there are two scenarios:

(a) The tooth may have been avulsed and lost at the time of injury.
(b) The tooth has been avulsed, found, but not replanted.

24.5.1 The Tooth Has Been Avulsed and Lost at the Time of Injury

Deciding on whether to maintain the resulting space or facilitate closure often involves multi-disciplinary treatment planning and warrants referral, particularly in patients under the age of 18 years [27]. Local referral pathways will differ, but

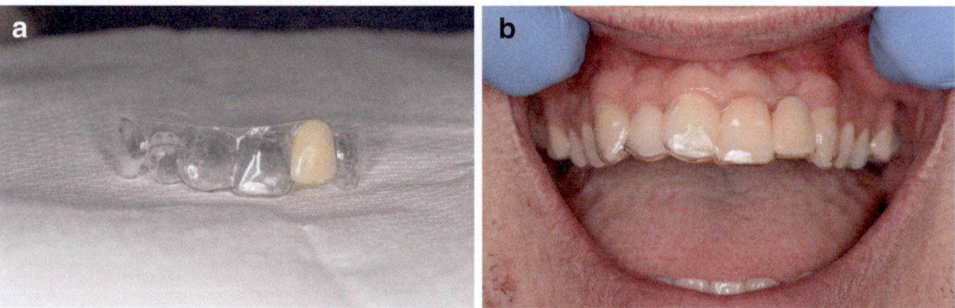

Fig. 24.6 (**a**) Missing tooth 22 required a quick solution to maintain aesthetics and space. An impression was recorded, along with occlusal relation and a shade for a composite fabricated tooth to be provided in an Essix retainer. Figure **b** shows the Essix retainer in situ

referral to a joint paediatric, orthodontic and restorative clinic is prudent where possible.

Whilst awaiting assessment on such a clinic, it is important to consider how to manage the edentulous space so that adjacent teeth do not drift and/or over erupt, further complicating the clinical challenges. In both adults and children, management of the space will depend on several factors, including cooperation, patient motivation, the condition of the remaining dentition and oral hygiene.

Removable appliances such as a single-tooth removable partial denture or a vacuum formed Essix retainer (Fig. 24.6) with a composite fabricated tooth are relatively quick and easy options [28]. These require limited cooperation, provided an intra oral scan or an impression can be recorded. Removable options are particularly useful for growing patients, where changes in gingival margins and skeletal growth require dynamic, adaptive aesthetic and functional treatment strategies.

24.5.2 The Tooth Has Been Avulsed, Found, But Not Replanted

There are occasions when a patient may attend over 48 h after avulsion having had no replantation. There may be situations where replantation can still be attempted; however, several days after injury this is often not possible. An immediate bridge can be fabricated using reinforced composite and the crown of the avulsed tooth as a natural pontic [29]. Figure 24.7 shows a case managed in this way. This can be a useful short to medium-term solution, providing an aesthetic result whilst definitive treatment planning is carried out. Alternatively, a removable partial prosthesis can be quickly made. Whatever option is chosen, the primary objectives remain the same: retain space, soft and hard tissues; restore aesthetics and function.

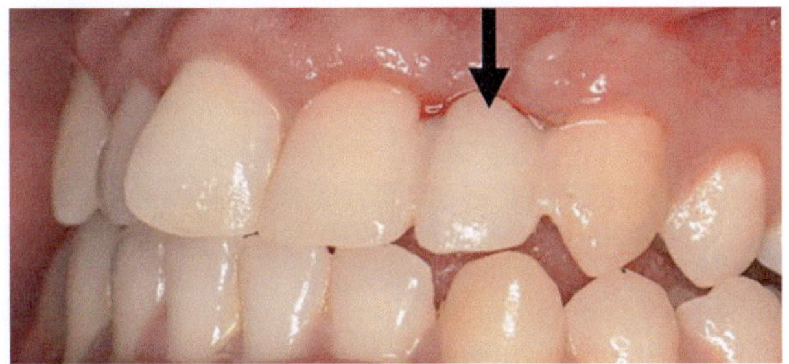

Fig. 24.7 Tooth 22 was avulsed, and the patient attended medical A&E with the tooth; however, it was not replanted. The patient was assessed dentally several weeks after injury, when the patient handed the avulsed tooth to the dentist. The edentulous 22 space was provisionally restored using the avulsed tooth crown. To do this, the root was removed, and the pulp contents were drilled out using a high-speed hand piece. The endodontic access cavity and resected root end were restored with composite resin and the tooth cemented to the adjacent teeth (after etching) using a composite resin. This provisional measure allowed ongoing monitoring of the adjacent traumatised teeth to better assess their prognosis prior to definitively replacing tooth 22

24.6 Planning for the Future

Patients sustaining TDIs are more likely to sustain TDIs again in the future, which should be considered when treatment planning. Preventive regimes include screening patients for participation in hobbies likely to result in collision or contact sports injury and recommendation of a mouthguard, accordingly. Custom fit mouth guards are more effective than both 'stock' and 'boil and bite' mouth guards, when made appropriately [30]. A uniform thickness of between 3 and 4 mm covering all teeth along with extension into the gingival sulcus is recommended.

In general, cases where several teeth have been involved in a TDI are more challenging and may need multidisciplinary specialist input. Medically, there are few conditions, which complicate TDI management in children, adolescents and adults. Medications may impact treatment outcomes. Bisphosphonates, for example, may reduce the success of dental implants [31]. Social factors of relevance to tooth restoration and/or replacement following TDI include tobacco use. In the case of dental implants and more invasive dental care, smoking affects healing [32] and is a risk factor for periodontal disease, which may affect treatment outcomes and the prognosis of restorative rehabilitation [33, 34]. Alcohol, although not directly impacting on the management of TDI (unless the patient is intoxicated at the time of presentation and cannot give consent), is associated with higher rates of TDIs [35]. Conversations with patients about alcohol intake can be challenging, particularly if consumption appears higher than the recommended maximum intake guidelines. Professional advice and signposting may be appropriate if alcohol was involved at the time of the TDI. Advice delivered as a 'brief intervention' appears effective [36].

Dental trauma primarily affects maxillary incisors, which are in the aesthetic zone. Over time, tooth discolouration following TDIs may present and require investigation and management. Teeth that have been displaced and replanted or repositioned can present with aesthetic problems in patients with thin phenotypes and higher smile lines. These cases may need specialist input.

24.6.1 TDIs in Children and Adolescents (Growing Patients)

TDI management may be complicated by levels of cooperation, and treatment needs to be staged with regard to growth and development. Following a TDI in a younger patient, the healing potential of the dental pulp is much higher in teeth with immature, open apices. This allows a variety of techniques to preserve teeth to be used, such as pulpotomy (full or partial), apexogenesis and revalcularisation, which can be attempted if functioning pulp or pulp-like tissue can be retained. If vitality is lost, apical barrier formation using MTA is possible (Fig. 24.8a, b) [37].

TDI tooth loss, or the development of an ankylosed tooth in a growing patient, can be very challenging from an aesthetic and functional perspective. A comprehensive approach is needed for assessment, potentially on a multidisciplinary clinic. Clinicians will assess caries risk [38], periodontal risk and malocclusion, along with screening for anomalies, such as molar incisor hypomineralisation, ectopic teeth and hypodontia.

If one or more dental implants are being considered after growth has ceased, early assessment by a restorative dentistry specialist is recommended in relation to treatment options, potential implant site preparation (e.g. by decoronating teeth with replacement resorption) and management of expectations of what may or may not be achievable.

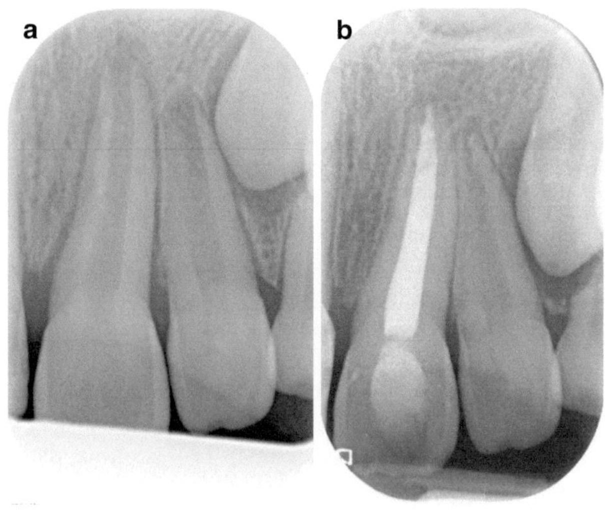

Fig. 24.8 (**a**) Showing tooth 21, which became non-vital in an 8-year-old girl. This has an open apex and was managed by formation of an apical barrier using MTA. Figure **b** shows completed root canal which was obturated using thermoplastic gutta percha

24.6.2 TDIs in Adults

In patients with closed apex teeth, the pulp may not survive the dental trauma because of rupture, severing or stretching of the neurovascular bundle. Certain injuries make the need for endodontic treatment in closed apex teeth more likely. These include root fractures with coronal segment displacement, intrusion, extrusion and lateral luxation [3]. It is important that as part of overall treatment planning, caries, periodontal risk and occlusion are assessed. The overall restorative status of adjacent teeth must be considered if a TDI affected tooth is lost or likely to be lost. For example, adjacent teeth may be appropriate bridge abutments or be of reduced prognosis themselves, requiring consideration within the overall treatment planning.

The majority of teeth affected by TDIs are anteriorly placed, within the aesthetic zone, and therefore are required to be preserved or replaced. Rarely, posterior teeth are affected, and in this situation, the shortened dental arch approach may be appropriate and is case-dependent.

24.7 Are Dental Implants the Answer?

Implants are a valuable tool for definitively replacing a tooth, but not a panacea. There are situations where implants are not suitable (Fig. 24.9). Trauma to the permanent dentition can occur at any age, with a reported higher incidence in the 10–12-year age group; [39, 40] this age is below the minimum recommended age of 18 years for considering dental implant placement [41]. Guidelines, although recognising a high success rate of 92–98% (implants present for 10 years or more), acknowledges factors that adversely affect implant prognosis. These include suboptimal oral hygiene, unstable periodontal disease, smoking/tobacco usage, parafunction, unstable occlusion and uncontrolled diabetes [32–34].

A minimum age of 18 years is recommended for dental implant placement because if placed in a growing patient, an occlusal discrepancy results as the patient continues to grow whilst the implant remains fixed in position, as an ankylosed tooth would. This results in issues such as a disparity in the incisal level and gingival margin levels [42]. Modification may be needed at a later stage to address aesthetic and functional implications but will have cost implications [43]. It appears that preserving traumatised teeth for as long as possible to delay implant placement may offer benefits in terms of aesthetics and cost.

Some TDI injuries are accompanied by loss of soft tissue and bone. This can complicate and/or preclude implant use. Treatment duration, multiple surgical procedures and frequency of appointments may not appeal to all patients. Figure 24.9 illustrates such a case.

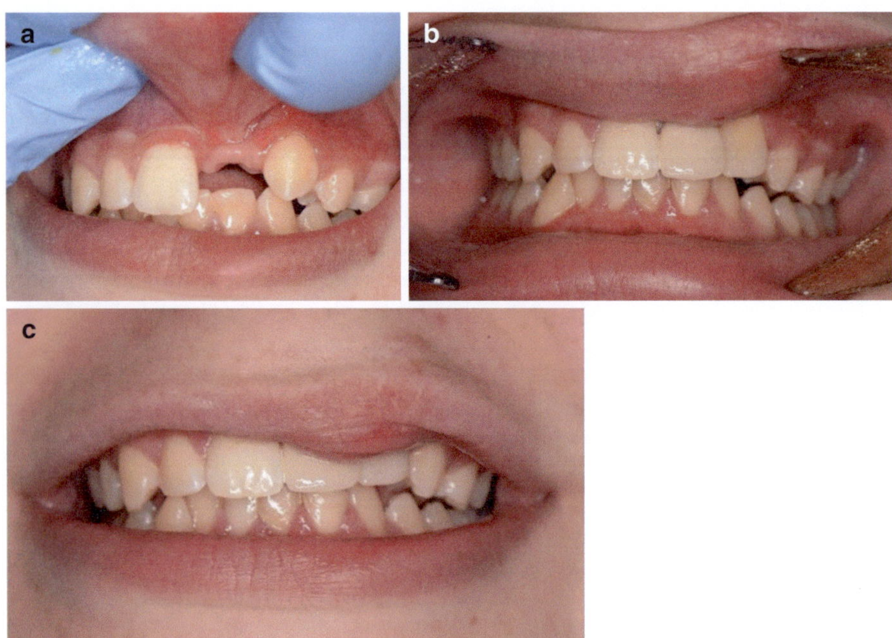

Fig. 24.9 (**a**) This 16-year-old patient lost teeth 21 and 22 in a TDI, and a significant amount of horizontal bone loss has occurred. A TDI-related scar affects the movement and appearance of the upper lip. The patient did not want to undergo surgical or orthodontic treatment, and an alternative strategy was developed. The images show the restoration of the dentition using a combination of resin-retained bridgework and composite resin restoration. The patient did not want to undergo bone augmentation, scar revision or implant placement. Following joint paediatric orthodontic and paediatric restorative clinics, a diagnostic wax up was undertaken. (**b**) Tooth 23 was reshaped with composite to resemble tooth 22. (**c**) Tooth 11 was used for an abutment for a resin-retained bridge (tooth 22 being the pontic). No tooth structure was removed to achieve this treatment, and the procedures are reversible should the patient wish to consider implants in the future. Unlike implant placement, this treatment was achievable before skeletal maturity, and the patient was able to dispose of the removable partial prosthesis they found uncomfortable

24.8 Conclusion

Dental trauma management can be challenging. Using a methodical evidence-based approach to the diagnosis, management and follow-up may enhance patient outcomes. Ongoing research is continually strengthening the evidence base for treatment strategies. Resources such as the IADT guidelines [3], which are reviewed and evolve, are recommended tools to refer to.

Going forward, developments in bioactive materials may provide alternative, more conservative, regenerative treatment modalities. Stem cell research may impact the management and outcomes of TDIs in the future. Until then, the key issues for the diagnosis, management and sequelae of TDIs for clinicians have been summarised here and in the preceding articles [1, 2].

Follow-up for early recognition of problematic TDI sequelae is important, and for more serious problems, such as replacement resorption, onward referral is advisable. Many TDIs, particularly in growing patients, benefit from multidisciplinary involvement at an early stage, whilst teeth, even if of a guarded or hopeless outlook, are still in situ.

References

1. Seeballuck C, Dolan SK, Kilgariff J. Getting it right at every stage: top tips for traumatic dental injury review: part 1. Br Dent J. 2024;236:82–6.
2. Seeballuck C, Dolan S, Kilgariff J. Top tips for the immediate management of dental trauma. Br Dent J. 2022;233:8–12.
3. International Association of Dental Traumatology. 2020 IADT Guidelines for the evaluation and management of traumatic dental injuries. https://www.iadt-dentaltrauma.org/for-professionals.html. Accessed Jun 2023.
4. Kilgariff JK, Fairless M. Displacement injuries: assessment and management. Prim Dent J. 2023;12:47–56.
5. Sobczak-Zagalska H, Emerich K. Best splinting methods in case of dental injury—a literature review. J Clin Pediatr Dent. 2020;44:71–8.
6. Todd S. How flexible is your trauma splint? BDJ Student. 2020;27:50.
7. Rao A, Rao A, Shenoy R. Splinting—when and how? Dent Update. 2011;38:341–6.
8. Cehreli ZC, Lakshmipathy M, Yazici R. Effect of different splint removal techniques on the surface roughness of human enamel: a three-dimensional optical profilometry analysis. Dent Traumatol. 2008;24:177–82.
9. Djemal S, Shah M. Avulsion injuries: assessment and management. Prim Dent J. 2023;12:57–63.
10. Scottish Government. Oral Health Improvement Plan. 2018. https://www.gov.scot/publications/oral-health-improvement-plan/. Accessed Nov 2023.
11. Park C. Oral and dental aspects of child abuse and neglect. Centre for Excellence for Children's Care and Protection; 2014. https://www.celcis.org/application/files/1515/3745/9870/oral-and-dental-aspects-of-child-abuse-and-neglect.pdf. Accessed Nov 2023.
12. Royal College of Paediatrics and Child Health. Child protection evidence. Systematic review on oral injuries. 2014. https://childprotection.rcpch.ac.uk/wp-content/uploads/sites/6/2020/05/child_protection_evidence_-_oral_injuries.pdf. Accessed Nov 2023.
13. General Dental Council. Focus on Standards. Standard 8.5. https://standards.gdc-uk.org/pages/principle8/principle8.aspx. Accessed Nov 2023.
14. Dunbar L. Did Not Attend v Was Not Brought. Dental nursing. 2019. https://www.dental-nursing.co.uk/features/did-not-attend-v-was-not-brought. Accessed Nov 2023.
15. Royal College of Paediatrics and Child Health. Child protection evidence—dental neglect. 2014. https://childprotection.rcpch.ac.uk/child-protection-evidence/dental-neglect-systematic-review/. Accessed Nov 2023.
16. Scottish Dental Clinical Effectiveness Programme. Practice Support Manual. Child protection. https://www.psm.sdcep.org.uk/content/ethical-practice/child-protection/#:~:text=All%20dental%20team%20members%2C%20as%20providers%20of%20care,safeguarding%20children%20and%20young%20people%2C%20and%20vulnerable%20adults. Accessed Nov 2023.
17. Harris J. Safeguarding children: noticing dental neglect. BDJ Team. 2018;5:18202. https://doi.org/10.1038/bdjteam2018202.

18. Simons D, Pearson N, Dittu A. Why are vulnerable children not brought to their dental appointments? BDJ Team. 2016;3:16156. https://doi.org/10.1038/bdjteam2016156.
19. Kirby J, Harris J. Development and evaluation of a 'was not brought' pathway: a team approach to managing children's missed dental appointments. Br Dent J. 2019;227:291–7.
20. Bücher K, Neumann C, Thiering E, Hickel R, Kühnisch J. Complications and survival rates of teeth after dental trauma over a 5-year period. Clin Oral Investig. 2013;17:1311–8.
21. Humphris G, Crawford JR, Hill K, et al. UK population norms for the modified dental anxiety scale with percentile calculator: adult dental health survey 2009 results. BMC Oral Health. 2013;13:29. https://doi.org/10.1186/1472-6831-13-29.
22. Wong HM, Humphris GM, Lee GT. Preliminary validation and reliability of the modified child dental anxiety scale. Psychol Rep. 1998;83:1179–86.
23. Lee JY, Divaris K. Hidden consequences of dental trauma: the social and psychological effects. Pediatr Dent. 2009;31:96–101.
24. Porritt JM, Rodd HD, Baker SR. Childhood dental injuries: a resiliency model of adaptation. Int J Paediatr Dent. 2015;25:267–81.
25. Porritt JM, Rodd HD, Baker SR. Parental quality-of-life impacts following children's dento-alveolar trauma. Dent Traumatol. 2013;29:92–8.
26. Rodd H, Noble F. Psychosocial impacts relating to dental injuries in childhood: the bigger picture. Dent J (Basel). 2019;7:23. https://doi.org/10.3390/dj7010023.
27. Alani A, Austin R, Djemal S. Contemporary management of tooth replacement in the traumatized dentition. Dent Traumatol. 2012;28:183–92.
28. Chopra S, Bansal P, Bansal P. Essix appliance: an innovation modification for use as temporary bridge—a case report. J Adv Med Dent Sci Res. 2020;8:184–6.
29. Raj R, Mehrotra K, Narayan I, Gowda TM, Mehta DS. Natural tooth pontic: an instant esthetic option for periodontally compromised teeth—a case series. Case Rep Dent. 2016;2016:8502927. https://doi.org/10.1155/2016/8502927.
30. Sliwkanich L, Ouanounou A. Mouthguards in dentistry: current recommendations for dentists. Dent Traumatol. 2021;37:661–71.
31. Sulaiman N, Fadhul F, Chrcanovic BR. Bisphosphonates and dental implants: a systematic review and meta-analysis. Materials (Basel). 2023;16:6078. https://doi.org/10.3390/ma16186078.
32. Silverstein P. Smoking and wound healing. Am J Med. 1992;93:S22. https://doi.org/10.1016/0002-9343(92)90623-j.
33. Apatzidou DA. The role of cigarette smoking in periodontal disease and treatment outcomes of dental implant therapy. Periodontol 2000. 2022;90:45–61.
34. Devlin A, Fee P. How do different levels of smoking affect dental implants? Evid Based Dent. 2021;22:28–9.
35. Magno MB, Nadelman P, Leite KLDF, Ferreira DM, Pithon MM, Maia LC. Associations and risk factors for dental trauma: a systematic review of systematic reviews. Community Dent Oral Epidemiol. 2020;48:447–63.
36. Kaner EF, Beyer FR, Muirhead C, et al. Effectiveness of brief alcohol interventions in primary care populations. Cochrane Database Syst Rev. 2018;2018:CD004148. https://doi.org/10.1002/14651858.CD004148.pub4.
37. Van Gorp G, Declerck D. Long-term outcome of endodontically treated traumatized immature upper incisors. J Endod. 2023;49:1106–19.
38. Office for Health Improvement and Disparities, Department of Health and Social Care, NHS England, and NHS Improvement. Delivering better oral health: an evidence-based toolkit for prevention. Updated 2021. https://www.gov.uk/government/publications/delivering-better-oral-health-an-evidence-based-toolkit-for-prevention. Accessed Oct 2023.
39. Goswami M, Aggarwal T. Prevalence of traumatic dental injuries among 1- to 14-year-old children: a retrospective study. Int J Clin Pediatr Dent. 2021;14:467–70.

40. Kovacs M, Pacurar M, Petcu B, Bukhari C. Prevalence of traumatic dental injuries in children who attended two dental clinics in Targu Mures between 2003 and 2011. Oral Health Dent Manag. 2012;11:116–24.
41. Dabar U, Shahdad S, Ashley M et al. Guidance on the standards of care for NHS-funded dental implant treatment. Royal College of Surgeons of England, Faculty of Dental Surgery; 2019. https://www.rcseng.ac.uk/dental-faculties/fds/publications-guidelines/clinical-guidelines/. Accessed Mar 2024.
42. Thilander B, Ödman J, Lekholm U. Orthodontic aspects of the use of oral implants in adolescents: a 10-year follow-up study. Eur J Orthod. 2001;23:715–31.
43. Bohner L, Hanisch M, Kleinheinz J, Jung S. Dental implants in growing patients: a systematic review. Br J Oral Maxillofac Surg. 2019;57:397–406.

Part IV

Periodontology

Periodontal Tips for Primary Care 25

Ewen McColl

Learning Points

- Recognise the multifaceted multifactorial nature of periodontal disease and how treatment approaches have to be catered for each individual case.
- Appreciate the importance of communication and motivation in improving periodontal outcomes.
- Understand how managing risk factors in tandem with periodontal instrumentation optimises treatment results.

25.1 Periodontal Medicine as a Treatment Approach

Periodontitis is a chronic multifactorial inflammatory disease associated with dysbiotic plaque biofilms and characterised by progressive destruction of the tooth-supporting apparatus, which may ultimately result in tooth loss [1]. The balance between the oral microbiome and the host's immune-inflammatory response defence is a fine one, and central to preventing any imbalance is to give the patient the necessary information and tools to manage their own oral hygiene on a daily basis.

Gaining this cooperation is key, and many of my top tips relate to the patient's role in a shared approach between clinician and patient in improving and maintaining oral hygiene. This approach also fits with twenty-first-century 'personalised medicine', which puts the patient at the centre of everything, and takes into consideration that the risk status of each patient differs. With regard to periodontitis, this individual risk status explains why some patients have significant periodontal destruction, whilst others have very little when exposed to similar bacterial challenge, as this is due to their individual immune responses to that challenge.

E. McColl (✉)
Peninsula Dental School, Plymouth, UK
e-mail: ewen.mccoll@plymouth.ac.uk

E. McColl, A. Alani (eds.), *Practical Tips in Clinical Dentistry*, BDJ Clinician's Guides, https://doi.org/10.1007/978-3-031-90355-7_25

Behavioural change can be time-consuming, and the tips will hopefully help dental team members in primary care to be as efficient with their time as possible, accepting the time constraints and fiscal challenges that may present in primary care, particularly with regards to management of periodontal conditions [2].

However, with an increasing awareness of the relationship between periodontal disease and systemic health, patients may be more receptive to changing behaviours to address their periodontal condition.

The aim of this short article is to present some clinical tips the author has found useful in managing periodontitis, which will hopefully benefit colleagues. As a proviso, many tips have been gleaned from colleagues and adapted to my own practice (including 18 years as a specialist periodontist) with communication the key. They have worked for me and my patients but will, of course, need some adaptation to each individual clinician's and patient's circumstances, with good communication always at the heart of managing our patients' oral health. I often reflect on ten things I wish somebody had told me at dental school that they never did—this would have saved me a lot of trial and error in practice, and I hope some of the below will be as helpful to colleagues as it has been to me.

25.1.1 Changing Behaviour to Optimise Outcomes

The British Society of Periodontology S3 guidelines and flow chart (BSP UK Clinical Practice Guidelines for the Treatment of Periodontal Diseases) [1, 3] highlight the importance of patient-performed oral hygiene in managing periodontitis. Similarly, the CGDent *Standards in dentistry* document [4] highlights the importance of oral hygiene to all aspects of dentistry. The Scottish Dental Clinical Effectiveness Programme (SDCEP)Guideline—Prevention and Treatment of Periodontal Diseases in Primary Care [5] provides many useful practical tips for managing periodontitis in primary care, with improvement in the patient's own oral hygiene at the core of disease management.

A **designated** oral hygiene (OH) specific session to go over all aspects of oral hygiene, allowing the patient to demonstrate what they currently do and what will be needed to improve, is time very well spent in my opinion. In discussing oral hygiene with our patients, the importance of interdental cleaning and supporting the patient to adopt this to become as routine as brushing is essential if disease is to be controlled.

It is important to explain to a patient the fact that interdental cleaning whilst more challenging is as crucial as brushing but can take time. That is, *like cleaning a car—the outside is easier than inside, with the inside requiring more time, and more specific cleaning implements, just like interdental cleaning!*

Much like with diet sheets, bespoke oral hygiene sheets can be developed and utilised to motivate patients to link their oral hygiene improvement to their own treatment goals (rather than our goals), which in the patient's case may be unrelated to control of periodontitis, i.e. to have restorations replaced to improve aesthetics. This may motivate patients to achieve their oral hygiene goal and clinically will also ensure the correct treatment strategy prior to moving to more advanced restorative care.

At the designated OH session, disclosing helps patients visualise areas they are missing, and a try-in of sizes of interdental brushes can be important, i.e. *like sweeping a chimney—if the brush doesn't touch the sides, then it will have little effect.*

Behaviour change [6] is, of course, a challenge on many occasions, and the BSP document highlights the engaging and non-engaging patient in recognition of the fact that despite our best efforts, for many reasons, patients may not be able to optimise oral hygiene and thus the compromises this may bring in optimising outcomes. It is important from a medico-legal perspective that this lack of progress is documented [7] to highlight that we have tried, even if unsuccessful in changing behaviour in relation to oral hygiene.

25.1.2 Reducing Risk Factors

As alluded to above, wider awareness of the importance of the mouth as a window to the rest of the body can be emphasised to patients who often find this makes sense, as they can visualise change, i.e. a reduction in inflammation and bleeding on brushing. For example, the importance of smokers being given smoking cessation advice can be brought into context when explaining to patients the impact of smoking on healing and vascularity of periodontal soft tissues [8]. This can help explain the wider effects, i.e. once you stop smoking, the tissues elsewhere will also start to heal and recover.

Similarly, I have had a number of patients over the years with poor periodontal conditions whom I have referred to their GP for diabetes testing, and this has led to a diagnosis of Type 2 diabetes. This emphasis on the importance of oral health to general health often improves motivation and patients' willingness to take on board the wider health message, when they appreciate the significance of controlling periodontal health to general health [9].

25.1.3 Instrumentation: Don't Blame Your Tools If You Don't Maintain Them

Non-surgical periodontal therapy works [10], but as with any other areas of dentistry if you don't have the correct instruments for the job or don't maintain them, the outcomes will be much less likely to be successful. Ultrasonic instruments for effective supra- and subgingival instrumentation should be well maintained, a variety of tips should be available and the instruments should be checked to ensure effectiveness. Don't just pick up any instrument and hope for the best. I know I used to!

It is similar to hand instruments. It is crucial to understand the ergonomics of the instruments not only for your and the patient's comfort but also to ensure effective root surface debridement, i.e. tooth/area-specific instruments. For effective root surface debridement, instruments must be maintained and sharpened accordingly. Take the time to study and understand the instruments you use, and the benefits to your patients and your own professional satisfaction of a job well done will be a virtuous cycle for all concerned.

25.1.4 You've Done the Hard Part!

Whilst in many cases the subgingival instrumentation (root surface debridement/ subgingival professional mechanical plaque removal [PMPR]) can be the most demanding stage of treatment from both the patient's and the clinical team's point of view, it is crucial that this hard work is not lost by absence of appropriate recall, review and effective maintenance regime. Patients, in my experience, are receptive to a maintenance recall when they are educated on its importance in maintaining their hard-won periodontal health, i.e. *much as when an engine has an overhaul, the future servicing is crucial if a similar recurrence of engine failure is not to reoccur.*

In my experience, the maintenance component, as with every other stage of treatment, is of equal importance and should not be overlooked. This stage is essential to not only reinforce oral hygiene but to adapt OH to any changes to dental anatomy, restorations, implant placement or changes with patients' manual dexterity [11, 12]. Similarly, the bespoke maintenance regime should target sites specifically with PMPR or root surface debridement where there are any signs of worsening of periodontal parameters. Recall intervals should be adapted to the patient's circumstances, and the visit is more than a quick scale and polish but a key stage on a lifelong journey in the management of the patient's periodontal condition.

The above tips are clearly not a compendium of managing periodontal disease, and for this, the British Society of Periodontology has many reference sources offering a wealth of advice for screening, diagnosing and treating periodontal diseases in primary care. The above provides some top tips I hope readers will find useful in managing primary dental disease, which is crucial to all aspects of restorative dentistry and, increasingly, our patients' general health.

25.2 Conclusion

With progress in knowledge on periodontal disease mechanisms, management has evolved into an approach where instrumentation and reducing risk factors provide the best outcome. Interaction at the interpersonal level plays a key role in a collaborative approach to motivate patients in becoming invested in their treatment.

References

1. West N, Chapple I, Claydon N, et al. BSP implementation of European S3 - level evidence-based treatment guidelines for stage I-III periodontitis in UK clinical practice. J Dent. 2021;106:103562. https://doi.org/10.1016/j.jdent.2020.103562.
2. Roberts-Harry E. Guidelines are not standards. Br Dent J. 2021;230:688.
3. British Society of Periodontology and Implant Dentistry. BSP UK version of the S3 Treatment Guidelines for Periodontitis. https://www.bsperio.org.uk/professionals/bsp-uk-clinical-practice-guidelines-for-the-treatment-of-periodontitis. Accessed 5 Jan 2022.
4. Moles D, Tredwin C, McColl E, Witton R, Burns L. Standards in dentistry. 2nd ed. London: Faculty of General Dental Practice (UK); 2018.
5. Scottish Dental Clinical Effectiveness Programme. Prevention and Treatment of Periodontal Diseases in Primary Care. June 2014. https://www.sdcep.org.uk/published-guidance/periodontal-management/. Accessed Jan 2022.
6. Carra MC, Detzen L, Kitzmann J, Woelber JP, Ramseier CA, Bouchard P. Promoting behavioural changes to improve oral hygiene in patients with periodontal diseases: a systematic review. J Clin Periodontol. 2020;47:72. https://doi.org/10.1111/jcpe.13234.
7. Hadden AM. Clinical examination and record keeping. London: Faculty of General Dental Practice (UK); 2016.
8. Ramseier CA, Woelber JP, Kitzmann J, Detzen L, Carra MC, Bouchard P. Impact of risk factor control interventions for smoking cessation and promotion of healthy lifestyles in patients with periodontitis: a systematic review. J Clin Periodontol. 2020;47:90. https://doi.org/10.1111/jcpe.13240.
9. Sanz M, Ceriello A, Buysschaert M, et al. Scientific evidence on the links between periodontal diseases and diabetes: consensus report and guidelines of the joint workshop on periodontal diseases and diabetes by the International Diabetes Federation and the European Federation of Periodontology. J Clin Periodontol. 2018;45:138–49.
10. Suvan J, Leira Y, Sancho FMM, Graziani F, Derks J, Tomasi C. Subgingival instrumentation for treatment of periodontitis. A systematic review. J Clin Periodontol. 2020;47:155. https://doi.org/10.1111/jcpe.13245.
11. Slot DE, Valkenburg C, Van der Weijden GAF. Mechanical plaque removal of periodontal maintenance patients—a systematic review and network meta-analysis. J Clin Periodontol. 2020;47:107. https://doi.org/10.1111/jcpe.13275.
12. Costa FO, Lages EJP, Cota LOM, Lorentz TCM, Soares RV, Cortelli JR. Tooth loss in individuals under periodontal maintenance therapy: 5-year prospective study. J Periodontal Res. 2014;49:121–8.

26 Practical Tips for Effective Use of Periodontal Instruments in Primary Care

Morag Powell, Ruth Potterton, and Ewen McColl

Learning Points

- Understand the indications, aims and objectives of periodontal instrumentation.
- Recall the indications for utilisation of hand or mechanised instruments and the relative advantages and disadvantages of each.
- Understand the core principles of instrumentation and how different instruments require specific clinical techniques to ensure effectiveness.

26.1 Introduction

Stabilisation of primary disease is a key pillar of successful treatment, and in addition to managing caries, managing periodontal disease is a crucial component of a successful treatment plan. The recent European Federation of Periodontology (EFP) S3 level clinical practice guidelines (CPG) [1] are evidence-based clinical guidelines providing recommendations to treat periodontitis. Crucial to successful implementation of these recommendations is delivering behavioural change and non-surgical instrumentation. Often, this is given passing attention with insufficient time allocated to behaviour change in treatment planning. Similarly, poorly maintained periodontal instruments and equipment not used to their full utility or design can lead to poorer outcomes for patients. In this article, we provide tips on how to

M. Powell
Dental Therapy and Hygiene, Peninsula Dental School (University of Plymouth), Derriford Dental Education Facility, Plymouth Science Park, Plymouth, UK

R. Potterton
Community Based Dentistry Peninsula Dental School (University of Plymouth), Derriford Dental Education Facility, Plymouth Science Park, Plymouth, UK

E. McColl (✉)
Peninsula Dental School, Plymouth, UK
e-mail: ewen.mccoll@plymouth.ac.uk

E. McColl, A. Alani (eds.), *Practical Tips in Clinical Dentistry*, BDJ Clinician's Guides, https://doi.org/10.1007/978-3-031-90355-7_26

meet these guidelines with best practice, borne from years of experience in optimising instrument utilisation, including an update on instruments which may facilitate patient care, and operator satisfaction.

26.2 Building Foundations for Optimal Treatment Outcomes

The treatment for stages I–III of periodontitis is delivered in a stepwise approach, each with different interventions [1]. This approach is broken down into four distinct steps, which clinicians move through sequentially, commencing with the first step of building foundations for optimal treatment outcomes prior to undertaking subgingival professional mechanical plaque removal (PMPR).

In this initial step, the focus is on control of the supra biofilm by the patient, with behavioural change interventions and risk factor control. The PMPR element within this step can be completed by various approaches including toothbrushing, hand instrumentation, ultrasonic instrumentation, traditional polishing and air polishing. The aim of this step is to identify and remove supra biofilm and calculus deposits which in turn will allow patients to carry out their personal homecare plan of toothbrushing and interdental cleaning that has been designed for them by their clinician.

26.3 Identification of Biofilm

The application of disclosing solution (Fig. 26.1) at each appointment during step one aids the patient in recognising the mature and cariogenic plaque that remains on the tooth surface after they have performed their homecare routine. Behaviour change interventions are targeted specifically to areas highlighted by the solution, with patients instructed using the Oral Health TIPPS [2] method of Talk, Instruct, Practise and Plan with personalised homecare plans created based on these findings. SMART goals are agreed and set with patient, with the expectation of the patient achieving them by the next appointment. Once a reduction of 50% of plaque and bleeding scores is achieved, the patient is then deemed as 'engaging', allowing progression to the next step of treatment. If goals are not achieved, then further

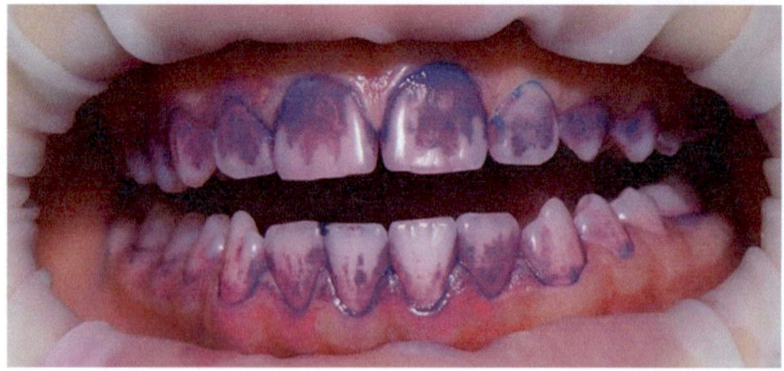

Fig. 26.1 Disclosing solution applied as part of the behaviour change intervention. Image courtesy of EMS

behaviour change interventions will be required prior to proceeding onto the next step of treatment.

An efficient method of removing this stained biofilm is with an air polishing device (APD). Current literature suggests that there is no significant difference in treatment outcomes when using APD compared to conventional techniques in the treatment of periodontal disease; however, it does identify a difference in patient comfort levels and professional treatment time when compared to hand instrumentation and ultrasonic scalers [3]. Therefore, the use of an APD can be an efficient and popular method of removing supra biofilm.

There are various types of powders available for use with APDs including glycine, erythritol and sodium bicarbonate. Glycine and erythritol powders have mostly superseded the use of sodium bicarbonate powders in general practice, with both powders reported in the literature as having improved patient comfort and less abrasiveness on the tooth surface. The use of APDs is technique sensitive and it is recommended that clinicians attend formal training prior to using on a patient.

Once the biofilm is successfully removed, the clinician's focus can then turn to the removal of supragingival calculus deposits and other plaque-retentive factors. APDs are unable to remove calculus deposits, and therefore, the options available for this include hand or ultrasonic instrumentation.

26.4 Supragingival Hand Instrumentation

There are a wide range of different supragingival scalers that can be used for supragingival PMPR. The fundamental difference between instruments used for supragingival and subgingival PMPR is that supra instruments have a tip and are therefore sharp at this point and should not be used subgingivally, and subgingival instruments have a rounded toe, designed this way to reduce trauma to the subgingival tissues. When viewed in cross section, the instruments are either triangular (sickle scaler) or semicircular (curette).

Sickle scalers have an anterior design, with H6/H7 being used as standard in undergraduate training, and a separate posterior design such as S204 or M23 scaler which allows for extended reach to the posterior regions. These instruments have two cutting edges which are set at a 90-degree angle to the lower shank of the instrument. However, the instruments are not used at this 90-degree angle as they require to be tipped slightly towards the tooth to an approximately 80-degree angle to reduce trauma to the gingival tissues. In addition to this angulation, only the anterior first third of the instrument should be engaged and adapted to the tooth surface, again to reduce trauma and increase patient comfort during the procedure [4].

Correct seating positions, posture and positioning of the patient are fundamental in enabling a clinician to achieve the correct periodontal instrumentation technique whilst maintaining a neutral body posture. Right-handed clinicians are best positioned between 8 and 1 o'clock on the clock face, with left-handed clinicians best positioned between 11 and 4 o'clock on the clock face [4].

The patient's head should sit between the hands of the operator when their elbows are tucked into their sides and their forearms parallel to the floor. For instrumentation in the lower arch, the patient's chin should be towards the chest allowing for the mandibular occlusal plane to be as parallel to the floor as possible. For the upper arch, the patient's chin should be raised upwards, allowing for the maxillary occlusal plane to be perpendicular to the floor.

The correct instrument grasp is the modified pen grasp which allows for precise control of the instrument and good tactile sensory feedback [5]. This grasp will not look the same for every clinician as it requires to be adapted based on hand size and finger length; however, adopting this grasp will lessen musculoskeletal stress to the clinician's fingers during instrumentation [4]. The handle selection of the instrument is also significant, with ergonomic handle designs recommended to reduce muscle load and pinch force. Two of the main risk factors for carpal tunnel syndrome in clinicians are the consistent use of a non-neutral wrist position and repetitive excessive pressure applied during pinch forces that occur during instrumentation. It is recommended that clinicians relax the fingers of the grasp between each instrument stroke to help prevent repetitive injuries [4, 6].

26.5 Ultrasonic Instrumentation

The two main options of ultrasonic technology available to use for both supra- and subgingival PMPR are magnetostrictive and piezoelectric. The literature advises that there is no significant difference in clinical outcomes when compared, and therefore, the choice of equipment used is generally the clinician's preference.

Ultrasonics convert electrical energy to mechanical energy in the form of vibrations. Taking Dentsply Sirona Cavitron Ultrasonic Scaling System as an example, their 25 K and 30 K inserts vibrate at 25,000 cycles and 30,000 cycles/s, respectively.

Whether the clinician opts to use a magnetostrictive, piezoelectric or a sonic scaler is often down to personal preference or availability within the primary care setting. There are many differing interchangeable tips/inserts to choose from varying in diameter, shape and length (depending upon unit manufacturer) to complete the required periodontal treatment, and as such, it is important to have a wide ranging and suitable selection. Whichever ultrasonic equipment is used, it is of vital importance to facilitate effective treatment, and the operator is aware of the selected tip movement (e.g., elliptical, linear, orbital/elliptical) and which surface(s) of the tip is 'active' when in use. Clinicians will be practised in their dexterity and know only a light pen grasp, using gentle 'featherlike' pressure, and small overlapping strokes is required.

In Cavitron tip selection, a common misunderstanding is that the thicker, heavier diameter inserts or Cavitron Powerline Ultrasonic Inserts cannot be used subgingivally.

Cavitron ultrasonic inserts:

Powerline: Moderate to heavy deposits sub and supra PMPR.

Slimline: Light to moderate deposits sub and supra PMPR.

30% thinner than Powerline inserts allowing for improved subgingival access.

Thinsert: Biofilm removal and light calculus deposits sub and supra PMPR.

47% thinner than Slimline inserts.

EMS piezon inserts:

Perio slim (PS): Can be used both sub and supra in 95% of areas.

Perio slim L&R: Used up to 8 mm in depth providing complete accessibility to all tooth surfaces.

Ultrasonic setup:

- Flush handpiece for minimum of 2 min (at the beginning and end of the day or after any significant period when it has not been used) and for at least 20–30 s between patients [7].
- Select appropriate tip or insert (if using insert (magnetostrictive) ensure handpiece chamber is filled with water first).
- Adjust water flow and appropriate power setting before commencing treatment.
- Adapt the working part of the tip to the tooth surface, and during activation, keep the ultrasonic tip in motion at all times. Power levels and water flow may need adjusting throughout the operative procedure especially if interchangeable tips/inserts are used to obtain the required outcome.

Ultrasonic tips will wear from use over time but cannot be sharpened back to optimum condition. A 1 mm loss of the tip will result in a 25% loss of efficiency, and a 2 mm loss will result in 50% loss of efficiency, which often leads the clinician to apply more pressure or increasing the unit's power during the procedure. This has the potential to cause inefficient PMPR and can lead to patient discomfort. To ensure continued efficiency of ultrasonic insets/tips, use a 'wear guide' frequently (Fig. 26.2). Wear guides are available from the manufacturer of the mechanical scaling unit being used (Fig. 26.3).

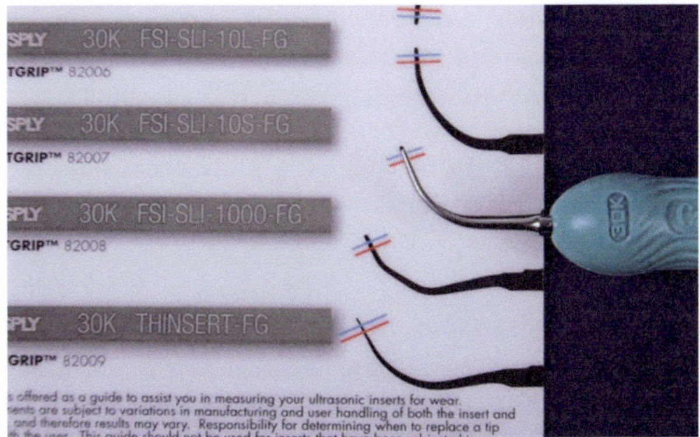

Fig. 26.2 Cavitron wear guide. Image courtesy of G. Malone, Dentsply Sirona

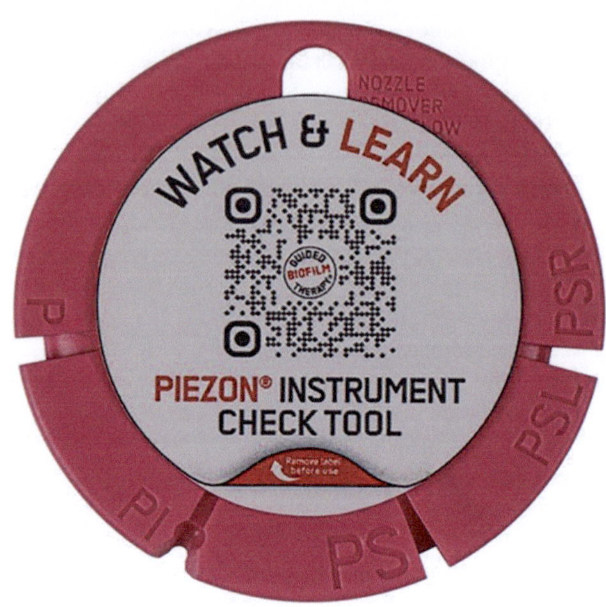

Fig. 26.3 Piezon instrument check tool. Image courtesy of EMS

26.6 Subgingival PMPR

Sanz et al. [1] advise within the S3 guidance on Step 2 that the current available evidence demonstrates that outcomes of periodontal treatment were not dependent on the type of instrument employed. This evidence was considered strong and consistent, advising that there was no clinically or statistically significant differences observed between the different types of instruments. However, they did highlight that there may be an ethical dilemma in that a patient's preference may conflict with a clinician's preference and due consideration should be given to this.

In addition to this, Suvan et al. [8] advise that subgingival instrumentation is an efficacious treatment in reducing inflammation, probing pocket depth and number of diseased sites in patients affected by periodontitis and that this effect was consistent, irrespective of the choice of instrument (sonic/ultrasonic vs. hand) or mode of delivery. Therefore, subgingival PMPR can either take the form of hand instrumentation, ultrasonic instrumentation or a blended method of both techniques with consideration given to the patient's preference and delivered with quadrant or full mouth treatment options.

26.7 Subgingival Hand Instruments

Subgingival hand instruments can either be universal or area specific in design. These instruments use slightly different techniques due to the differing angles of their cutting edges. The shank of both instruments can vary in length, with a shorter shank designed for use in shallow pockets and longer shanks designed for use in deep pockets. In addition to this, shank design can be rigid for removal of heavy deposits or flexible for removal of small to medium deposits of calculus.

26.8 Universal Curettes

These come in a variety of designs including Langer, Columbia, Barnhart and McCalls. Universal curettes have two cutting edges, inner and outer, which both sit at 90° to the lower shank (Fig. 26.4). Similarly to the sickle scaler, the universal curette requires the lower shank to be tilted towards the tooth during instrumentation, to allow the instrument to be used at 70- to 80-degree angle. It should be noted that for use in the anterior regions, only the outer cutting edge of the instrument is used. For correct technique in this area, clinicians should ensure that the lower shank is titled across the tooth, which in turn only allows for the outer cutting edge to be engaged on the root surface.

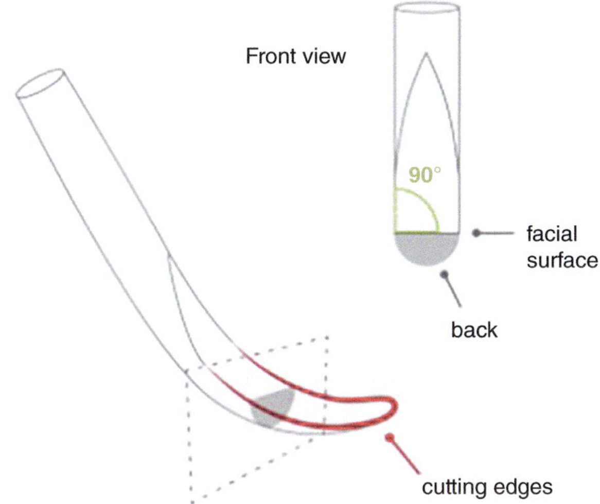

Fig. 26.4 Universal curette with two cutting edges. Image courtesy of Deppeler

26.9 Area-Specific Curettes

Area-specific curettes are, as their name suggests, used in specific areas on each tooth. Much like the universal curettes, they also come in a variety of designs including Gracey curettes, Kramer-Nevis and Turgeon Series. The most common area-specific curette used during undergraduate training in the United Kingdom is the Gracey curette series.

Area-specific curettes are designed with a cutting edge set at a 70-degree angle to the lower shank, on the working end of the instrument (Fig. 26.5). This angulation tilts the face of the instrument, giving it a lower and upper cutting edge. It is only the lower cutting edge of the working end of the instrument that is used for periodontal instrumentation.

Within the Gracey series, there are a total of nine different designs, ranging from a Gracey 1/2 through to a Gracey 17/18, providing the best adaption to complex root anatomy (Fig. 26.6) [9]. As the numbers of the series increase, as does the bend in the shank which allows for more reach in the posterior regions of the mouth. The Gracey 17/18 has the deepest bend in the shank allowing for use in the distal aspects of posterior molars. It should be noted that not all instrument brands follow the same colour-coding system, and clinicians are advised to gain an understanding of the number of the instrument used in each area and not the colour of the instrument.

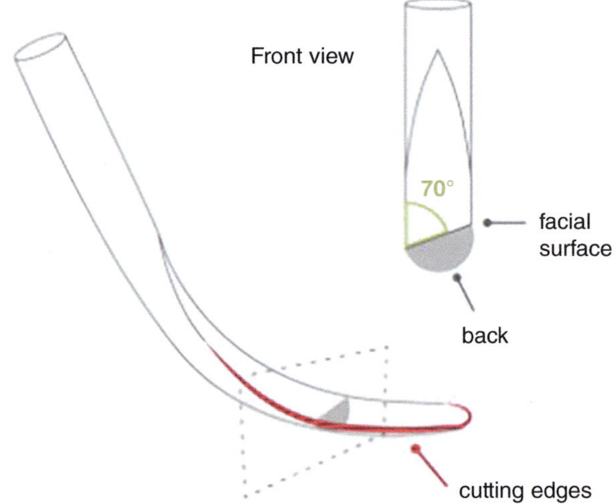

Fig. 26.5 Area-specific curette with one cutting edge. Image courtesy of Deppeler

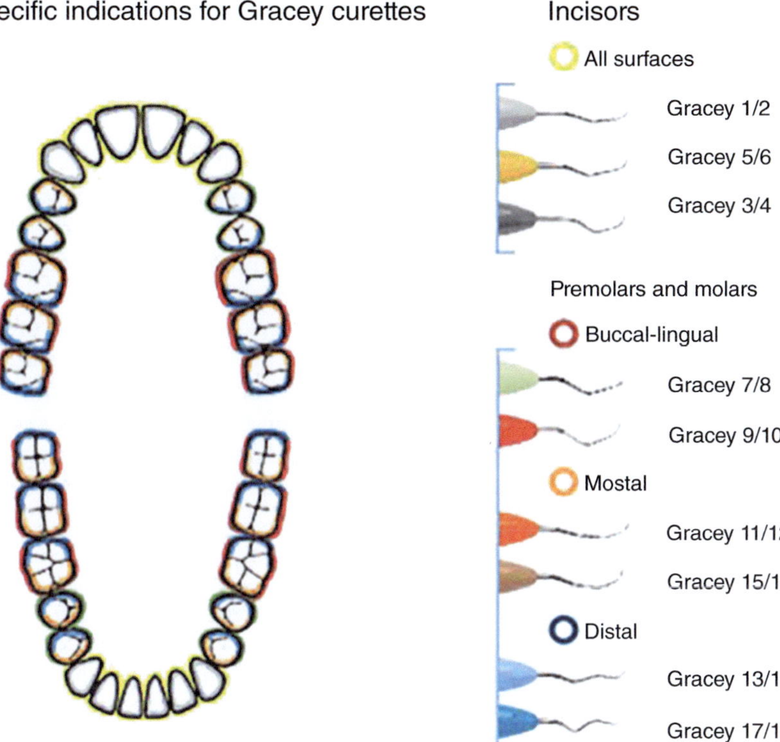

Fig. 26.6 Full gracey series. Image courtesy of LM Dental

26.10 Technique for Using Universal and Area-Specific Curettes: 3As

Whilst both instruments have differing degrees of their cutting edges, they are both used with the same technique of adaptation, angulation and activation in an instrument stroke.

Adaptation is the first step of an instrument stroke, where the clinician adapts the anterior first third of the cutting edge of the instrument to the root surface and feels engagement of this area of the instrument with the root surface of the tooth. Angulation is when the clinician angles the lower shank of the instrument to allow for correct instrument stroke. For a universal instrument, the lower shank requires to be titled towards the tooth to allow for an approx. 80-degree angle, and for an area-specific instrument, the lower shank requires to be parallel to the long axis of the tooth as the required angle of 70° is already present in the cutting edge. When each of these steps are correctly in place, this then allows for the clinician to take an activation stroke to remove the calculus. As with all periodontal instrumentation, a fulcrum should be used for stability and control, and these can be either intra or extra oral [4].

26.11 Calculus Detection: Periodontal Explorer Probes

Periodontal explorer probes are an excellent tool to identify calculus deposits on the root surface, surface irregularities, deficient restorative margins, excess cement and carious areas [9]. There are a variety of designs of these probes available from most periodontal instrument manufacturers. A popular periodontal explorer is the EXD 11/12, which has a similar shank design in terms of shape to that of the 11/12 Gracey curette. The shank on this instrument is very thin and flexible in design in comparison to a standard Gracey shank, allowing for excellent tactile feedback when assessing root surfaces of deep pockets for residual calculus deposits.

26.12 Sharpening and Monitoring Instrument Wear

Hand instruments need to be sharp to remove deposits effectively and efficiently, preventing trauma to soft tissues; improve quality of results and treatment outcomes; and provide the patient with a more comfortable experience and are less demanding for the clinician. Periodontal instruments will dull through the rounding of the cutting edge after 15–45 instrument strokes [10]; therefore, they require to be sharpened on a very frequent basis. Dull cutting edges will result in burnished calculus (a calculus deposit where only the top part of the calculus has been removed, leaving a 'burnished' deposit behind), increased lateral pressure and pinch force on use leading to musculoskeletal issues, and increased operator time to perform good-quality PMPR [4].

Cutting edges of the instruments can be assessed both visually and manually by using a plastic sharpening testing stick. Visually, a dull cutting edge of an instrument will reflect the light due to the rounding of the cutting edge, whereas a sharp cutting edge will not reflect the light when it is placed on it. When assessing the sharpness of the cutting edge manually by using a test stick, the cutting edge of a sharp instrument will 'bite' the surface when it is sharp, and therefore, if this does not occur and the instrument does not engage with the testing stick, the instrument is identified as needing sharpening. Some of the more modern instrument ranges have been designed with a coating that requires less sharpening than standard stainless-steel instruments, in addition to ranges of instruments that do not require to be sharpened at all. It is important to note that once a non-sharpen instrument becomes dull, it must be replaced as it is not able to be sharpened.

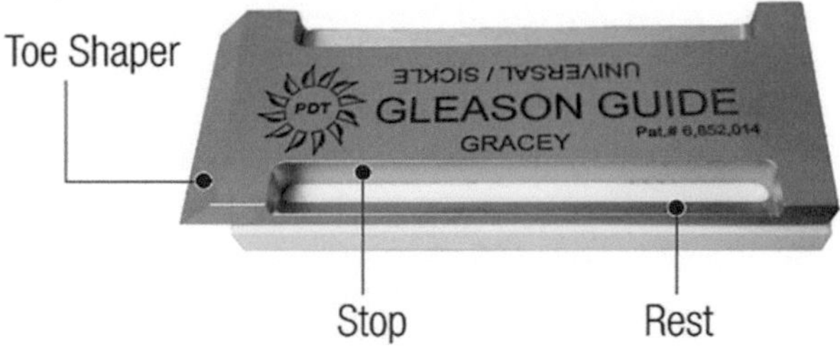

Fig. 26.7 Gleason guide. Image courtesy of PDT dental

When sharpening instruments, it is important to ensure that the angle of the cutting edges of the instrument is preserved; therefore, it is recommended to use a sharpening device that has both universal and area-specific angles predetermined such as the Gleason guide (Fig. 26.7) to sharpen the instruments with.

26.13 Implant Instrumentation

The EFP have recently published guidance on the multidisciplinary treatment of peri-implant diseases. This S3 level clinical practice guideline focuses on best practice interventions required to prevent the development of peri-implant disease or their recurrence and to treat patients with dental implants following the development of peri-implant diseases [11]. At the time of writing, this guidance advises that it is unknown which specific PMPR regime is the most effective in reducing the risk of recurrent peri-implantitis. However, it does advise that based upon the periodontal literature and indirect evidence, the following:

26.14 Dental Implant Biofilm Removal

For this specific intervention, guidance advises the use of titanium or stainless-steel curettes, ultrasonic/sonic instruments, rubber cups or brushes, and APDs with glycine powder or erythritol alone or in combination.

26.15 Peri-implant Mucositis Treatment

For the treatment of mucositis, the recommendation from current guidance is that ultrasonics with plastic tips or APDs with glycine powder or titanium curettes or chitosan brushes *may be considered* as a single mode of PMPR. Clinicians should be aware that this guidance advises against the use of APDs in combination with conventional PMPR—curettes, ultrasonics or both, and that they should only be used as a single mode of treatment for peri-implant mucositis.

26.16 Non-surgical Management of Peri-implantitis

A stepwise approach is also advocated for the treatment of peri-implantitis, with the aim of controlling peri-implant biofilms and inflammation along with submarginal instrumentation. In patients with peri-implantitis, it is recommended to perform non-surgical supra- and submarginal instrumentation with titanium or stainless-steel curettes and/or ultrasonic/sonic devices. It is important to note that it does not recommend the use of APDs for non-surgical submarginal peri-implant instrumentation. Literature advises that cases of subcutaneous emphysema have been reported after the use of APDs during submarginal instrumentation and therefore these clinical practice guidelines only consider the use of APDs for biofilm control or as a stand-alone treatment for peri-implant mucositis [11].

26.17 Titanium Instrument Hand Instruments

Titanium instruments are made from the same titanium alloy as implants and abutments and are available in various designs including sickle scalers and curettes. These titanium instruments have the benefit that they can also be sharpened which is advantageous for both calculus and excess cement removal. The literature acknowledges that titanium, graphite and plastic implant scalers were all within safe limits in regard to damage to the implant surfaces; however, this surface can become contaminated with trace elements that plastic, graphite or stainless-steel scalers leave behind [12]. Therefore, titanium curettes are the instrument of choice for hand instrumentation.

26.18 Ultrasonic Implant Tips

The three recommended materials used with ultrasonic implant tips are polyether-ether-ketone (PEEK) used with piezoelectric, Ultem (polyetherimide, PEI) used with magnetostrictive and titanium alloy used with piezoelectric [12]. All three of these materials are deemed safe to use, in terms of damage to the surface of implants, for PMPR in both titanium and ceramic implants [10].

26.19 Conclusion

As with any instrument used in clinical dentistry, following instructions for use and understanding the full utility of the instrument will not only optimise outcomes for patients but improve comfort and safety for the operator. In this short article, we have highlighted key considerations for optimising instrument use in the management of periodontitis, which we hope will be of benefit to busy clinicians.

Practical tips are intended as a series of experiential tips rather than a compendium of the evidence.

References

1. Sanz M, Herrera D, Kebschull M, et al. Treatment of stage I–III periodontitis—the EFP S3 level clinical practice guideline. J Clin Periodontol. 2020;47(Suppl 22):4–60. https://doi.org/10.1111/jcpe.13290.
2. SDCEP. Prevention and treatment of periodontal diseases in primary care. 2014. Available https://www.sdcep.org.uk/published-guidance/periodontal-care/. Accessed August 2023.
3. Martins O, Costa A, Silva D. The efficacy of air polishing devices in supportive periodontal therapy: clinical, microbiological and patient-centred outcomes. A systematic review. Int J Dent Hyg. 2023;21:41–58.
4. Gehrig JS, Sroda R, Saccuzzo D. Fundamentals of periodontal instrumentation and advanced root instrumentation. Burlington: Jones & Bartlett Learning; 2020.
5. Canakci V, Orbak R, Tezel A, Canakci CF. Influence of different periodontal curette grips on the outcomes of mechanical non-surgical therapy. Int Dent J. 2003;53:153–8.
6. Dong H, Loomer P, Barr A, Laroche C, Young E, Rempel D. The effect of tool handle shape on hand muscle load and pinch force in a simulated dental scaling task. Appl Ergon. 2007;38:525–31.
7. NHS England. HTM 01–05: decontamination in primary care dental practices (2013 edition) chapter 6 dental unit water lines. Available https://www.england.nhs.uk/publication/decontamination-in-primary-care-dental-practices-htm-01-05/. Accessed August 2023.
8. Suvan J, Leira Y, Moreno F, Graziani F, Derks J, Tomasi C. Subgingival instrumentation for treatment of periodontitis. A systematic review. J Clin Periodontol. 2020;47:155–75.
9. Newman G, Laughter L, Essex G, Elangovan S. Newman and Carranza's clinical periodontology for the dental hygienist. Missouri: Elsevier; 2021.
10. Balevi B. Engineering specifics of the periodontal curet's cutting edge. J Periodontol. 1996;67:374–8.
11. Herrera D, Berglundh T, Schwarz F, et al. Prevention and treatment of peri-implant diseases—the EFP S3 level clinical practice guideline. J Clin Periodontol. 2023;50:4–76. https://doi.org/10.1111/jcpe.13823.
12. Wingrove S. Peri-implant therapy for the dental hygienist. Hoboken: Wiley; 2022.

Part V

Oral Surgery

Practical Tips for Oral Surgery

27

Kamran Ali and Ewen McColl

Learning Points

- To understand the need to comprehensively assess the patient prior to any oral surgery procedure and the need to obtain valid consent.
- To appreciate the need to have the appropriate instruments available and to utilise these correctly during treatment.
- To recognise the need for post-operative management of the patient once treatment is completed to ensure minimisation of any further morbidity or complications.

27.1 Introduction

As extractions will make up the majority of oral surgery procedures in primary care, this article focuses on practical tips for performing extractions in a safe and predictable manner, with minimal trauma to the hard and soft tissues. The ultimate aim of all these measures is to improve the experience of patients undergoing extractions.

K. Ali
Oral Surgery, Qatar University College of Dental Medicine, Doha, Qatar

Faculty of Health, Plymouth University, Plymouth, UK

E. McColl (✉)
Peninsula Dental School, Plymouth, UK
e-mail: ewen.mccoll@plymouth.ac.uk

E. McColl, A. Alani (eds.), *Practical Tips in Clinical Dentistry*, BDJ Clinician's Guides, https://doi.org/10.1007/978-3-031-90355-7_27

27.2 Patient Preparation

Patient preparation is crucial to ensure safety, and although tooth extractions can usually be accomplished without complications, it is best to err on the side of caution. Overestimation of tooth extractions often leads to gratitude whilst underestimation may result in embarrassment and medico-legal consequences.

- Obtain a thorough patient assessment and evaluate any risks of tooth extractions due to comorbidities such as cardiovascular or hepato-renal disease, diabetes, immunosuppression and concomitant medications such as blood thinners and anti-resorptive drugs [1, 2]. Do not hesitate to discuss your treatment plan with the patient's GP if there are any concerns regarding patient's medical status.
- Carry out a thorough clinical assessment to evaluate access to the tooth, its position in the arch and condition of the crown, and note any adjacent restorations which may be at risk of damage during instrumentation for tooth extraction. Consider an appropriate radiograph to obtain a good view of the peri-radicular region and identify anatomical challenges (dilaceration, hypercementosis, accessory roots, ankylosis, concrescence and proximity to antral floor or inferior alveolar/mental nerve, etc.) [3].
- Obtain a valid patient consent through shared decision-making. Whilst patient reassurance is paramount, it is equally important to moderate expectations, clearly explain potential risks and resist the temptation to promise too much!
- Always consider use of surgical safety checklist to minimise human errors resulting in wrong tooth extractions [4].

27.3 Select Appropriate Instruments

A variety of instruments may be used for undertaking tooth extractions including forceps, luxators and elevators. It seems sensible to arrange all instruments which may be possibly required prior to the procedure. Fetching additional instruments during the procedure is time-consuming and makes nurses feel pressurised. Moreover, it may compromise cross-infection control due to the need to get instruments from drawers and frequent changing of gloves, etc. In addition, the dentist may be perceived by the patient to be struggling due to repeated need for additional instruments. Indeed, oral surgeons lay out all the instruments on the surgical tray prior to commencing the procedure!

27.4 Prioritise Access

Good access and vision of the surgical site is fundamental to performing any operative procedure including tooth extractions and requires appropriate positioning of the operator and the patient, adequate retraction of soft tissues (lips, cheeks, tongue, etc.) and excellent lighting conditions throughout the procedure. Whilst the need for good access is obvious, we have often observed clinicians using a position of mechanical disadvantage to approach the patient and ignoring poor soft tissue retraction and lighting especially when dealing with difficult extractions. Unfortunately, this attitude only makes the procedure more challenging and adds to the stress and frustration of the dentist (and the patient!). It is best to focus on maintaining a clear access and vision to the operative site throughout by appropriate positioning, good soft tissue retraction, ensuring unimpeded passage of light and effective suction.

27.5 Use Your Instruments Correctly

Notwithstanding the wide variations in the difficulty levels of tooth extractions encountered in clinical practice and different approaches used by clinicians, it is often helpful to commence tooth extractions with luxators. Unless ankylosed, teeth are anchored in the alveolar bone by the periodontal ligament. Luxators have a sharp blade and can be used as periotomes to sever the periodontal fibres with minimal force. When used appropriately, luxators can often make tooth extractions a straightforward job, almost! Next, elevators such as Coupland's can be used to elevate the tooth by engaging it with the elevator blade near the cemento-enamel junction on the buccal aspect. Rotation of the elevator along its long axis may allow elevation of the tooth along its path of withdrawal. Finally, the correct forceps can be used to displace and deliver the tooth securely.

Some of the generic principles applicable during extraction with any type of instruments include:

- Protect the airway securely with a tongue depressor and use high-volume suction; this is especially important using elevators as tooth fragments may be dislodged into the airway with potentially adverse consequences.
- Use the non-dominant hand effectively to retract the soft tissues; support the alveolus (and mandible) to minimise the risk of bone fracture and to obtain tactile feedback during tooth movements.
- Never lean on the patient—*no knees on the patient's chest please!*
- Use a buccal approach and avoid working across the arch.
- The extraction instrument must rest only on the tooth to be extracted without any impingement on the soft tissues and avoid any force on adjacent teeth or restorations.
- Avoid excessive apical force on maxillary posterior teeth in close proximity to the antral floor and mandibular molars in close proximity to the inferior alveolar nerve.
- Always use a controlled force and see what the tooth wants to do! If the tooth is stubborn and no movement is achieved, re-evaluate the radiographs to rule out anatomical variations (dilaceration, hypercementosis, ankylosis, accessory roots, etc.). Consider a surgical approach if within the competency of the operating dentist; otherwise, it may be best to stop the procedure and consider a specialist referral.

27.6 Provide Good Post-Extraction Management

Several measures are required to achieve uneventful healing following a tooth extraction [5].

- After a successful tooth extraction, avoid the temptation to place a bite pack within the next microsecond! Palpate the socket walls to rule out the presence of any sharp bone and smooth with a bone file or rose-head surgical bur if required. Look carefully down the socket and use saline irrigation and suction to clear away any debris in the socket and reduce the microbial load. These measures are important to ensure uncomplicated healing of the extraction socket.
- Achieve haemostasis prior to discharging the patient and never send the patient home with a bite pack in situ. A pressure pack placed directly over the extraction socket and held securely with the bite for 10 min is usually adequate to achieve haemostasis. Patients must avoid talking to the dentist/nurse during this time as it may compromise haemostasis. Patients on blood thinners may require additional local measures to achieve haemostasis [1].
- Provide written and verbal post-extraction instructions regarding pain control, postoperative bleeding, oral hygiene, diet and things to avoid (smoking, alcohol, heavy exercise). Patients must be instructed to avoid active spitting/rinsing for at least 24 h after extractions as it may dislodge the blood clot in the socket, compromise healing and possibly risk development of alveolar osteitis.
- Provide an emergency contact number and arrange a follow-up for complicated extractions.

Finally, dentists may consider additional training to develop their extraction skills specially to master safe and effective use of luxators and elevators and to carry out surgical tooth extractions. It may be worth exploring opportunities to work some sessions at local oral surgery units in primary and secondary care or local dental schools. Given the opportunity, such exposure may provide invaluable experience to dentists interested in improving their oral surgery skills.

References

1. Toole J, McKenna G, Smyth J. Managing patients at risk of medication related complications requiring dental extractions in primary care. Prim Dent J. 2020;9:54–8.
2. Wilmott S, Yates J, Pretty IA. Dental extractions in primary care for patients at risk of MRONJ. Br Dent J. 2021. https://doi.org/10.1038/s41415-021-3674-8.
3. Hupp MR, Ellis JR, Tucker E. Contemporary oral and maxillofacial surgery. 6th ed. Missouri: Elsevier; 2008. p. 92–112.
4. Dargue A, Fyfe E, French K, et al. The impact of wrong-site surgery on dental undergraduate teaching: a survey of UK dental schools. Eur J Dent Educ. 2021;25:670–8.
5. Sambrook PJ, Goss AN. Contemporary exodontia. Aust Dent J. 2018;63(Suppl 1):S11–8.

Optimising Surgical Flap Design for Oral Surgery

28

Jim Carey, Ayisha Davies-House, and Ewen McColl

Learning Points

- To understand the need to plan flap design in advance of treatment taking into account the nature of treatment, anatomical factors and method of closure.
- To gain knowledge of good practice in incising and raising flaps to maximise access for treatment.
- To appreciate the importance of wound closure and suturing on the overall care of the patient.

28.1 Introduction

Surgical flap design and management is something general dental practitioners may have to consider on a regular basis, often at the most inopportune of moments when time pressures are at their greatest. There are few clinicians who have not been faced with the prospect of raising a flap for a surgical extraction when time is short, and the need to be as efficient and effective as possible is essential. This chapter refers to buccal flaps that are more likely to be carried out in primary care.

Improving surgical flap design and management helps to produce predictable results, assists healing, improves patient comfort and decreases complications. It should be noted however that when carrying out any surgical technique, access and

J. Carey
Peninsula Dental School (University of Plymouth), Derriford Dental Education Facility, Plymouth Science Park, Plymouth, UK

A. Davies-House
Peninsula Dental Social Enterprise, Plymouth, UK

E. McColl (✉)
Peninsula Dental School, Plymouth, UK
e-mail: ewen.mccoll@plymouth.ac.uk

E. McColl, A. Alani (eds.), *Practical Tips in Clinical Dentistry*, BDJ Clinician's Guides, https://doi.org/10.1007/978-3-031-90355-7_28

vision should be optimal, and an awareness of vital structures is paramount to limit adverse complications.

In this chapter, we discuss techniques and tips to optimise flap design and management that, based on our experience, will improve outcomes for patients and hard-pressed clinicians.

28.2 Flap Design

Designing a flap is key to successful dentoalveolar surgery and as such should not be underestimated. A well-designed flap will give good access to allow the surgery to be completed whilst protecting important anatomical structures and facilitating healing of the surgical site. A poorly designed flap risks complications including poor healing and potential long-term harm.

28.3 Preserve Important Structures

(a) Avoid incisions over or near to foraminae, blood vessels or nerve pathways.

A sound working knowledge of anatomy is essential to flap design. A misplaced incision could cause avoidable complications such as bleeding or nerve damage. Think of the anatomy beneath the surface when planning your flap. For example, one must not extend a relieving incision down between the lower premolars due to the risk of damage to the mental neurovascular bundle.

(b) Maintain the integrity of papillae, fraenae and other structures.

It is important to preserve the soft tissue anatomy both to aid closure and to ensure that those structures are maintained following healing. Interdental papillae should be included within the flap and must not be bisected or transected. Incisions should not be placed across fraenae.

(c) Anticipate aesthetic concerns.

If a flap is planned in the anterior region, be mindful as to how much gingival display the patient exhibits when talking and smiling. In the presence of a 'gummy smile', one might design a flap whereby incisions and hence resultant scars are less immediately apparent.

28.4 Anticipate Complications

(a) Bony defects and cysts.

Placing an incision over a lesion will complicate its removal and compromise healing. Plain radiographs are invaluable but can be anatomically misleading. Additionally, a radiograph taken several months ago may not show the current extent of a defect, granuloma or cyst. It is also vital to plan for any additional defect resulting from necessary bone removal to remove the roots and/or lesion completely. Ensure that ample allowance is made for any bony defect beneath soft tissue such that any incision is placed at a safe distance lateral to the defect margins. The wound margins must rest on sound, uncompromised bone; otherwise, there is a significant risk of wound breakdown and poor healing.

(b) Oro-antral communication (OAC).

If an OAC is a significant risk, plan your flap design accordingly such that it could be modified if required to close the OAC. If unsure, or management of this complication would fall beyond your skill set, seek specialist advice and refer.

28.5 Design for Good Access

1. Ensure access to the surgical site is sufficient.

   Access is essential. Poor access can lead to excessive retractive force and tearing of the soft tissues. Ensure the extent of the flap allows sufficient access with gentle retraction. Whilst it is desirable to raise only as much tissue as required, healing will occur over the same time period regardless of flap size (Fig. 28.1).
2. Plan for extension.

   Design bearing in mind how the flap could be extended to improve access if required. If an envelope alone is insufficient, where would the relieving incision(s) best be placed? A relieving incision can also be extended if safe to do so.

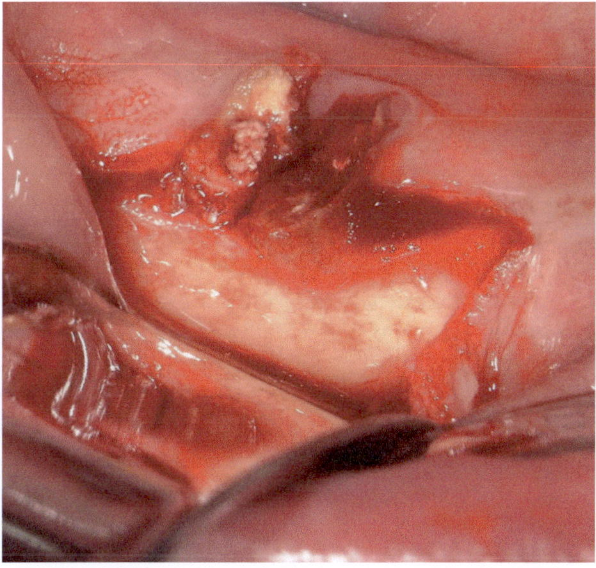

Fig. 28.1 Envelope flap for LR7 roots, with no adjacent teeth, allowing sufficient access for surgical removal

28.6 Make Controlled Incisions

1. Feel before you cut.

   Palpate firmly to ensure relieving incisions will be placed over sound bone. Surface anatomy can be visually misleading. What appears to be firm may be soft tissue overlying a tissue space containing key structures. Palpation will confirm the presence of bone and reassure the operator before scalpel placement.
2. Handle the scalpel properly.

   Hold the scalpel as one would a pen and with the forefinger extended along the top of the handle. Use appropriate finger rests, ensuring that you do not slip.
3. Intra-crevicular incisions.

   These may be made using near vertical 'walking' or sawing movements of the scalpel into the gingival crevice around the cervical margins of the teeth. Resist any temptation to turn the blade in the papilla—this will transect the latter. The blade should approach the mesial and distal aspects of each papilla by insertion at their respective sides. That is, the scalpel must to be removed and repositioned to incise each side of the papilla. Intra-crevicular incisions may need to be recapitulated.
4. Plan any relieving incision with care.

   Place relieving incisions carefully and firmly down to bone in one smooth movement. Avoid recapitulating these whenever possible because it will be very challenging to follow the same line of incision. Keep the incision over the alveolus, within the attached mucosa. Do not extend any relieving incision into the free mucosa nor too deeply into the sulcus.

28.7 Raise a Full-Thickness Flap

1. Loosen any gingivae and papillae.

   A flat plastic, curved Warwick-James, or similar, may be used to loosen the papillae and gingivae. The tissues can be tenaciously attached and will easily tear if pulled. Press against the bone whilst turning the instrument gently rather than attempting to 'pull'. Similarly, microsurgical instruments and papilla-specific elevators, such as the Buser elevator, can be very helpful in initial flap management (Fig. 28.2 and Table 28.1).
2. Find the plane beneath periosteum.

   It is important to raise the periosteum fully with the overlying mucosa. This may be easier to find initially via any relieving incision. Push underneath the periosteum with the tip of the periosteal elevator pointing *towards* the bone. Again, do not attempt to pull the flap off the alveolar bone because it will tear, or you may 'button hole' through the flap. Raise the flap from the bone in this manner ensuring that the full thickness of muco-periosteum is released and raised. Poorly raised or macerated periosteum will cause excessive pain and inflammation and slower healing in the post-operative phase.

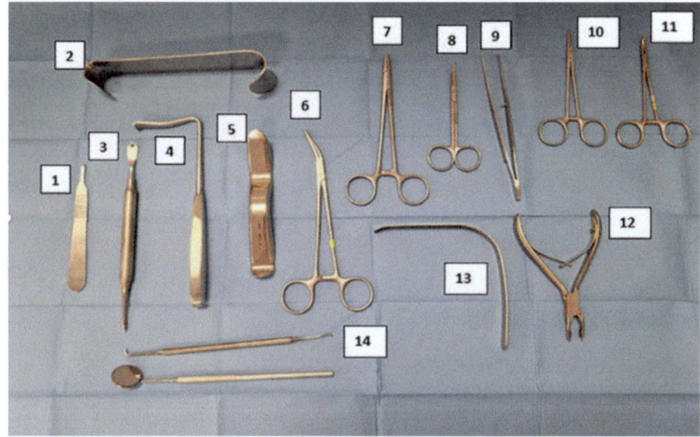

Fig. 28.2 Emergency oral surgery kit

Table 28.1 Instruments in the emergency oral surgery kit (depicted in Fig. 28.2) and their uses

Number	Instrument name	Instrument role
1	Number 3 scalpel handle	Handle to a number 15 scalpel blade
2	Kilner cheek retractor	Used to retract the cheek during suturing
3	Periosteal molt elevator	Aid to raising a mucoperiosteal flap
4	Bowdler henry rake retractor	Mucoperiosteal flap retractor
5	Minnesota retractor	Mucoperiosteal flap retractor
6	Toothed fickling forceps	Used to pick up tooth/bone fragments
7	Needle holder	Used to hold the suture needle
8	Suture scissors	Used to cut sutures
9	Gillies toothed tissue forceps	Used during suturing to hold the mucoperiosteal flap
10	Straight mosquito clip	Used to remove soft tissue fragments
11	Curved mosquito clip	Used to remove soft tissue fragments
12	Rongeur bone nibbler	Used to remove sharp alveolar bone
13	Lack tongue depressor	Used to keep the tongue away from the operative field for protection
14	Mitchell trimmer	Aid to raising a mucoperiosteal flap, used to curettage and debride tissue

3. If the flap is tethered.

   If small points are tethered when raising the flap, gentle retraction with a periosteal elevator can aid in identifying any point of gingival attachment which may be released via careful incision.

28.8 Reposition the Flap with Care

1. Use landmarks.

   Suture anatomical landmarks, such as papillae, first. This will aid correct repositioning of the flap for closure. For more extensive flaps, it may be helpful to start with the landmarks towards the middle of the flap to ensure correct alignment.

2. Take an appropriate ‘bite’ of tissue.

   For intra-oral relieving incisions, the bite is usually 3–5 mm. It is important to ensure the suture doesn’t pull through the delicate tissue whilst still apposing the tissue accurately. The needle should be rotated through the tissue, following its curve, to ensure it does not cut through. The wound margins should be slightly everted.
3. Avoid excessive tension.

   Sutures should hold the tissue gently back in place. Too much tension may cause the suture to pull through the tissue. Excessively tight sutures will result in pain and potential tissue necrosis due to swelling during the post-operative phase.
4. Tighten and knot carefully.

   An appropriate surgeon’s knot should be used, with 3–5 mm of tail end remaining after the knot to avoid unravelling. The knot should be tightened without over-tightening the suture itself. If a suture is too loose and the knot locked tight, it may be appropriate to cut the suture out and replace it. Similarly, if the suture appears to be too tight, or incorrectly positioned, it is perfectly reasonable to remove and reposition it. Bear in mind that multiple re-attempts at suturing may be challenging because the intra-oral soft tissues are delicate.

28.9 It Is Better to Stop if You Are Getting into Trouble

No matter your level of experience, there are always occasions when the unexpected can happen. If things are not going to plan, stop and reassess. If the situation is moving beyond your skill set, listen to your gut feelings. Close with sutures, explain the situation to your patient, review and refer as needed. It is far better to abandon a procedure than to cause serious complication or irreparable harm.

28.10 Conclusions

The need to carry out a surgical extraction in primary care often arises at the most inopportune of moments, when the adrenaline levels of patient, clinician and nurse often rise accordingly. The practical tips in this chapter if followed will offer you the chance of success. Raising the flap sufficiently to allow appropriate vision and access is key. Having a surgical kit on standby will prevent much anxiety, and as always, further ongoing training and mentoring will help to optimise outcomes for patients and clinicians alike.

Managing Oral Surgery Complications in Primary Care

29

Jennifer Sawyer, Araz Ahmed, Jim Carey, Ewen McColl, and Claire Moss

Learning Points

- Appreciate that complications within oral surgery should be anticipated, mitigated and managed effectively.
- Understand the importance of consent when describing risks of oral surgery procedures.
- Recall the methods of managing various oral surgery complications and the need for follow-up and further management or referral if required.

29.1 Introduction

In the previous chapter, we have discussed measures to optimise oral surgery outcomes [1, 2]. Even when these tips are applied meticulously, surgical complications may arise and can present when least expected. Primary care clinicians may have to manage such complications during an often-busy patient list, so in this short paper, we discuss tips that clinicians may find useful in managing such complications.

J. Sawyer · J. Carey
Oral Surgery, Peninsula Dental School (University of Plymouth), Derriford Dental Education Facility, Plymouth Science Park, Plymouth, UK

A. Ahmed · C. Moss
Peninsula Dental School (University of Plymouth), Derriford Dental Education Facility, Plymouth Science Park, Plymouth, UK

E. McColl (✉)
Peninsula Dental School, Plymouth, UK
e-mail: ewen.mccoll@plymouth.ac.uk

E. McColl, A. Alani (eds.), *Practical Tips in Clinical Dentistry*, BDJ Clinician's Guides, https://doi.org/10.1007/978-3-031-90355-7_29

29.2 Surgical Preparation: Anticipate the Complication

'By failing to prepare you prepare to fail' [3]. Preoperative assessment and planning are crucial to the success of any surgical intervention. In identifying potential risks and complications preoperatively, they may be planned for and often mitigated.

Complications may be classified as pre-, intra- or post-operative, or as surgical, medical or patient related. A thorough medical history, clinical exam and radiographic assessment should allow the dentist to anticipate and therefore minimise the risk of intraoperative surprises such as bleeding due to known coagulopathies, difficulty in surgical access or challenging root morphology. Similarly, identifying those with marked dental anxiety or a history of difficult extractions will help to inform treatment planning. If a patient reports a history of excessive bleeding or challenging extractions, it is wise to be mindful that history tends to repeat itself. Preoperative preparation is essential; ensure that all necessary (including potentially necessary) equipment and instruments are readily available. Make sure that you have surgical handpieces, luxating instruments, suture kits, haemostatic agents, etc., readily available and this will significantly reduce intraoperative stress for you, your nurse and your patient. Having a prepared oral surgery complication kit may save time and limit stress levels should any complications arise.

29.3 Consent

The consent process should bring together the patient's presenting complaint, clinical findings, diagnosis and the treatment options in a discussion with the patient. An acute condition may mean that some form of treatment is required on the day a patient presents, if safe to do so in the practice setting. The gold standard for routine and elective treatment is that patients should have a period of time to consider any treatment options discussed, along their associated risks and benefits. This means treatment is normally carried out at an appointment subsequent to that initial discussion. This is particularly important where the risk of a significant complication may be anticipated. Surgical-, medical- and patient-specific risk assessment is key in the consent process. Those predictable or potential risks should be clearly identified so that both you and the patient are prepared to manage them should they arise. This in turn forms part of the informed consent process. Consider your patient holistically; for example, if their work is public facing, they may require more time away from that role after surgical treatment. Similarly, if they are about to jet off for a scuba diving holiday, it might not be the best time to remove an upper tooth with a significant risk of oro-antral communication.

It is wise to provide your patient with a clear post-operative care plan, in advance of any proposed treatment, including anticipated analgesic requirements; likelihood and probable duration of any trismus, bruising or swelling; and guidance on when and how to seek urgent or emergency assistance should it be required.

29.4 Risk Assessment and Management of Common Complications

29.4.1 Root Fractures/Crown Fractures

Often but not always predictable, we all recognise the distinctive 'snap' heard when a crown or root fractures during extraction. Should this occur, do not panic; stop, reassess and plan your next course of action.

Risk factors: Curved, bulbous, lengthy or dilacerated roots; heavily restored and non-vital teeth; dense or sclerotic bone; cementoma; poor surgical technique.

Management: Identify known risk factors preoperatively. In the event of a coronal or root fracture, consider your visibility and access. If you are unsure what remains and where, consider an intraoperative periapical radiograph to reassess the situation. Consider whether the retained fragment is sufficiently small and pathology-free to be left in situ (<3 mm or the apical 1/3 of a root may be acceptable) or whether it requires retrieval. If you decide to retrieve the root remnant, consider the proximity of adjacent structures (such as the antrum, mental nerve, inferior alveolar nerve, implants), the access, visibility and your surgical competence. If lacking in the later, seek support from a colleague and include a basic surgical skills course in your personal development plan (PDP).

1. Ensure that you have good lighting and that you and the patient are positioned to optimise visibility and access. Surgery should be undertaken standing. Be prepared to move around your patient as you work to maintain optimal access and visibility throughout.
2. Ensure excellent local anaesthesia. Particularly if you've been struggling for a while, the local anaesthetic may be wearing off. Top up the anaesthesia if necessary, bearing in mind the total dose administered.
3. Consider soft tissue access. Is a soft tissue flap required to visualise the retained fragment and/or to access it? If raising a flap, ensure that it is a full-thickness mucoperiosteal flap, remembering the principles of flap design. Within reason, a large flap will heal as well as a small one and will provide better access and visibility. A larger flap will have a better blood supply and be easier to retract than a thin finger of mucosa. This is particularly true for those who infrequently raise flaps.
4. If bony access is required, a flap must be raised, the soft tissues retraced and a gutter cut around the roots using a surgical handpiece (reverse exhaust, self-irrigating, high torque and excellent tactile feedback). Carefully run the bur vertically parallel and adjacent to the root (but not into the root) to form a gutter which will provide an application point and path of extraction. Be vigilant to protect adjacent teeth, soft tissues and vital structures. Soft tissue retractors such as a Minnesota, Bowdler-Henry rake, Lacks and Kilner are essential to protect the soft tissues at the operative site and to prevent trauma.
5. Once the tooth has been delivered, it can be tempting to immediately turn your attention to wound closure. However, meticulous debridement will reduce the

risk of postoperative pain, infection and bony sequestra. Ensure that the bone margins are smooth and that all debris including loose bone fragments have been removed. Irrigate the socket and under the flap, copiously, with sterile saline or water. Ensure that your assistant allows the saline to pool, helping any debris to float upwards, before aspirating it away. Repeat as required until the area is clean.

6. Reposition the flap and close with resorbable sutures (e.g., 4–0 or 3–0 Vicryl Rapide is standard).
7. Confirm haemostasis before discharging the patient with a comprehensive post-operative care plan which includes adequate analgesia and emergency contact numbers. If there are concerns about the risk of post-operative complications, a review appointment or telephone call should be scheduled. Patients do feel well cared for if there is a follow-up.

29.4.2 Oro-Antral Communication (OAC)

A hole into the antrum is a risk with some upper premolars and molars. These do not need to be intimidating if managed appropriately. If the risk of a sizeable OAC is considered very high, then it may be prudent to seek advice or specialist referral.

Risk factors: Lone standing upper molars, pneumatised antra, sclerotic bone, older patients, >50% of the root(s) overlying the antrum, discontinuity of the PDL space/lamina dura, poor surgical technique, presence of antral pathology (Fig. 29.1).

Management: Preoperative risk assessment. If considered high risk, consider an elective surgical approach and design the flap such that it could be advanced in the event of an OAC.

If an oral antral communication is suspected, gently suction over the socket with good light to confirm if present. Never push the suction to the apical region or probe because this risks creating or enlarging a hole or rupturing intact sinus lining which would otherwise aid healing. Performing a Valsalva manoeuvre (a 'nose-blowing' test) is also now contraindicated for the same reasons. If you suspect but cannot

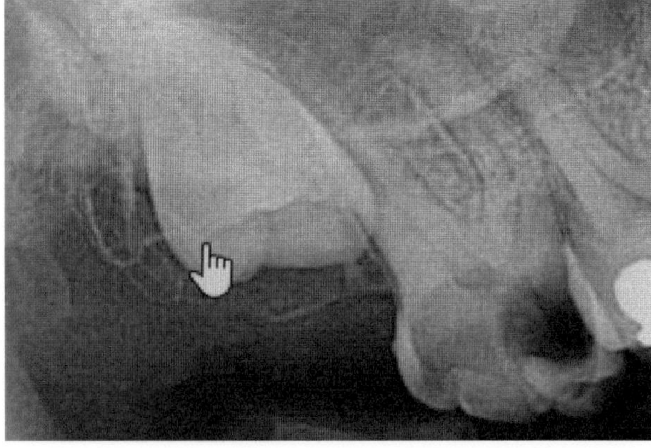

Fig. 29.1 Preoperative radiograph showing a grossly carious 17 adjacent to an unerupted 18. The antral floor appears to lie about halfway down the roots of the 17

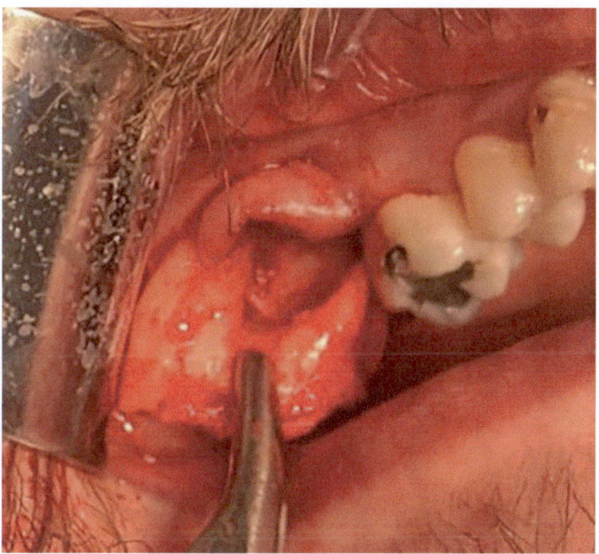

Fig. 29.2 Extraction of the 17 and 18 with the tuberosity attached

confirm an OAC, it may be prudent to advise the same post-operative behaviour as if there were an OAC (Fig. 29.2).

A communication ≤4 mm has a reasonable chance of healing on its own [4], if the patient follows the post-operative care instructions. Ensure that there is a stable clot in the socket before discharging the patient with a follow-up appointment and antral care instructions (no nose blowing and sneeze with mouth open for 2 weeks). Consider prescribing ephedrine nasal drops, for the affected side, and antibiotics.

If there is a larger OAC (≥5 mm), and you are skilled in the technique, you may wish to perform a buccal advancement flap to obtain primary closure. However, this should not normally be attempted unless you are clearly competent to do so. That is, you should have enhanced skills or specialist training in oral surgery. In the event of a larger OAC, where you are not competent and confident to safely close it, a phone call to your local oral surgeon/oral and maxillofacial surgeon will yield good advice on how best to manage and refer. These patients will normally need to be seen quite quickly. In some circumstances, you may be advised to have a cover plate or suck-down splint made urgently by your local lab: These may be used as an emergency measure in cases where onward referral is required for definitive repair (Figs. 29.3, 29.4, and 29.5).

29.4.3 Tuberosity Fractures

Most tuberosity fractures can be avoided with careful planning and good technique. However, they can occur even with the correct technique.

Risk factors: Lone standing molars, older patients, pneumatised antra, ankylosed teeth, poor surgical technique.

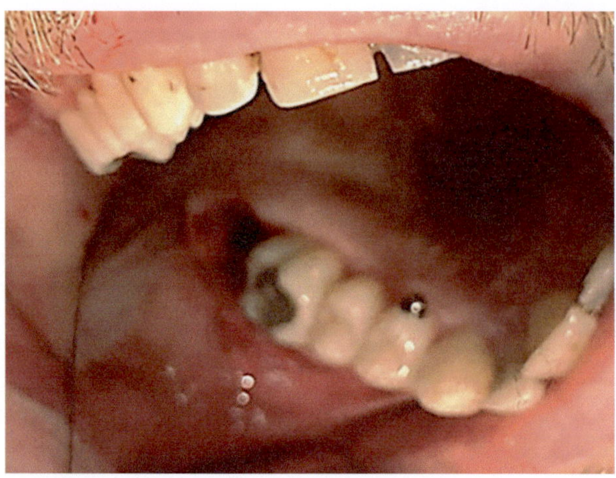

Fig. 29.3 Intra-oral photograph of the 17 and 18 OAC

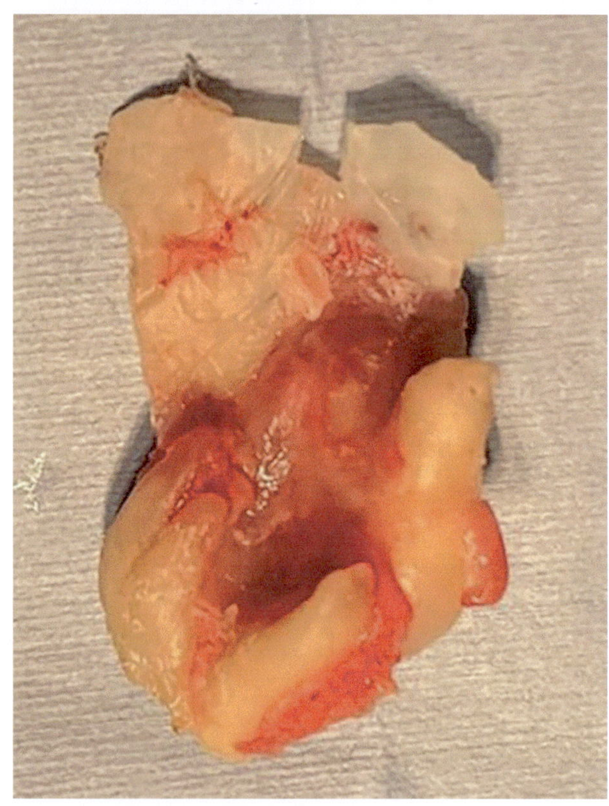

Fig. 29.4 17 and 18 with the tuberosity attached

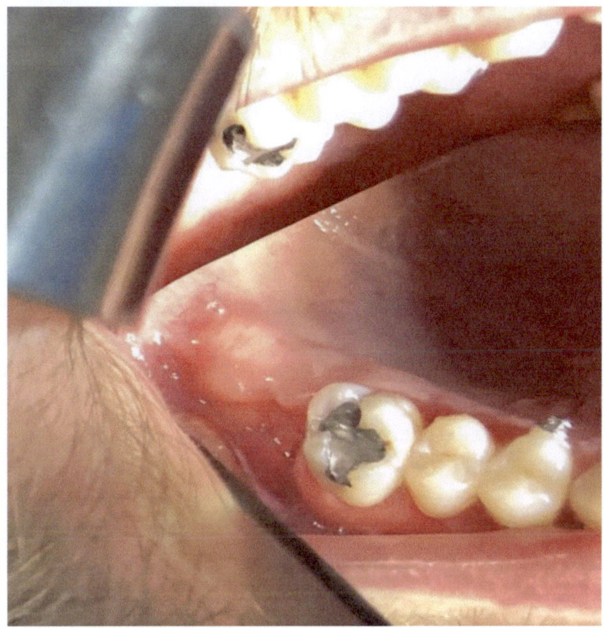

Fig. 29.5 Three weeks post-operatively. OAC repaired at the time of surgery

Management: Consider an elective surgical approach, if within your competency, if the patient is deemed at high risk of fracture.

In the event that you suspect a tuberosity fracture, stop and reassess the situation. Small, insignificant fractures may be confined to the distal alveolus without involving the entire tuberosity or the antrum. Very small alveolar fractures may be safe to carefully dissect and remove with the tooth. A palatal mucosal tear is a clear sign of a tuberosity fracture and likely indicates a more significant fracture. If the tooth can be readily separated from the bone, it may be appropriate to do so—unless it would form an essential part of a splint. If the tooth cannot be readily separated from the bone, reposition and splint, either with composite and wire or with a suck-down splint. Larger fractures involving the body of the tuberosity should be splinted and allowed to heal before the tooth is surgically removed, at a later date (>6 weeks later, often by a specialist). If you are unsure as to how to proceed, you should seek urgent advice from your local oral surgery team (Fig. 29.2).

Mucosal tears should be sutured and haemostasis ensured. If the fracture involves the antrum, then an antral care plan should be followed (no nose blowing/sneeze with mouth open for 2 weeks, antibiotics, ephedrine). The patient should receive adequate analgesia and a follow-up appointment.

29.4.4 Post-Operative Bleeding

Bleeding is often, although not always, predictable. Careful assessment and management will allow most bleeding to be readily controlled with simple measures.

For those where bleeding is predictable due to medication, such as Direct Oral Anticoagulants (DOACs), and other antiplatelet or anticoagulant medications, follow appropriate guidance such as that issued by SDCEP [5].

Bleeding is classified as primary (intraoperative), reactionary (within 24 h, usually as the vasoconstrictor effect in the local anaesthetic is wearing off) and secondary (7–10 days post-operatively, often associated with infection).

Should a patient present with a post-operative bleed, it is therefore helpful to determine when the surgery took place and when they started to bleed.

Risk factors include anticoagulant or antiplatelet drugs, haemophilia, thrombocytopaenia, underlying bone marrow disease and severe liver disease (deranged clotting) and injury to tissues and vessels intraoperatively.

Management: Hopefully, at-risk patients will be identified preoperatively via a targeted history and appropriate measures can be taken to reduce the risk of significant bleeds. However, should a patient present with a post-operative bleed, the following is helpful:

1. Under good light and suction, identify the bleeding site, evacuating any large clots if necessary. Apply firm pressure to the bleeding site with damp gauze for at least 10 min as timed by a clock. In the meantime, set up local anaesthetic with a vasoconstrictor (e.g., 2% lidocaine with 1:80,000 adrenaline) for local infiltration, a suture set with 3–0 or 4–0 resorbable suture (e.g., Vicryl Rapide™) and haemostatic agent (e.g., Surgicel, Gelatamp or Hemocollagene, and many more).
2. If the socket is still bleeding, administer local anaesthetic, identify the bleeding site (bone/mucosa/vessel), place the haemostatic material of choice and place one or more sutures (e.g., mattress suture) to constrict the mucosa over the bone margins and to hold the haemostatic agent in situ. Reapply a damp swab with firm pressure. It may be helpful to hold it yourself to ensure that consistent, firm pressure is applied. Re-check the socket after at least 10 min. If bleeding has arrested, monitor the patient for at least another 10 min to ensure satisfactory haemostasis.
3. If the bleeding is still not settling, call the local oral surgery or oral and maxillofacial surgery department for further advice. The patient may require further investigations and advanced support.

29.5 Post-Operative Pain

All patients should be advised regarding appropriate and adequate post-operative analgesia. Most simple extractions and paediatric patients can be managed with simple analgesia such as paracetamol and ibuprofen [6]. These work well together when given at therapeutic doses. Post-operative pain is best controlled by administering analgesia before the local anaesthetic wears off and if taken regularly for the first 48 h.

Options for analgesia in primary care include paracetamol, NSAIDs such as ibuprofen, opioids (dihydrocodeine) or over the counter co-codamol. Patients requiring high or increasing levels of analgesia should be reassessed clinically to determine the cause of pain (swelling, infection, alveolar osteitis). In secondary care, codeine or tramadol may be prescribed for those undergoing more extensive procedures, in addition to appropriate simple analgesia.

Never underestimate the power and relief to the patient of providing a local anaesthetic block ± infiltration, especially one of the longer acting local anaesthetics (e.g., bupivacaine 0.5%), to help break the pain cycle and allow time for the oral analgesics to take effect.

Pre-warn patients with known TMD or chronic pain syndromes that symptoms may worsen for a period post-operatively but should settle with time. This will alleviate worry for the patient and reduce the demand for additional appointments.

29.6 Alveolar Osteitis (Dry Socket)

Dry socket is an all too familiar complication and, whilst often predictable, all patients should be warned of this risk, including those who are at higher risk of developing it.

Risk factors: Surgical extraction, mandibular extraction, difficult or traumatic extraction, smokers, female.

Management: Patients tend to present 3–4 days post-operatively with a history of worsening, severe, aching/throbbing pain that may radiate along the jaw. Analgesia may provide limited relief. The peri-socket mucosa may be inflamed and the socket devoid of coagulum. There is often food debris in the socket.

1. Offer local anaesthetic; many patients are happy to proceed without.
2. Under good light, irrigate the socket with sterile saline or water. A wide bore needle on a 20 ml syringe is effective, as is a Monoject-type curved-tip plastic syringe. Continue to flush the socket until all debris is removed.
3. Gently place a small volume of Alveogyl [7] in the socket. Never pack it in.
4. Re-discuss the post-operative care instructions, including analgesia, smoking cessation and emergency contact details. It is also not uncommon, with a severe dry socket, to need to re-irrigate the socket within a few days and reapply a dressing.

29.7 Conclusions

Complications following oral surgery procedures are regularly encountered, no matter your level of experience. Following these tips will hopefully assist clinicians in reducing the risk and managing such complications effectively in a primary care setting. However, always remember that you can stop and seek advice if you are encountering a situation beyond your clinical comfort zone.

References

1. Carey J, Davies-House A, McColl E. Top tips for optimising surgical flap design in primary care. Br Dent J. 2023;234:138–40.
2. Ali K, McColl E. Oral surgery: top tips for primary care. Br Dent J. 2023;232:196–7.
3. Franklin B. Forbes quotes. Available https://www.forbes.com/quotes/1107/. Accessed May 2023.
4. von Wowern N. Closure of oroantral fistula with buccal flap: Rehrmann versus Môczár. Int J Oral Surg. 1982;11:156–65.
5. Scottish Dental Clinical Effectiveness Programme. Management of dental patients taking anticoagulants or antiplatelet drugs. 2022. Available https://www.sdcep.org.uk/published-guidance/anticoagulants-and-antiplatelets/. Accessed October 2023.
6. Coulthard P. Post-operative oral surgery pain: a review. Oral Surg. 2008;1:167–77.
7. Septodont. Alvogyl information leaflet. Available https://www.septodont.co.uk/wp-content/uploads/sites/12/2023/03/IFU-alveogyl.pdf?x26140. Accessed May 2023.

Managing the Bleeding Patient in Primary Care

30

Claire Moss, Eithne Fyfe, and Ewen McColl

Learning Points

- To recall the haemostasis process
- To recognise the different types of post-operative bleeding
- To identify risk factors in post-operative bleeding
- To recall systemic factors that can increase post-operative bleeding tendency
- To understand a pathway for identifying and managing post-operative bleeding

30.1 Introduction

In previous oral surgery related top tips, we have discussed measures to manage oral surgery complications in primary care [1]. This short paper builds on from these tips and outlines specific strategies to manage the patient who has prolonged or abnormal bleeding following soft tissue surgery or exodontia, and provides management advice to anticipate, avoid and manage prolonged or excessive post-operative bleeding.

C. Moss · E. Fyfe
Peninsula Dental School (University of Plymouth), Exeter Dental Education Facility, Exeter, UK

E. McColl (✉)
Peninsula Dental School, Plymouth, UK
e-mail: ewen.mccoll@plymouth.ac.uk

E. McColl, A. Alani (eds.), *Practical Tips in Clinical Dentistry*, BDJ Clinician's Guides, https://doi.org/10.1007/978-3-031-90355-7_30

30.2 Haemostasis

There are three steps in the normal haemostatic process:

1. Vascular constriction
2. Platelet aggregation
3. Activation of the coagulation cascade to form a fibrin clot

30.3 Types of Post-operative Bleeding

There are three types of post-operative bleeding:

1. Primary bleeding occurs perioperatively due to the surgical intervention/trauma (and may be excessive or prolonged due to complicating local factors or systemic factors).
2. Reactionary bleeding occurs 2–3 h after surgery as the constrictor effects on the blood vessels of the adrenaline from the local anaesthetic diminish. This may also result from the patient not adhering to the post-operative instructions for wound care leading to disruption of the blood clot/coagulum.
3. Secondary bleeding occurs 7–10 days after surgery due to infection at the surgical site which becomes inflamed and hyperaemic.

30.4 Risk Factors for Post-operative Bleeding

Risk factors for haemorrhage can be considered in relation to timing of surgery [2].

1. Preoperative risk factors—for example, medical complications, anticoagulant or antiplatelet medication, hypertension
2. Perioperative risk factors—for example, traumatic extraction, soft tissue laceration, large vessel disruption, oral-antral communication, local vascular abnormalities or pathological lesions
3. Post-operative risk factors—for example, local infection or local pathology, retained root or mobile bone fragment, physical trauma to socket disrupting the clot or failure to follow post-operative instructions for wound care

30.5 Pathway to Manage a Patient with a Post-operative Haemorrhage

1. Check patient is systemically stable (observations/vital signs) whilst simultaneously controlling any active bleeding with temporary local measures (pressure packs).
2. Review medical history for details of medical conditions or medications contributing to preoperative risk factors.

3. Review the surgical notes and X-rays to highlight any perioperative risk factors.
4. Examine the surgical site to determine the source of the bleed, either soft tissue or bone.
5. Carry out steps to achieve definitive haemostasis systematically from simple to more complex strategies.
6. If haemostasis cannot be achieved, the patient should be transferred to emergency department (ED) for further management.

30.6 Is the Patient Systemically Well?

When a patient presents in primary care with a post-operative bleed, the most important consideration is the overall health and wellbeing of the patient. When did the bleeding start? Has it been continuous or intermittent? Try and get an understanding/estimation of how much blood has been lost by interrogating the history. Is this blood-stained saliva or persistent active bleeding? Has the patient managed to drink/eat/take other essential prescribed medications? Is there a risk of medical complications resulting from failure to take medications, particularly for a diabetic patient. Are they confused? Could they be dehydrated? Consider recording blood pressure to determine possible hypotension. If systolic blood pressure is below 100 mmHg and diastolic pressure below 60 mmHg and the heart rate (raised) tachycardic above 100 beats/min (even if the BP is normal) [2] or if you have any other concerns, try to stem the bleeding by packing and arrange urgent transfer to ED for further management.

30.7 Does the Patient Have a Known Medical Condition or Take Medication That Could Be Causing the Post-operative Bleeding?

If the patient is systemically stable, it is important to determine if there are any medical factors contributing to the post-operative bleeding. Though this is unlikely to alter the immediate strategies for bleeding cessation, it may explain the reasons for the abnormal bleeding and highlight specialties or medical professionals who will support future patient management.

30.7.1 Does the Patient Take Any Antiplatelet or Anticoagulant Medication?

A patient may be prescribed antiplatelets or anticoagulants if they have certain medical conditions such as atherosclerosis, cardiac arrythmias and ischaemic heart disease or have had a heart valve replacement. These medications are also prescribed prophylactically for prevention of stroke, deep vein thrombosis, pulmonary embolism or myocardial infarction. The medication might be taken long term and patients should be aware of the risks of increased bleeding following a surgical procedure.

30.7.2 A Medical Condition Affecting the Platelets, Either in Number or Function

Has the patient been diagnosed with ITP (idiopathic thrombocytopaenia) causing a low platelet count? An autoimmune disease? Bone marrow failure? Liver or kidney disease or HIV/aids? Has the patient recently undergone chemotherapy? Or do they have an inherited condition such as von Willebrand's disease or Bernard-Soulier syndrome?

30.7.3 A Medical Condition Causing Vascular Defects

Has the patient been diagnosed with rare inherited conditions such as hereditary haemorrhagic telangiectasia or Ehlers-Danlos syndrome which affect integrity and strength of blood vessels? Might the patient have vascular fragility either age-related or as a side effect of high steroid dose treatment for another condition?

30.7.4 A Coagulation Disorder

Does the patient have an inherited coagulopathy? Has the patient or family member been diagnosed with haemophilia A (factor VIII deficiency); Christmas disease (factor IX deficiency); factors V, X or XII deficiency; von Willebrand's disease (a coagulation and platelet disorder); or afibrinogenaemia? Does the patient have an acquired coagulopathy due to liver disease, renal disease, malabsorption, bone marrow failure or malignancy such as myeloma, leukaemia or bony metastasis?

30.7.5 Local Vascular Abnormality

Is there a local anatomical vascular abnormality or pathological vascular lesion such as a haemangioma?

30.7.6 A Suspected But Undiagnosed Bleeding Disorder

Does the patient have previous bleeding tendencies? Has the patient bled excessively in the past? Does the patient have a history of bruising? Does the patient have a family history of bleeding? Does the patient consume, now or in the past, excessive amounts of alcohol which might have caused damage to the liver resulting in a deficiency of clotting factors? Once bleeding has been controlled, consider contacting the GP outlining the post-operative complications and history so that the GP can arrange blood tests and onward referral for further investigations if appropriate.

30.8 Review of Surgical Notes

The surgical notes should be reviewed to determine if there is any surgical contributory factor for the bleeding such as details of retained root fragments, mobile bony fragments left in the socket or a fractured tuberosity that could cause infection and secondary bleeding. Assessment of the radiographs may indicate if the root apex was positioned near an anatomical structure likely to cause a post-operative bleed, such as the inferior dental neurovascular bundle, or if there was any local pathology that could represent hyperaemic inflammatory tissue.

30.9 Assess the Surgical Site

The surgical site should be assessed with good lighting, irrigation and suctioning. Any granulation tissue should be carefully debrided, large clots/coagula evacuated and the site inspected. This may require local anaesthetic for pain control. If the site continues to bleed, any sutures should be removed to enable the surgical site to be fully assessed to determine if the bleeding is from soft tissue or bone.

30.10 Bleeding From Soft Tissue

When managing a post-operative bleed, the simplest methods for haemostasis should be considered first and more complicated strategies, or those requiring less commonly available chemical agents should be used as a last resort.

30.10.1 Application of Pressure

Pressure should be applied to the bleeding site with a damp sterile gauze using digital pressure to the area for 15 min by either the patient or operator. It is worth noting that if the patient is partially dentate, the practice of biting against the gauze is not recommended as the absence of opposing teeth will reduce the pressure to the socket.

30.10.2 Vasoconstriction

Local anaesthetic with adrenaline, such as 2% lidocaine with 1:80,000 adrenaline, can be infiltrated around the bleeding site specifically to cause vasoconstriction to aid clotting; however, a reactionary bleed can occur when the vasoconstrictor effect diminishes.

Ethyl chloride or Endofrost can be sprayed on to a cotton wool roll and wrapped in sterile gaze and applied with pressure to the bleeding surgical site. It is important not to let the chemical agent directly contact the mucosa to avoid a chemical burn. This cold compress will also encourage vasoconstriction.

30.10.3 Suturing of a Socket (Fig. 30.1)

Placement of a horizontal mattress suture or a simple interrupted suture using a resorbable material such as a 3-0 or 4-0 Vicryl Rapide may be used in suturing. The aim of suturing is to reoppose the tissues to their original position prior to surgery, and unless an oral-antral communication has been created, the socket should remain

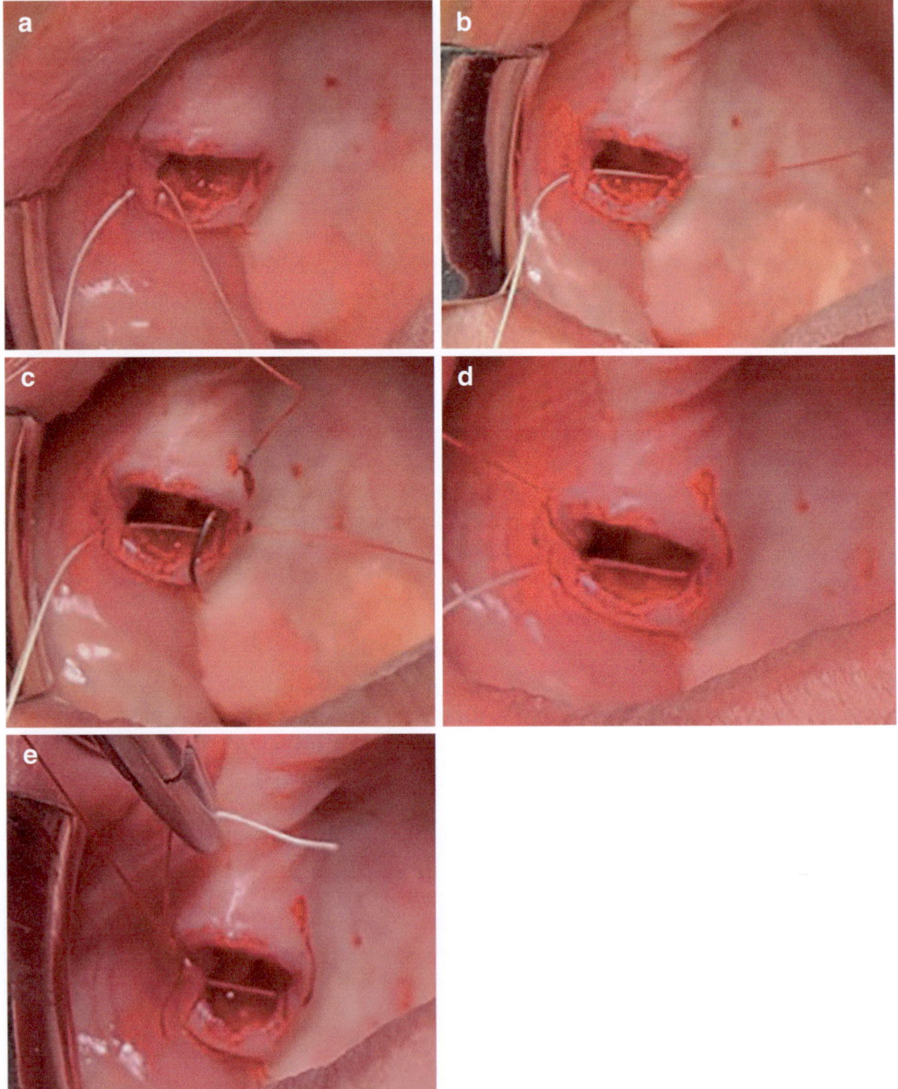

Fig. 30.1 (**a**–**e**) The sequential process of delivering a horizontal mattress suture to promote haemostasis

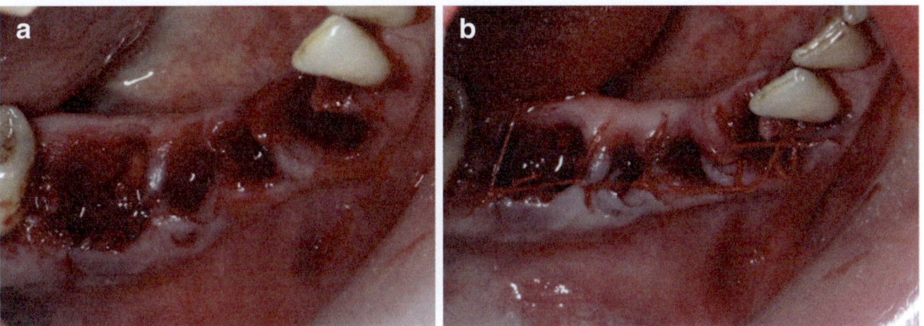

Fig. 30.2 (**a**, **b**) Continuous suture for approximation of multiple sockets

patent to avoid unnecessary tension on the tissues. Sutures can also support retention of any haemostatic dressing placed. Figure 30.2 shows continuous suture for approximation of multiple sockets.

With all suturing techniques, the position of the suture knot needs to be considered to avoid irritation to the lingual tissues or excessive trauma during mastication if positioned palatally. The specific resorption times of the suture material should be checked with the manufacturer as resorption times following straightforward exodontia require no longer than 10 days to avoid debris and food build-up around the sutures, leading to inflammation or local infection.

Suturing may be used alone or with a haemostatic dressing material. It can be challenging to avoid dislodging the haemostatic dressing whilst suturing, and in the case of Surgicel placement, it is often easier to tuck the Surgicel into the socket after it has been sutured.

30.10.4 Haemostatic Dressing Materials

The most commonly used material is Surgicel which is a plant-derived oxidised cellulose polymer that breaks down when placed on an open wound and stimulates the production of thrombin and fibrinogen, promoting coagulation of the blood to form a clot/coagulum. Surgicel has additional reported bactericidal properties, but when introducing any foreign body to a surgical site, there are risks of complications and tissue reactions.

Collagen sponges such as Hemocollagene work also to promote coagulation. They have the advantage like the resorbable gelatine sponge Gelfoam of being a three-dimensional matrix that can be cut down to shape to fit a socket and act as a physical haemostat; however, these sponges are made from animal products, bovine and porcine material and therefore may be unsuitable for some patients due to religious or ethical concerns.

30.10.5 Chemical Haemostatic Agents

If the above processes have been followed and the patient continues to bleed post-operatively, the use of chemical haemostatic agents should be considered.

Tranexamic acid works as an effective antifibrinolytic to prevent fibrin breakdown. It can be prescribed in tablet form, in liquid form for injection or made up by hospital pharmacy as a mouthwash. The tablet form is not useful in this praxis, and unfortunately, the mouthwash is unstable and so patients with a known bleeding disorder should be prescribed the mouthwash in advance by a hospital haematologist or oral surgeon with a request to hospital pharmacy to prepare the mouthwash for collection the morning of surgery. The logistics of tranexamic acid mouthwash preparation make this difficult to dispense for emergency patients and so patients with a post-operative bleed in primary practice can instead use tranexamic acid for injection, which comes in 5 ml glass ampules of concentration 100 mg per 1 ml. Drops can be applied to sterile gauze and used as a pressure pack to the area, or the liquid drawn up into a fine disposable syringe and dripped directly into the socket. The tranexamic acid should be left in the socket for as long as possible before either suctioning or allowing the patient to swallow the small volume of liquid.

Silver nitrate is a powerful chemical cauterising agent and for the purposes of oral surgery comes in a stick form with 95% silver nitrate at the tip of a plastic stick that is effective in delivering the chemical to bleeding soft tissues which might be difficult to access. This is particularly useful for haemostasis in regions difficult to suture such as after a punch biopsy in the palate. After the bleeding has stopped, the area should be gently swabbed with saline on a gauze to deactivate the chemical to prevent damage to surrounding tissues.

Ferric sulphate 15.5% comes as an astringent solution to be used with gingival retraction cord and acts as a haemostatic agent to reduce bleeding from inflamed mucosa. It is not routinely used for post-extraction haemostasis.

Bleeding from a specific identifiable vessel is a less likely complication from exodontia presenting in primary care and is more likely to occur following more extensive oral and maxillofacial surgery in a hospital setting. Strategies to tie off/ligate vessels and use of diathermy are beyond the remit of this paper, which is aimed at the primary care setting; however, it is worth noting that the placement of deep sutures to incorporate an identifiable vessel can be effective in achieving ligation and local control.

30.11 Bleeding from Bone

The site of the bleed in the bone should be explored to assess if the bleeding is from a vessel traversing the bone or from the bone itself.

Small bleeding sites from the cancellous bone may be managed by burnishing, using a Mitchell's trimmer to mechanically compress the bone.

Care needs to be taken around a bleeding vessel in the socket as this is likely to indicate the proximity of a nerve to the surgical site. In some cases, the inferior alveolar nerve in the inferior dental canal with its associated artery may be in contact with the apices of the lower molar teeth increasing the risk of a post-extraction bleed from the socket. Bone wax can be used as a mechanical tamponade to stem the bleeding [3] and thereby facilitating clot formation. Horsley's bone wax contains a sterile mixture of white beeswax with isopropyl palmitate, a palm oil-based emollient, with moisturiser and thickening and antistatic agent. Bone wax is non-resorbable and some of the reported complications include interference with healing and infection, and therefore, some clinicians carefully remove the wax after bleeding has stopped.

30.12 To Anticipate and Avoid Bleeding in the Future

1. Preoperatively: Follow the SDCEP Guidelines (2022) [4] for managing patients taking antiplatelets or anticoagulants with specific preoperative and post-operative instructions for patients taking direct oral anticoagulants (DOACs), warfarin or other vitamin K antagonists, injectable anticoagulants, antiplatelet drugs and antiplatelet and anticoagulant combinations. Where indicated, liaise with medical colleagues to ensure management in the primary care setting is appropriate.
2. Perioperatively: Take steps to reduce bleeding such as placement of sutures or haemostatic agents post-operatively for patients taking antiplatelets or anticoagulants or who have any other known systemic or local factors that could cause prolonged or excessive bleeding.
3. Post-operatively: Emphasise to the patient the importance of following the post-operative instructions.

30.13 Conclusions

Abnormal excessive bleeding can occur post-operatively in patients with known medical conditions causing coagulopathies or in patients with undiagnosed conditions. Post-operative bleeding may occur as a side effect of prescribed antiplatelet or anticoagulant medication or may result from a surgical complication. The above paper provides a comprehensive strategy for patient management with initial patient assessment, to confirm that they are systemically stable, then medical and surgical site assessment to aid in diagnosing the cause of the bleed. Procedures to aid haemostasis starting from the most straightforward to more complicated strategies have been presented with clinical tips; however, if haemostasis cannot be achieved, then the patient should be transferred to an ED preferably with an on-site maxillofacial unit for further investigations and management.

Acknowledgements With thanks to Dr Jane Parker, Specialist Oral Surgeon at Whittington Health NHS Trust, for collaboration with clinical photographs (Fig. 30.1).

With thanks to Dr David Parmenter, Oral Surgery Specialty Doctor at King's College Hospital, for clinical photographs (Fig. 30.2).

References

1. Sawyer J, Ahmed A, Carey J, McColl E, Moss C. Top tips for managing oral surgery complications in primary care. Br Dent J. 2023;235:672–5.
2. McCormick NJ, Moore UJ, Meechan JG. Haemostasis part 1: the management of post-extraction haemorrhage. Dent Update. 2014;2014(41):290–6.
3. Das JM. Bone wax in neurosurgery: a review. World Neurosurg. 2018;2018(116):72–6.
4. Scottish Dental Clinical Effectiveness Programme, editor. Management of dental patients taking anticoagulants or antiplatelet drugs. 2nd ed. Dundee: Scottish Dental Clinical Effectiveness Programme; 2022. Available https://www.sdcep.org.uk/published-guidance/anticoagulants-and-antiplatelets/. Accessed April 2024.

Part VI

Removable Prosthodontics

Removable Prosthodontics: Fundamentals of Success

31

L. Blakely, W. A. V. Beare, and Ewen McColl

Learning Points

- Understand the need for a stable oral environment with good oral hygiene measures and absence of plaque-associated disease prior to denture construction
- Recall a methodical sequence of designing a partial denture incorporating stability, support and retentive features
- Recognise techniques in making the denture less plaque retentive
- Understand the techniques in impression making for partial dentures to ensure the definitive cast is adequate for denture construction
- Recall the various aspects that need checking at the metal try-in stage
- Appreciate a logical sequence to jaw registration and recording

31.1 Introduction

The advent of dental implants to replace missing teeth and an increase in adults retaining teeth into old age [1] may mean that partial denture provision is not as regularly carried out as was the case 30 years ago. However, for many reasons, this does not necessarily mean that an intact dentition will survive a lifetime, and

L. Blakely
Spring Hill Specialist Dental Centre, Tavistock, Devon, UK

Derriford Dental Education Facility, University of Plymouth, Plymouth Science Park, Plymouth, UK

W. A. V. Beare
Derriford Dental Education Facility, University of Plymouth, Plymouth Science Park, Plymouth, UK

E. McColl (✉)
Peninsula Dental School, Plymouth, UK
e-mail: ewen.mccoll@plymouth.ac.uk

E. McColl, A. Alani (eds.), *Practical Tips in Clinical Dentistry*, BDJ Clinician's Guides, https://doi.org/10.1007/978-3-031-90355-7_31

provision of partial dentures remains a key skill in a dentist's armamentarium of treatment options.

For many patients, a partial denture will meet entirely their functional and aesthetic needs though it has been estimated that 30–50% of these prostheses are not worn [2]. Clearly, despite the intended benefit, these patients must perceive there to be no functional or aesthetic advantage in wearing the denture [3].

An often-heard complaint is the denture was uncomfortable or inconvenient leading to rejection. This results in a disappointing outcome for both patient and clinician and reinforces negative perceptions about removable partial dentures (RPDs) on both sides. To mitigate this disappointment, dentists should apply not just evidence but pragmatism and full consideration of the patient's wishes when considering dentures as a treatment option. In many cases, replacing all missing teeth may be neither necessary nor desirable, and limiting treatment goals may be more sensible. A problem-solving approach should be used for tooth replacement decisions [4] and patient made fully aware of risks and benefits of tooth replacement so that provision of a denture is patient-led [3], with the patient fully cognisant of how treatment or no treatment may impact on their oral health. For example, the shortened dental arch (SDA) may be considered as the most sensible option if this can meet aesthetic and functional demands rather than considering more extensive tooth replacement [3].

When discussing risk/benefits with the patient, the detrimental effect of RPDs on plaque formation is well known, with the most significant increase in plaque accumulation due to lower dentures with a lingual plate design [5]. The wearing of a partial denture can additionally result in an increased incidence of caries and periodontal breakdown [6, 7], so picking the correct treatment modality for the correct patient is crucial.

Many patients understandably initially prefer and seek a fixed option for tooth replacement, but through the process of assessment of the patient and an understanding of the feasible options, it may lead the patient to the choice of a removable solution.

It is the authors' experience that with patient education and understanding, considered design planning and control of clinical stages, it is possible to provide a denture that is comfortable, functional and aesthetic and gives the patient confidence. The dentures should integrate well with the remaining dentition so that the wearer can become unaware of the denture in the mouth.

In this series, we discuss practical tips based on the authors' (cumulatively over a century!) experience of providing partial dentures that we hope will benefit all clinicians embarking on partial denture provision. The series starts with an analysis of fundamentals linked mainly to cobalt chrome dentures, in part 2 acrylic dentures and part 3 managing challenging free end saddles.

31.2 Is the Patient's Mouth RPD Ready?

There is good evidence that metal framework dentures with appropriate design and maintenance can function well [8] and much of the potential harm can be mitigated by focusing on hygienic principles of RPD design [9].

Fortunately for our patients, there is a large body of evidence that further tooth loss is not inevitable, and meticulous oral hygiene can offset the potential harmful sequelae of wearing an RPD [8].

The often-quoted adage 'that it is better to preserve what remains than replace that which is lost' is still very pertinent.

- Prior to making an RPD, educate the patient about the potential for further tooth loss if oral hygiene is not of a good standard so that the patient understands the risks of wearing a denture.
- Recommend the care of a hygienist; individualised oral hygiene guidance is of great benefit.
- Provide diet advice to minimise sugar frequency and prescribe fluoride toothpaste where indicated.
- Complete all other required treatment, such as caries control, periodontal therapy, endodontics and restorations before constructing the denture. However, considering design of the denture at an early stage can facilitate provision of helpful features in the restorations such as suitable space for rests, undercuts for clasps and guide planes.

Apart from a denture replacing teeth in a space visible to the patient, there is no evidence that a particular design increases patient acceptance of a denture [10].

The design principles suggested are those that appear to work well with successful patient acceptance and long-term stability when reviewed in practice. They are based on a consensus opinion of prosthodontic specialists [11] and the evidence that supports the importance of focusing on hygienic principles of design [9].

31.3 Design the Design!

In contemporary removable prosthodontics, the state-of-the-art denture combines hygienic design principles and good biomechanics. This cannot be achieved if the design is delegated to the laboratory [12]. The clinician must be in control of deciding the design for the bespoke denture that is best for the individual patient.

Initially plan what you think is the best denture for the patient by looking at the cast, taking note of any obvious design challenges such as markedly tilted teeth, etc. Plan a design incorporating the necessary components in the simplest hygienic form.

- Follow a logical sequence of design, deciding on which teeth to replace, which may not be all that are missing. Determine optimal saddle extension. Then plan support, direct retention, reciprocation, major connector shape and need for any indirect retention.
- Survey the primary cast or ask the technician to survey the cast if you are unable to do so yourself. The technician has great expertise in the technical aspects of your design, and a teamwork approach can be very helpful at this stage.

- The survey will help determine the best path of insertion and if the design will be possible. It will show if there is a need for tooth modification to achieve the ideal design at the chosen path of insertion, and the available undercuts for clasp positioning (this can be modified).
- Discuss the proposed denture design with the patient. This is both helpful if the patient has not had a denture before and if the proposed new denture will be a different design to the existing denture. Patients tend to find this interesting and appreciate the thought that has gone into the making of their denture.
- Tooth modification will improve denture stability and avoid occlusal problems. Modifications include:
  - Rest seat and gully preparation, to make space for the minor connectors, clasps and rest seats to fit over the occlusal surfaces without propping the occlusion.
  - Guide planes give a specific path of insertion that can reduce the number of clasps required. Additionally, modifying the path of insertion can avoid compromising aesthetics with 'black triangles' on anterior saddles.
- Additive tooth preparation using composite resin to exaggerate cingulum shape to improve support for rest seats or produce undercuts for clasps.
- Tooth modifications can be planned and trialled on the primary cast. This allows you to see how much preparation you need, which can be difficult in the mouth. The cast can then be an aide-memoire for mouth preparation.
- Indirect restorations can have these modifications built in providing the denture is designed in advance and sufficient space is allowed when preparing the tooth.
- An occlusal registration or tooth try-in will be needed prior to crown preparation, either to match the porcelain shade or if the prepared tooth is the posterior occlusal contact (Fig. 31.1). The occlusal registration or try-in can then be transferred to the crown cast to ensure accurate articulation.
- Long-span anterior saddles will require a tooth try-in to establish tooth position for retention tags/backings and may affect decisions in the denture design.
- Ensure the denture design is finalised and all tooth preparation completed before recording the master impression.

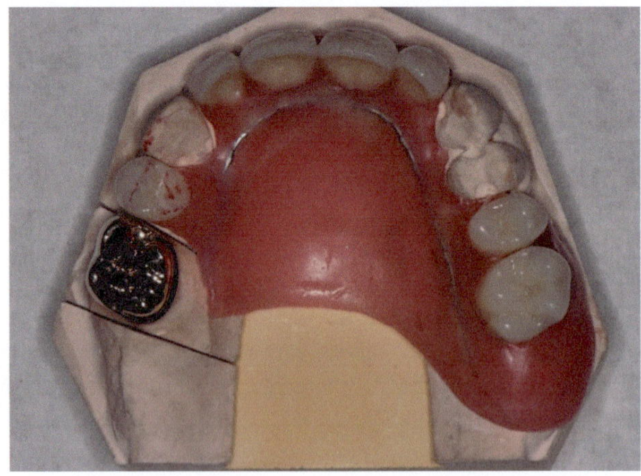

Fig. 31.1 Tooth try-in to establish anterior tooth position and convey required occlusion for fabrication of cast crown. Photograph Linda Blakely

31.4 Design for Hygiene

The weight of evidence is that the survival of the remaining teeth in the presence of RPDs is biological rather than mechanical (Fig. 31.2). This forms the basis of the Scandinavian approach to RPD design and provision [13].

Covering the gingival margins has a detrimental effect on periodontal health [7].

The focus when designing a denture should be on hygienic principles, which interfere as little as possible with plaque control and do not damage the oral tissues, in accordance with modern concepts of preventative dentistry [9].

- Avoid unnecessary gingival coverage.
- 3 mm rule: This is essential to reduce the risks of periodontal inflammation. The denture should have 3 mm or more clearance of the denture base and connectors from the teeth [14, 15]. This minimises plaque collection near the gingiva, allows saliva flow and gives access for interdental brushes with the denture in situ. This will be adjacent to premolars and molars and will not compromise aesthetics.
- To achieve the designed gingival clearance, the working cast will need careful blocking out, and good communication with the technician is essential.
- Simple and hygienic design of major connector that joins the saddles directly to keep clear [15] of gingival margins, maintaining 3 mm rule.
- In the upper, a mid-palatal strap and modifications work well.
- In the lower, the best options for hygiene are lingual bar, dental bar or sub-lingual bar.
- Lingual plate design is not hygienic and pose the highest risk to the remaining teeth and periodontal health.
- Two clasps only (one each side) are preferable.
- Connect cingulum rests laterally from the saddle and use horizontally approaching minor connectors and reciprocators to avoid covering the gingiva [15].
- Avoid using the baseplate/major connector for reciprocation. This covers the gingiva.

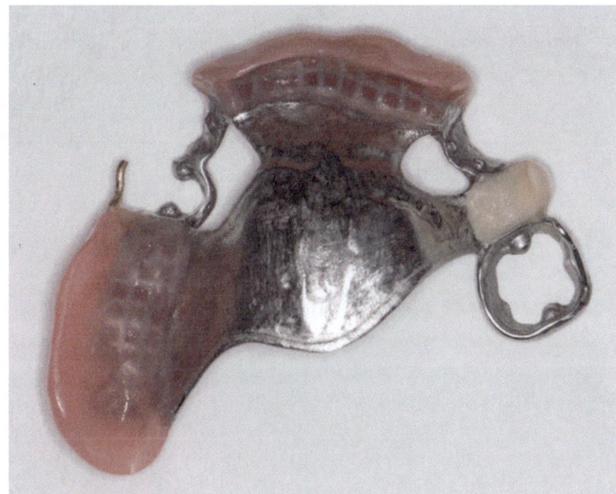

Fig. 31.2 RPD with good tooth and tissue support, hygienic major connector with horizontal minor connectors kept clear of the gingivae, two clasps for retention

31.5 Design for Stability and Comfort

Good biomechanics are essential to give the denture stability in function. If the denture is comfortable and less like a foreign body in the mouth, it is easier for the patient to adapt and accept the denture.

Good biomechanics also improve stress distribution and avoid trauma to the tissues.

- Support saddles optimally with rests; this includes anterior saddles.
- Rest seat preparation will improve the stability of the denture, control the loading on the teeth, prevent the teeth moving away from the framework and indicate to the laboratory the position for the rests. Preparing space for rest seats avoids occlusal interferences and further occlusal adjustment.
- Aim for four well-distributed areas of support (tooth or mucosal support).
- Provide good retention to resist displacement. Ideally, only two clasps are used, so their position needs careful planning to be effective. The use of guide surfaces facilitates use of fewer clasps. On premolars and canines, casts occlusally approaching clasps do not work in the longer term as there is not enough length for flexibility. Use a cast I-bar or a wrought clasp (stainless steel or gold).
- Ensure the clasp is reciprocated (see mouth preparation).
- If using C-clasps on single standing molars, ensure there is sufficient encirclement from the active clasp and reciprocating arm to prevent the tooth escaping from the clasp assembly. An alternative, the ring clasp will give better encirclement.
- The major and minor connectors, rests and bracing components should be rigid to control stress to abutments and tissues.
- The denture should not interfere with the patient's intercuspal position (ICP). Maintain guidance on natural teeth where possible.
- There should be simultaneous contact on closure with natural and denture teeth.
- The framework should have a good fit and be passive when seated to avoid pressure on the teeth.

Finally, review the overall design for simplicity and that the design conforms to hygienic principles and discuss with the patient.

31.6 Clinical Tips

31.6.1 Primary Impressions

Impressions are required that show good detail of the teeth and the alveolar ridges with a record of full sulcus depth to survey and plan the denture as well as for fabrication of accurate custom trays.

- Standard stock trays often do not allow for seating over the teeth with suitable adaption over the edentulous areas and palate, and sufficient extension into the sulci. Trays frequently require modification.
- This is easily achieved using inexpensive putty or compound over the edentulous span and palate in the upper. Trim away any material that has spread over the teeth for ease of reinsertion and to allow a thickness of alginate of at least 4 mm around the teeth to allow the material to deform elastically on removal. Warmed baseplate wax can also be added to the rim of stock trays to give extension to full sulcus depth adjacent to teeth or into lingual sulcus.
- Apply adhesive for an alginate wash ensuring it has dried before loading the alginate, avoiding overfilling the tray, reseat the tray back down to the putty and border mould.

31.6.2 Planning the Space

This is an important and often overlooked stage of the process. Deciding on the adjustments necessary at the outset as part of RPD provision is preferable to what may appear to the patient as unplanned post-insertion adjustments.

Using the primary casts, assess the occlusion and anything that may make the denture more challenging.

- Ensure there are no blips on the cast; this can add millimetres of inaccuracy when articulating the casts.
- If there are not enough remaining teeth to locate the casts accurately, preliminary rims will be needed. This will be the case with most distal extension saddles.
- Decide if there is an acceptable and stable ICP, and if it is best to conform.
- If the habitual ICP is compromised due to loss of vertical dimension, mandibular deviation and over-erupted teeth, this will often require a further aspect of treatment planning for restoration of occlusion in centric relation at an appropriate vertical dimension and suitable occlusal plane.
- If the denture is simply treated as gap filling exercise within an unfavourable occlusion, there will be a significant compromise on space for denture components, achieving a good occlusion and a stable denture.

31.6.3 Mouth Preparation

Small adjustments to the teeth can greatly improve the stability, function and comfort of the denture.

- Prepare rest seats—to create space for the rest to avoid an occlusal interference, blend with tooth contour and improve axial loading of the abutment.
- Bonded composite cingulum rests are useful on teeth with thin enamel (lower incisors/canines) and greatly improve support for lingual and dental bars where

good support is challenging in the lower arch. Bonded composite rest are reliable if placed under optimum bonding protocol [16].

- Bonded composite can be added on buccal surfaces to improve undercuts for clasp retention. This is best over a wide area and adjusted to provide appropriate depth of undercut (0.25 mm for cast chrome, 0.5 for wrought clasps).
- To achieve effective reciprocation, the tooth may need modification to provide a wider surface, so contact is maintained on the tooth preventing movement of the tooth as the clasp leaves the undercut.
- Guide surfaces limit path of insertion/displacement; this allows the use of fewer clasps. The fit and stability of the framework will be better. Take care not to encroach on 3 mm rule by preparing the guide surface within 3 mm of the gingiva.
- Prepare guide surfaces before rest seats.
- Prepare gullies to allow clasp arms to exit, to give space for occlusal approaching clasps (especially with worn dentitions). Opposing cusps may also need adjustment to create space.
- If crowns are required that will be in contact with the denture base, plan to incorporate rest seats, guide planes and undercuts in the crown, to work with denture design.

31.6.4 Secondary Impressions

It is important that the impression is accurate and captures the detail of the teeth, any preparations and correct sulcus depths.

- Use a rigid spaced custom tray.
- Use either lab-fabricated or chair side-added stops. This allows the required space to be maintained, the tray to be relocated to same position and held without movement during border moulding and whilst the final impression sets to avoid deformation of the impression material. Avoid positioning the stops over teeth with rest seat preparations for a more accurate impression.
- Check extension in sulcus depth and around frenal attachments giving 3 mm space for impression material.
- Interdental spaces should be blocked with soft wax or bite registration material to prevent the impression tearing. Check this material is not covering where the denture framework will contact.
- Do not overfill the tray with impression material and ensure tray is seated back down to the stops.
- Remove the set impression carefully to avoid distortion; breaking the seal on the distal aspect can help with this.
- Carefully inspect the impression for the absence of air blows and drags and that the detail of the mouth preparations has been recorded.

31.6.5 Occlusal Registration

In the authors' experience, this is a frequent cause of inaccuracies both for planning the denture and fabrication.

- Use hard base rims if possible; this is particularly helpful for the lower rim.
- Use full palatal coverage of rim for stability during registration, even if the final major connector will have less coverage.
- When anterior teeth are missing, trim the rim for correct incisal level and lip support. Where lower incisors are present, the palatal aspect of the upper rim should be reduced to allow closure at the correct vertical dimension whilst maintaining the wax for the incisal position as the guide for tooth setup.
- Using the warmed wax squash-bite approach is highly likely to introduce errors as the mucosally supported rim sinks into the tissues and possibly distorts. The articulated casts will not be in the same relationship as in the patient's mouth.
- Trim the rims so the opposing teeth cusps very lightly touch the rim without displacement or create a 1 mm gap. Use location notches if appropriate. A low viscosity material is used to finalise the registration. Tempbond or ZoE work well. Automix bite registration materials need to be used with care to avoid errors as there is a tendency for the material to extrude between opposing teeth. Ensure that the rims do not become displaced during registration and maintain gentle contact on the chin to avoid the patient opening as the registration material sets.
- Place the casts into the rims and check the record is the same as seen in the mouth. Automix registration material often needs trimming to ensure the opposing cusps are fully seated.

31.7 Try-In

The framework should seat fully with a positive, passive location, not rock or interfere with the patient's occlusion.

- If the framework does not fit, use fit-check silicone or powder occlusal spray to identify where the framework is binding and adjust. Take care when adjusting to avoid opening up space between the framework and teeth which would allow food ingress in function.
- A common area to cause binding is on the marginal ridge next to the rest seat.
- After adjustment if the framework does not fit acceptably, check any mouth preparations for sharp angles, adjust and retake the master impression.
- Once the framework is assessed as satisfactory, rims can be attached if a definitive jaw registration is required or proceed to a wax try-in of the teeth.

31.8 Fit and Review

- Use light-bodied silicone to check for over-extension for potential pressure areas on the fit surfaces of saddles. Carefully adjust the acrylic where it protrudes through the silicone.
- Allow time to demonstrate and ensure the patient is able to insert and remove the denture and not to use the clasps to remove the denture.
- Explain to the patient what to expect in terms of being aware of the denture, transitory effect on speech, possible increase in salivation and the time it may take to adapt. A forewarned patient is more likely to take any issues in their stride and less likely to react negatively to the denture.
- Give instruction on how to keep the denture clean.
- The intricate shape of chrome frameworks can be tricky to clean, particularly around the internal aspect of clasp assemblies. Large size interdental brushes are perfect for this.

31.9 Ongoing Care

Appointments with the hygienist are invaluable to reinforce oral hygiene measures to maintain gingival health which is essential for long-term prognosis of the remaining dentition [11].

Disclosing a denture and abutments can be very instructive to show the patient how they are managing and where to clean more effectively.

The denture should be reviewed at regular intervals, to ensure the fit remains good and there are no problems.

31.10 Conclusion

- Apply a problem-based approach to RPD provision.
- Get the mouth RPD ready and gift your patient a state-of-the-art denture combining hygienic design and good biomechanics.
- Successful RPD provision is a team effort between patient, clinician, hygienist and technician.
- Maintain the mouth and denture—It should not be fit and forget; encourage the patient to return for reviews and appropriate maintenance.

References

1. Adult Dental Health Survey. Oral health in the United Kingdom 1998. London: Palgrave Macmillan; 2000.
2. Graham R, Mihaylov S, Jepson N, Allen PF, Bond S. Determining 'need' for a removable partial denture: a qualitative study of factors that influence dentist provision and patient use. Br Dent J. 2006;200:155–8.
3. Allen PF, Jepson NJ, Doughty J, Bond S. Attitudes and practice in the provision of removable partial dentures. Br Dent J. 2008. https://doi.org/10.1038/bdj.2007.568.
4. Öwall B, Käyser AF, Carlsson G. Prosthodontics. In: Principles and management strategies. London: Mosby-Wolfe; 1996.
5. Addy M, Bates JF. Plaque accumulation following the wearing of different types of removable partial denture. J Oral Rehabil. 1979;6:111–7.
6. Tuominem K, Ranta PI. Wearing of removable partial dentures in relation to dental caries. J Oral Rehabil. 1988;15:515–20.
7. Zlatarić DK, Celebić A, Valentić-Peruzović M. The effect of removable partial dentures on periodontal health of abutment and non-abutment teeth. J Periodontol. 2002;73:137–44.
8. Petridis H, Hempton TJ. Periodontal considerations in removable partial denture treatment: a review of the literature. Int J Prosthodont. 2001;14:164–72.
9. Öwall B, Budtz-Jörgensen E, Davenport J, et al. Removable partial denture design: a need to focus on hygienic principles? Int J Prosthodont. 2002;15:371–7.
10. Jepson N, Thomason JM, Steele J. The influence of denture design on patient acceptance of partial dentures. Br Dent J. 1995;178:296–300.
11. Davenport JC, Hammond P, de Mattos MG. The acquisition and validation of removable partial denture knowledge. II. Design rules and expert reaction. J Oral Rehabil. 1996;23:811–24.
12. Davenport JC, Basker RM, Heath JR, Ralph JP, Glantz PO, Hammond P. A clinical guide to removable partial denture design. London: BDJ Books; 2000.
13. Thorén M, Gunne J. Textbook of removable prosthodontics – the Scandinavian approach. Copenhagen: Munksgaard Danmark; 2012.
14. Yeung AL, Lo EC, Chow TW, Clark RK. Oral health status of patients 5–6 years after placement of cobalt-chromium removable partial dentures. J Oral Rehabil. 2000;27:183–9.
15. Stilwell CE. Revisiting the principles of partial denture design. Dent Update. 2010;37:651–712.
16. Janus CE, Unger JW, Crabtree DG, McCasland JP. A retrospective study of resin-bonded cingulum rest seats. J Prosthodont. 1996;5:91–4.

32 Acrylic Removable Partial Dentures

L. Blakely, W. A. V. Beare, and Ewen McColl

Learning Points
- Understand aspects of acrylic partial dentures that make them inherently more likely to result in plaque retention and tooth loss.
- Appreciate methods in minimising comorbidity in acrylic partial denture design and construction.
- Recall design features that are important for retention, stability and support.

32.1 Introduction

To provide a suitably strong denture, Acrylic Removable Partial Dentures (ARPDs) are inherently bulkier and have greater tissue coverage, resulting in a more plaque-retentive denture that may contribute to increased caries incidence and periodontal breakdown, with subsequent tooth loss [1]. The majority of ARPDs provided are mucosal borne, with potential for occlusal load to be transmitted directly to the underlying tissues, damaging the supporting structures.

The risk of prosthesis failure through biologic damage is higher with ARPDs, as adhering to hygienic principles is more challenging. Whilst not ideal, we will discuss ways of mitigating risk to the patient's oral health when providing ARPDs.

L. Blakely
Spring Hill Specialist Dental Centre, Devon, UK

Derriford Dental Education Facility, Plymouth Science Park (University of Plymouth), Plymouth, UK

W. A. V. Beare
Derriford Dental Education Facility, Plymouth Science Park (University of Plymouth), Plymouth, UK

E. McColl (✉)
Peninsula Dental School, Plymouth, UK
e-mail: ewen.mccoll@plymouth.ac.uk

E. McColl, A. Alani (eds.), *Practical Tips in Clinical Dentistry*, BDJ Clinician's Guides, https://doi.org/10.1007/978-3-031-90355-7_32

Traditionally, ARPDs have been used as interim prostheses to maintain appearance and function immediately after extractions or as part of a stabilisation phase whilst other restorative and periodontal treatment is carried out, before providing a definitive prosthesis. Additionally, with a failing dentition, APRDs can be used as a transitional trainer denture, allowing ease of additions to the denture and a period of adaption prior to the final complete denture.

In clinical practice, far more acrylic dentures are made than chrome framework dentures, and a significant proportion of these dentures are intended as definitive dentures [1]. Additionally, for many patients, an ARPD may be chosen as a cost-effective treatment option.

32.2 Upper Acrylic Dentures

Good design of an ARPD should aim to minimise the disadvantages of this type of denture. This, combined with good oral hygiene, can allow an upper ARPD to function well over a prolonged period of time [2].

The classic 'Every' denture [3] was proposed when clinical observation noted that provision of partial dentures resulted in aggravating existing decay and periodontal infection and the belief that lateral loads on the remaining teeth caused damage to the supporting structures. Although this was based on an earlier understanding of the pathogenesis of dental disease, the design features advocated were the foundation for considering an approach to denture design that minimised the potential damage from wearing a denture.

The Every denture is a claspless design for upper-bounded saddle dentures. The saddles have wide embrasures and the baseplate is kept a minimum 3 mm clear of the remaining teeth [4]. This concept is a hygienic design. The drawback is that this denture design has no tooth support and does not include distal extension saddles.

The best approach is to use some of the design principles of the Every denture, combined with additional features to improve retention and support, so limiting iatrogenic damage [5].

When providing an ARPD, specific design decisions need to be made to ensure the denture is as hygienic a design as possible (Fig. 32.1). As there is less potential for tooth support, the denture base requires broad extension to distribute load and improve rigidity and strength.

The design should not be delegated to the laboratory but requires clear instruction and communication with the technician [6].

The design sequence and principles for planning components is the same as metal framework dentures.

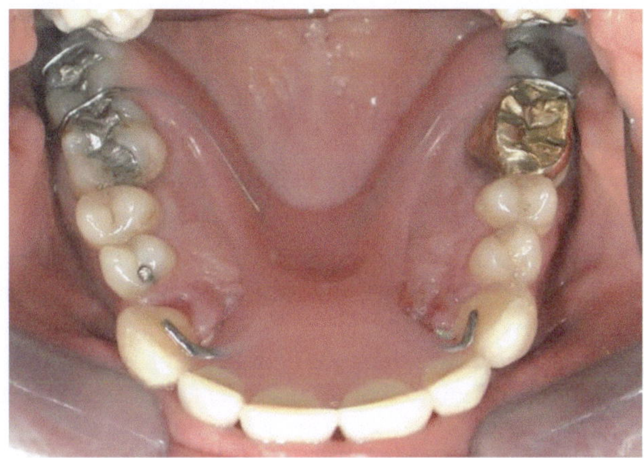

Fig. 32.1 Modern ARPD, made to hygienic principles with good support. (Image courtesy of Charlotte Stilwell)

32.3 Design for Support and Stability

- Optimise mucosal support by using a major connector that covers the centre of the palate. An area of 5 cm^2 in the midline of the palate remains stable, with no resorption recorded after many years post extraction [7]. This will provide longer-term stability.
- For distal extension saddle dentures, the amount of mucosal support should be increased.
- With distal extension saddle dentures, it is essential for both support and bracing that the saddle base extends to the hamular notch and full sulcus depth [8].
- With bilateral distal extension saddle dentures, the posterior border should extend to the post dam [8].
- Tooth support can be provided on anterior abutment teeth (canines, incisors) by extending the acrylic of the denture base onto the cingulum area. On posterior teeth, where the design indicates contact with the major connector, the acrylic should finish above the survey line [9].
- Support on posterior teeth can be from a rest made of half round stainless steel.
- Direct retention in the main comes from good adaption of the fit surface to the mucosa and the cohesive retention from saliva. Contacts between abutments and denture need to be tight but passive. The polished surfaces should be shaped to assist the patient to gain muscular control.
- Direct retention can be enhanced by preformed wrought wire clasps positioned to engage undercuts, either occlusal or gingival approaching, or a ring clasp (for lone-standing teeth). The clasps are embedded into the acrylic.

- Ball-ended clasps, C-clasps and Adams clasps that originate from the major connector can also be used and additionally provide some vertical support where they cross the teeth.
- Reciprocation for clasps is most effectively provided by the acrylic base plate that should finish on and above the survey line, except for ring clasps (self-reciprocating).
- Retention and stability can be enhanced by the use of guide planes (see part 1) and close contact between saddle and natural abutment teeth.
- Where the denture base contacts the natural teeth, ensure that acrylic collets finish above the survey line and have an accurate fit to help resist denture movement during loading and minimise the risk of 'gum stripping' [8].
- Indirect retention will improve denture stability. With bounded saddles, this can be achieved with baseplate extension on abutments taken onto the cingulum or finishing above the survey line. With bilateral distal extension dentures, extend the baseplate to use the remaining teeth (this also improves tooth support). The compromise is additional tissue coverage.
- The denture occlusion should not interfere with the patient's intercuspal position (ICP). The occlusion should be carefully planned and adjusted, aiming for light contacts in ICP, as heavy contacts will drive the denture down into the mucosa, causing discomfort and tissue damage.
- Maintain the natural tooth guidance and adjust the denture to avoid lateral interference that will create lateral stress and reduce stability [4].

32.4 Design for Hygiene

- Plan the design to leave as much gingival tissue uncovered, compatible with providing support and indirect retention.
- The denture base should be kept at least 3 mm clear of the gingival margins [8], except in areas where the major connector is providing cingulum rest support or reciprocation.
- With single-standing teeth between saddles, it may not be practical to have 3 mm clearance.
- Where the major connector joins a saddle, the acrylic should cross at 90° [8].
- Where the denture base contacts natural teeth, ensure that acrylic collets finish above the survey line and have an accurate fit to prevent food packing and periodontal damage [8].
- The denture base should have a pin-dam to minimise food ingress [8].

The traditional 'Spoon' denture, used to replace single or few anterior teeth, is not advised. Whilst this is a hygienic design, there is a risk of inhalation or ingestion. The size of the denture is an important risk factor for this serious adverse event [10]. A safer design is one modified to extend the major connector bilaterally to the palatal aspect of a molar and add wrought clasps.

An ARPD with a 'horseshoe' shape design should be avoided. This design combines extensive gingival coverage with support mostly provided by the alveolar ridges that will resorb over time. The risk is that as the denture sinks, the hard and soft tissues will be damaged; this can cause 'gum stripping'.

32.5 Lower ARPD

Due to the poor strength of acrylic, the major connector has to cover all the abutment surfaces and no clearance of the gingiva is possible. The lingual plate design results in significantly higher plaque deposition than other major connectors [11] with the potential for caries and periodontal inflammation (Fig. 32.2). There is less available tissue support to start with, and with alveolar ridge resorption, the saddle will 'sink' into the tissues and a higher risk, the denture will strip the gum away from the abutment teeth.

Consequently, lower ARPDs are only appropriate for interim or transitional dentures.

To minimise the potential damage during the interim phase, the following design features should be incorporated:

- Optimum tissue support for distal extension saddle dentures to include support from the buccal shelves, extension onto the retromolar pad.
- Wrought wire clasps for retention.
- Wrought wire rests for support. Modified ball clasps can also be used [2]. Tooth support is more effective with bounded saddles.
- Ball-ended clasps can be helpful providing vertical support for Class IV immediate replacement temporary dentures, where tissue support is extremely poor.
- Collets with a good fit around the remaining teeth and finishing above the survey line.

An often-omitted stage of denture construction is blocking out unnecessary undercuts and duplicating the cast prior to processing the denture.

Whilst this can increase fabrication costs, there will be considerable saving on the time of chairside adjustments. Multiple saddle dentures, with each saddle

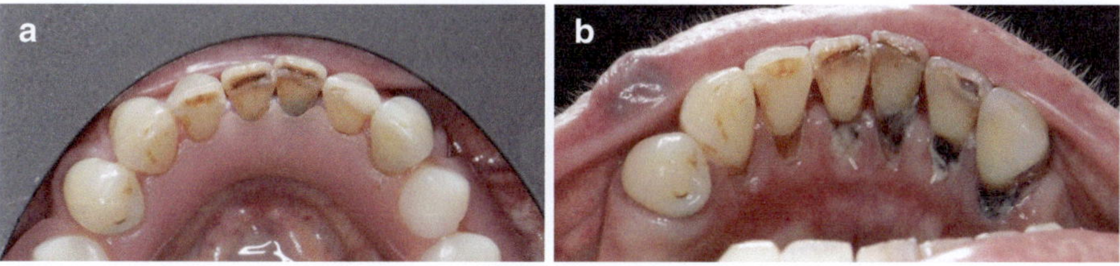

Fig. 32.2 **a & b** Caries and gum stripping caused by a poorly supported denture and a lingual plate with poor fit of collets. (Image courtesy of Linda Blakely)

having a conflicting path of insertion, can be quite time-consuming to fit. Inaccurate adjustments of the collets and denture base results in gaps between the denture and teeth resulting in food packing, reduced retention and stability, with increased potential for tissue damage [1]. This negates the benefits of the considered design. Blocking out the cast does give gingival relief, but this is not associated with a greater risk of deterioration in gingival health [12].

On fitting the denture, adjustment should be required to enable the denture to be seated, from the fit surface look for undercuts that conflict with the path of insertions, and carefully adjust. Do not adjust the occlusal aspect of any collets as this will open up a space between denture and tooth.

ARPDs may be more prone to causing sore areas. Use light-bodied silicone to check the fitting surface and flange borders, and carefully adjust where indicated.

Reiterate the value of continued hygiene support and review of the denture fit [2].

32.6 Conclusions

Whilst a poorly designed and constructed ARPD can compromise a patient's oral health, the ARPD remains an important modality for replacing missing teeth. Finance may preclude more complex replacement options, and for many patients, an acrylic denture may be the only option available, so incorporating our tips will hopefully increase the chance of a long-term successful outcome in such patients.

References

1. Walmsley AD. Acrylic partial dentures. Dent Update. 2003;30:424–9.
2. McCartney JW, Fisks S. The all-acrylic resin mandibular removable partial denture: design considerations. J Prosthet Dent. 1997;77:638.
3. Every RG. The elimination of destructive forces in replacing teeth with partial dentures. N Z Dent J. 1949;45:207–14.
4. Dyer M. The 'Every' type acrylic partial denture. Dental Pract Dent Rec. 1972;22:339–41.
5. Wilson VJ. Acrylic partial dentures—interim or permanent prostheses? SADJ 2009; 64: 434, 436–438, 440.
6. Davenport JC, Basker RM, Heath JR, Ralph JP, Glantz PO. Communication between the dentist and dental technician. Br Dent J. 2000;189:471–4.
7. Watt DM, MacGregor AR. Designing complete dentures. WB Saunders Co.; 1976.
8. Davenport JC, Basker RM, Heath JR, Ralph JP, Glantz PO. A clinical guide to designing removable partial dentures. BDJ Books; 2000.
9. Stilwell CE. Modern RPDs; a serious option. Schottlander course manual, 2006.
10. Jagger R. Swallowed and inhaled dentures—What's the problem? Dent Update. 2014;41:882–90.
11. Bates M, Addy JF. Plaque accumulation following the wearing of different types of removable partial dentures. J Oral Rehabil. 1979;6:111–7.
12. Orr S, Linden GJ, Newman HN. The effect of partial denture connectors on gingival health. J Clin Periodontol. 1992;19:589–94.

Distal Extension Saddle Dentures

33

L. Blakely, W. A. V. Beare, and Ewen McColl

Learning Points

- Understand the biomechanical challenge distal extension saddles represent to the natural dentition and especially the abutment unit.
- Understand design techniques to mitigate issues with the natural dentition and the support tissues in this pattern of edentulism.
- Appreciate the relative differences in the process of construction, delivery and maintenance that make distal extension saddle dentures different to other denture designs.

33.1 Introduction

The distal extension saddle (DES) denture presents a technically demanding challenge for dentists to construct and a challenge for patients to wear! Problems arise due to the differing response of teeth and mucosa to occlusal load and lack of tooth support and direct retention at the distal end of the saddle. This creates instability, with the potential movement leading to unfavourable stress on abutment teeth and supporting tissues. Movement of the denture will make the denture uncomfortable

L. Blakely
Spring Hill Specialist Dental Centre, Tavistock, Devon, UK

Derriford Dental Education Facility, Plymouth Science Park (University of Plymouth), Plymouth, UK

W. A. V. Beare
Derriford Dental Education Facility, Plymouth Science Park (University of Plymouth), Plymouth, UK

E. McColl (✉)
Peninsula Dental School, Plymouth, UK
e-mail: ewen.mccoll@plymouth.ac.uk

E. McColl, A. Alani (eds.), *Practical Tips in Clinical Dentistry*, BDJ Clinician's Guides, https://doi.org/10.1007/978-3-031-90355-7_33

to wear. Not surprisingly, DES dentures have a higher failure rate than bounded saddle dentures, and this failure rate is significantly higher for lower dentures [1].

Where a less-than-complete dentition can satisfy a patient's functional needs, many DES dentures are not worn [2].

Of relevance today are the risks of using DES removable partial dentures (RPDs) within the ageing population. This can cause a fourfold increase in new root caries in elderly patients compared with restoration with bridges [3]. A better option for older patients may be maintaining or improving an SDA (shortened dental arch) with simple fixed prostheses, including resin-bonded bridgework [4].

DES RPDs may be helpful in managing an extreme SDA and can provide improved stability for an upper complete denture [5]. The evidence does not support that DES can contribute to occlusal stability or improve masticatory efficiency [6, 7].

33.2 Clinical Tips

A decision to make a denture should be patient led with the patient understanding the time and effort required to learn to adapt to the challenges of this denture design.

If the denture is to be accepted, not be uncomfortable or the cause of damage to the remaining teeth and oral tissues, the design needs careful planning by the clinician. Do not leave design decisions to the laboratory. Considered design and tooth preparation can greatly improve the fit and stability of the denture. Unfortunately, over 70% of dentures are made without this benefit [8]. Following the fundamentals as described in part one of this series is crucial, in addition to the following tips which will help optimising the chances for success.

33.3 Design for Hygiene

- Do not cover or cross gingival margins wherever possible.
- Join connectors directly to the saddle and leave at least 3 mm clearance between connector and gingival margin [9].
- To achieve the required hygienic 3 mm clearance, and avoiding wrapping the components around the abutments, the cast will need careful blocking out.
- In the lower arch, the best options for hygiene are lingual bar, dental bar and sublingual bar.
- Dental bars are preferable where there is lower lingual gingival recession, and the sulcus is reduced. A dental bar avoids covering vulnerable root surfaces.
- Lower lingual plate designs are not hygienic and pose the highest biologic risk to the remaining teeth.

33.4 Design for Comfort and Stability

Good biomechanics aim to manage the high loads on the saddle and control the lateral and rotational loads in function.

All DES RPDs require greater tissue support than bounded saddle RPDs and should cover as wide an area as possible.

With all distal extension saddles, consider using the two abutments adjacent to the saddle to increase tooth support [9].

Direct retention will be more effective if the clasps are placed close to the saddle.

Unilateral distal extension RPDs will be significantly more stable if there is cross-arch support and ideally four widely distributed areas of support.

There should be simultaneous contact on closure with natural and denture teeth. Avoid heavy contacts on the saddle that cause movement by driving the DES into the tissues and lifting the chrome framework off the teeth.

Where possible, maintain lateral guidance on the natural teeth. Design the occlusion so there are light contacts in intercuspal position (ICP), but in lateral movement, the denture teeth are separated to avoid lateral force on the denture saddle. This may not be possible if the pattern of tooth loss is such that there are no natural tooth antagonists.

33.5 Upper

- Extend DES saddles to hamular notch and around the tuberosity for support, stability and bracing [10].
- A bilateral DES RPD should have greater tissue coverage, utilising the posterior palate, to provide sufficient support (Fig. 33.1). Extend the denture to the vibrating line. An acrylic post dam will enhance physical retention (as per complete denture) and facilitates a reline when required. This will also resist rotational movement around the clasp axis.

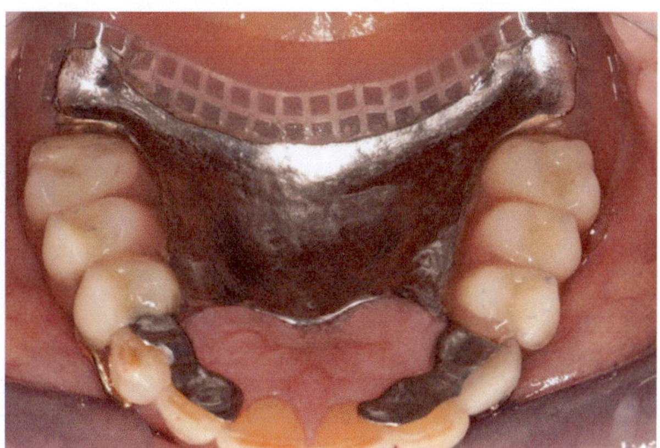

Fig. 33.1 Upper bilateral DES denture, showing extension to acrylic post dam, anterior palate uncovered and optimum tooth support with hygienic horizontally approaching minor connectors to join rests to the saddle. The chrome occlusal surface was to accommodate lower tilted molars. (Photograph Linda Blakely)

- Aim to avoid covering the anterior part of the palate if possible. This avoids interference with speech and is less irritating for the patient [10].
- With unilateral DES RPDs, a modified mid-palatal strap major connector in the vault of the palate is a good choice; it is a simple shape and can be made rigid.

33.6 Lower

- Optimum extension of the saddle base is essential! This should include coverage of the buccal shelves, and extension onto the retromolar pad, to gain stable support from non-alveolar bone. Full extension into the functional sulci will assist with bracing against lateral forces in function. The shape of the saddle base should be the same as the posterior part of a complete denture.
- Saddles should be adapted to the neutral zone and flanges contoured to assist muscular control.
- Reduce the width and length of the occlusal table. This reduces load on the ridge. Omitting the last molar creates space and allows the tongue and cheek to assist retention.
- Ensure good tooth support (see above). Rest seat preparation will give axial loading to the abutments and improve the stability of the denture.
- Guide planes also assist retention and stability of the denture; this small contribution can be helpful in the lower arch.
- Clasps on premolars and canines can be cast chrome I-bars or wrought clasps that can be gingival or occlusally approaching. Careful clasp tip positioning will, in addition to retention, help avoid the saddle moving distally away from the abutments.
- Avoid using a plate design/extension of saddle for clasp reciprocation; this is not hygienic.
- The mandibular major connector should be rigid [10]. Ensure there is sufficient thickness of chrome to achieve this.
- Dental bars combined with additive composite rests provide excellent overall support [9] for DES (Fig. 33.2). The fit of the dental bar over the composite rests will resist distal movement of the denture away from the teeth. The rests need to be shaped to share the same path of insertion.

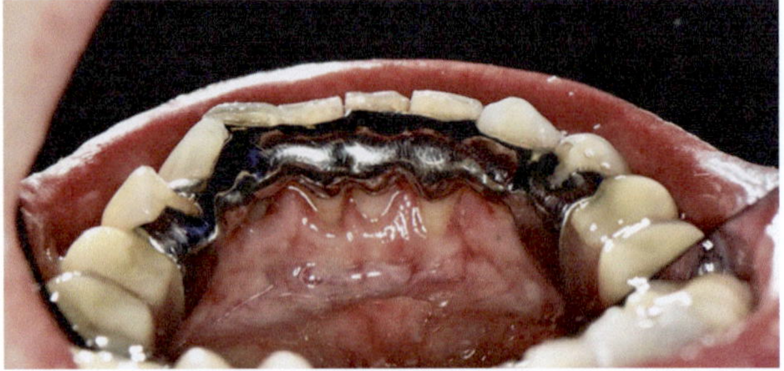

Fig. 33.2 Dental bar supported by composite rests at 10-year review. Bar is clear of gingival margins, and with ongoing hygiene care, the periodontal health has not deteriorated. (Photograph Linda Blakely)

- With longer spans of major connector, combine a dental bar and lingual bar to maintain rigidity with a hygienic design [9].

Due to the lack of a distal abutment, there will be more denture movement. This will be movement towards the ridge with displacement and compression of the tissue under occlusal loading, and movement away for the tissue when chewing sticky food.

Movement of the DES away from the tissues will occur around an axis between the clasp tips and it is usual to provide indirect retention to resist this.

The indirect retainer comprises a rest seat anterior to the rotation axis and as far away from it as practicable.

- Dental bars can provide ample indirect retention.
- Lingual bars and sublingual bars require an additional component to provide indirect retention. A hygienic option is to connect the indirect retention rest directly to the saddle with a horizontal approach. This avoids crossing the gingival margin and simplifies the design.
- The traditional Cummer arm indirect retainer covers the gingiva and, if placed on the tooth adjacent to the primary abutment, may not give the required 5 mm clearance between minor connectors, creating a food trap and tongue irritant [10].
- If the indirect retainer is placed on an anterior tooth, a rest seat should be prepared or added to avoid force on the inclined tooth surface resulting in unwanted tooth movement [10].

These rotational movements of the saddle in function can potentially impart undue stress on the abutment teeth. A design suggestion for minimising stress on the abutment is the RPI system (mesial occlusal rest, distal guide plane and I-bar). However, this cannot be used to mitigate shortcomings in the stability of the overall design, such as under-extended saddle bases and inadequate tooth support. More recent research indicates that if plaque control is good with no periodontal inflammation, and hygienic design principles applied with overall good support for the denture, then the forces on the abutments will not cause attachment loss [11]. This supports the need to ensure good plaque control at the outset and arrange appropriate ongoing hygiene care.

Traditionally, the altered cast technique, a two-stage technique, has been advocated as a method to record the differential support provided by teeth and the support that can be obtained from the more displaceable edentulous ridge. The aim was to improve load distribution and increase stability of the denture.

However, it has been found that a one-piece impression can offer base support equal to that of an altered cast impression technique. Achieving this depends on the quality of the definitive impression, fit of the framework checked under magnification and extension of the bases onto anatomic landmarks [12].

The authors find it easier to do this one-piece impression in two stages. This allows focus on recording the anatomic landmarks of the saddle separately (as per complete denture), and then subsequently recording the details of the teeth and tooth preparations.

A spaced tray with stops is fabricated on the primary cast. The extension is checked in the mouth and adjusted if necessary. The distal extension and lingual border are border moulded and then an impression made of the saddle area. Trim the set impression material to give 4 mm clearance from the teeth; this allows a suitable thickness for the wash impression material over the teeth and ease of reinsertion. A second stage wash impression will record the teeth and preparations. The tray can then be reseated to the same place and held firmly down over the saddle area whilst the border moulding is repeated and until the wash impression sets. This provides an undisplaced impression of the teeth and a displaced impression of the tissue of the distal extension. The authors prefer greenstick and medium-bodied silicone for the saddle/lingual area and a lighter-bodied silicone or alginate for the secondary wash.

33.7 Conclusions

As with all dentures, regular review is important to ensure that the denture is functioning well and oral hygiene remains good. Due to the potential for greater alveolar resorption in the mandible, the denture should be regularly assessed for saddle fit, and the need for reline, which will be more frequent. This will maintain denture stability and minimise tissue damage in the longer term.

References

1. Vanzeveren C, D'Hoore W, Bercy P, Leloup G. Treatment with removable partial dentures: a longitudinal study. Part 1. J Oral Rehabil. 2003;30:447–58.
2. Elias AC, Sheiham A. The relationship between satisfaction with mouth and number and position of teeth. J Oral Rehabil. 1998;25:649–61.
3. Jepson NJA, Moynihan PJ, Kelly PJ, Watson GW, Thomason JM. Caries incidence following restoration of shortened lower dental arches in a randomised controlled trial. Br Dent J. 2001;191:140–4.
4. Jepson NJA, Allen PF. Short and sticky options in the treatment of the partially dentate patient. Br Dent J. 1999;187:646–52.
5. Wöstmann B, Budtz-Jørgensen E, Jepson N, et al. Indications for removable partial dentures: a literature review. Int J Prosthodont. 2005;18:139–45.
6. Witter DJ, De Hann AFJ, Kayser AF, Van Rossum GMJM. A 6-year follow-up study of oral function in shortened dental arches. Part 1: occlusal stability. J Oral Rehabil. 1994;21:113–25.
7. Witter DJ, Cramwinckel AB, Van Rossum GMJM, Kayser AF. Shortened dental arches and masticatory ability. J Dent. 1990;18:185–7.
8. Nassani MZ, Devlin H, Tarakji J, McCord JF. Designing cobalt chromium removable partial dentures for patients with shortened dental arches—a pilot study. J Oral Rehabil. 2011;38:608–14.
9. Stilwell C. Revisiting the principles of partial denture design. Dent Update. 2010;37:682–90.

10. Davenport JC, Hammond P, de Mattos MG. The acquisition and validation of removable partial denture design knowledge. II. Design rules and expert reaction. J Oral Rehabil. 1996;23:811–24.
11. Haralambos P, Hempton TJ. Periodontal considerations in removable partial denture treatment: a literature review. Int J Prosthodont. 2001;14:164–72.
12. Frank RP, Brudvik JS, Noonan CJ. Clinical outcome of the altered cast impression procedure compared with the use of the one-piece cast. J Prosthet Dent. 2004;91:468–76.

Complete Denture Prosthetics: Core Principles

34

L. Blakely, W. A. V. Beare, A. Harris, and Ewen McColl

Learning Points

- Appreciate the importance of communication and dialogue when discussing the prospect of a new complete denture, taking note of specific cues that may provide insight into the problem.
- Understand ways in which modifications to the current denture, temporary or definitive, can inform the subsequent complete denture construction.
- Recall techniques in making an impression that is adequately extended with the requisite detail and anatomical features that will allow for baseplate creation.
- Recognise the key role jaw relations play in the creation of a successful complete denture and how best to register these once established.

34.1 Introduction

Edentulism can have a significant impact on a patient's ability to eat, speak and socialise effectively [1]. Complete denture prosthetics (CDP) refers to the body of knowledge and skills pertaining to the restoration of a patient's edentulous arches

L. Blakely
Spring Hill Specialist Dental Centre, Tavistock, Devon, UK

W. A. V. Beare
Derriford Dental Education Facility, Plymouth Science Park (University of Plymouth), Plymouth, UK

A. Harris
Peninsula Dental School (University of Plymouth), Derriford Dental Education Facility, Plymouth Science Park, Plymouth, UK

E. McColl (✉)
Peninsula Dental School, Plymouth, UK
e-mail: ewen.mccoll@plymouth.ac.uk

E. McColl, A. Alani (eds.), *Practical Tips in Clinical Dentistry*, BDJ Clinician's Guides, https://doi.org/10.1007/978-3-031-90355-7_34

with complete dentures [2]. It is a complex discipline where the art and science of dentistry combine and often presents many challenges to clinicians.

Whilst the majority of edentulous patients can expect an enhanced quality of life after the completion of conventional complete denture construction [3], 10–20% of patients report dissatisfaction [4]. Common complete denture referrals to secondary care often concern loose dentures related to resorbed mandibular ridges, complicated by high expectations and low coping ability [5]. Examination of such patients often reveals further compounding factors of incorrect base extension, poor adaptation of denture bases to tissues and inaccuracy of the retruded jaw registration.

This short article will hopefully provide primary care practitioners with helpful tips to avoid these common errors in complete denture prosthetics cognisant of the complexities involved.

34.2 Initial Consultation

The authors consider this the most important stage of CDP:

- Listen to the patient to gain understanding of their concerns, expectations, motivation and attitude to dentures as always being empathetic with insight into the patient's perspective is of benefit. Good clinical skills allied with effective communication skills have been associated with improved prognoses of complete denture treatment [6].
- A comprehensive history, thorough examination of the denture-bearing tissues and assessment of the denture design should follow. The clinician should ask: Is this a previously satisfactory denture that requires replacement? Or have there been a number of unsatisfactory dentures with this perceived fault? Identifying the fault and determining a treatment strategy to overcome this is crucial to success.
- Similarly, the clinician should establish: Is this a denture design fault that can be remedied with a different approach? Or a patient with reduced adaptive capacity (e.g., the 'frail elder'), a patient with unreasonable expectations or one who will never be happy with conventional dentures?

34.3 Therapeutic Diagnostics

This is a process of testing remedial changes prior to denture construction [7]. It aids the clinician in assessing the likely success of proposed alterations, improving patient understanding and aiding consent. The addition of baseplate wax to the patient's existing denture, moulded to the tissues at the proposed new extension, extending the upper denture to the vibrating line or the lower denture to the retromolar pads can demonstrate the precise extent of change and is helpful for the patient to perceive the improvement in retention and stability. This can be supplemented with a thin wash in light-bodied silicone to address any deficiency in fit surface.

Such diagnostic modification of dentures may be reversible or irreversible.

Other examples of reversible diagnostic changes are:

- Relining using a tissue conditioner to improve tissue adaption and extension.
- Using occlusal pivots to obtain even occlusal contact.
- Improving lip support and incisal position and increasing the occlusal vertical dimension (OVD) by adding baseplate or carding wax over the six upper anterior denture teeth and occlusal aspect of lower denture. A preliminary record of the proposed incisal position can be recorded with an Alma Gauge for future rim prescription.

Whilst the authors would not recommend carrying out irreversible alterations unless you are confident of the result, irreversible changes include:

- A chairside reline of the existing denture to improve extension.
- Removing lingual cusps of lower posterior teeth to improve tongue space and polished surface contour.
- Creating a mentalis groove.

Such changes will aid in formulating a diagnosis and dcvcloping a treatment plan. This in turn should lead to a discussion with the patient as to the likely success of the treatment. Document your findings and conversation with the patient and obtain consent for treatment.

34.4 Impression Taking

- Avoid making a denture on a primary cast; this is likely to combine errors of both under- and overextension, reducing retention, and cause instability. A primary impression should be overextended to record all the potential area of support for the denture and show the landmarks for customised tray fabrication. A muco-displacive impression material such as a condensation-cured silicone putty works well. It is sufficiently viscous to displace the tongue and record mylohyoid anatomy, as well as the full depth of the buccal sulci. The frena will require firm manipulation to give accurate reproduction.
- Developing a good primary impression may be seen as a valuable investment of time and is crucial in determining the quality of all subsequent stages.
- Whether designing a close fitting or spaced tray, draw the desired outline on the cast. This should ideally be 2–3 mm short of the sulcus to allow border moulding.
- To help resist distal displacement, the lower denture should cover the lower two-thirds of the retromolar pad. On the model, draw a line from this point at 45° to an imaginary line along the lower ridge crest extended buccally to the external oblique ridge. The special tray should not extend beyond this line to avoid displacement by the masseter. More recent work suggests providing a notch in the custom tray at the buccal base of the retromolar pad to relieve around the Someya

Sinew String, which can be observed in 10% of patients [8]. Design stub (vertical) handles to avoid displacing the lips, especially with the lower tray.
- Always check the tray in the mouth and adjust to ensure there is no overextension; this is most likely to occur around the frenal attachments and in the post mylohyoid fossa.
- Ask the lab to space the tray with one layer of modelling wax (1.25 mm thick) and to leave the wax in the tray. Trim away 4 mm of wax from the tray margin and border mould the tray. Remove the remaining wax before using light-body vinyl polysiloxane (VPS) impression material to record the impression.
- The authors prefer a spaced tray for silicone impressions. Close-fitting impression trays work well with ZnO Eugenol impression, but VPS impressions benefit from having more space for the material to flow.

The vast majority of retention for an upper denture is provided by the peripheral seal from the full depth and width of the posterior buccal sulcus around the tuberosity and from compression of the tissues in the post-dam area.

- Use separate stage border moulding with either VPS or green stick compound to capture this. Failure to capture the width of the sulcus results in a denture with a thin flange, missing the opportunity to use the cheek tissue to maximise the peripheral seal. Additionally, tissue compression by the post dam prevents the wash impression slumping away from the tissues during the setting. Having taken the trouble to capture the detail, after disinfection, use an indelible pen to mark the extent of the height and width of sulcus to be retained on the cast; this will guide the technician to retain the correct extension.

34.5 Jaw Relations

Obtaining the best-quality impression is the foundation for denture success, providing stable bases on which to record the jaw relationship. The purpose of occlusal registration is not just to record the vertical dimension but to shape the rims to communicate to the technician the position of the teeth for aesthetics and function.

- Ensure the rims are constructed on the more accurate master and not the primary cast.
- Reference the existing dentures to decide on aspects to keep or change, including information obtained via therapeutic diagnostics. Further information can be obtained from dentate photographs and biometric guides [9].
- Shape the upper rim first for aesthetics and good lip support. Be aware that placing upper teeth too far palatally will have an effect on lower tooth position and compromise denture stability.

- Align the upper rim to the naso-tragal line and inter-pupillary line. Check when the patient smiles the rim is harmonious with the lower lip.
- Lower teeth should be set over the ridge and in the neutral zone for stability. A common error is setting lower posterior teeth with lingual inclination and lower anterior teeth too far forward of the ridge.
- Respect the skeletal base relationship, as setting a Class 11 patient in a Class 1 setup will cause instability of the dentures. Class 11 patients often have an active mentalis muscle, and care is required in positioning the lower incisors. This may require either a horizontal space to allow the mentalis to contract without displacing the denture or retroclined teeth. The labial flange should not be bulky.
- If using conventional rims, at the start, trim the 'heels' from the distal aspect of upper and lower rims. This will greatly reduce inadvertent tipping of the rims and minimise occlusal errors.
- All patients require bilateral simultaneous contact on closure. Carefully trim the rims to achieve this at the chosen OVD. Ensure adequate freeway space has been provided, taking several measurements to confirm. Rehearse closure into centric relation (CR) with the patient. A line can be marked on the rim to assess reproducibility. Reproducibility shows you have found centric relation.
- When difficulty recording the retruded record is anticipated, remove the lower denture on arrival or place a cotton wool roll between the dentures. This allows some deprogramming to occur. Use the 'Fish' exercise and ask the patient to open and close without the lower denture in place as fast as they can; encourage maximum opening each time. When the patient's muscles have been exhausted, manipulate them into their retruded contact position (RCP) and record your jaw relationship. An alternate means of deprogramming is to use 'occlusal pivots' as a therapeutic diagnostic on the old dentures. Roughen up the occlusal surfaces of the lower first and second premolars on each side of the denture. Add some composite bond to the rough surface and a mound of composite on it. Have the patient close up gently in RCP so they indent the composite with no other tooth contact. Cure the composite with the patient in this occlusal position. Smooth and polish the mound, removing excess composite but ensuring there is even contact on both left and right sides. Allow the patient to wear the denture for a few days. Most patients will benefit from increased stability of the lower denture as the even contact on closure will reseat the denture correctly on its supporting tissues.
- Care should be taken to avoid increasing the vertical dimension. Cut four V-shaped notches in each rim. Wax is notoriously unreliable as a registration material so use a bite registration paste. Place some silicone adhesive on the lower rim and Vaseline on the upper rim. This allows you to check the reproducibility of your recording. Once completed, replace the rims on the casts and check that they seat correctly, removing any spare plaster that gets in the way but taking care not to trim the denture extensions.

34.6 Managing Resorbed Lower Ridges

The reduced area of support, proximity of muscle attachments to the ridge crest and thinning of mucosa may contribute to a patient complaint of loose and uncomfortable dentures.

- Manage the patient's expectations at the outset by explaining about the difficulties of making a stable and comfortable denture. Advise fixative will in all likelihood be needed. Fixative is helpful in the days after fit to minimise small unfamiliar movement that can be irritating.
- Consider a neutral zone impression to improve the denture stability. This technique combined with meticulous border moulding will greatly improve denture stability.
- Consider reducing the OVD to reduce load on the ridge. Reduce the size of the occlusal table, using narrow teeth, reducing length by leaving off last molar and avoiding loading the distal ridge incline.
- At the 'Fit' appointment, explain comprehensively about what to expect during acclimatisation to the new dentures. Include the likelihood of sore areas, transitory altered speech, increased saliva production and learning a new chewing pattern.
- A useful tip is to use a light-bodied silicone wash to identify potential area of pressure that will cause soreness under the denture. This can eliminate many sore areas before they occur.
- Always check the occlusion for even, bilateral contact and no slide between retruded contact and denture ICP, before adjusting any of the fit surface. A good proportion of soreness can come from occlusal errors causing denture movement.

Once treatment has been completed, encourage the patient to return for regular reviews to have a soft tissue examination. Additionally, timely relines can help maintain functional dentures before replacement dentures are required.

34.7 Conclusion

Complete denture construction has been described as an art form rather than a science. An awareness of patient's expectations needs to be balanced against the presenting anatomical challenges and the scope for the patient to acclimatise to a complete denture prosthesis. The key aspects of optimal impression making, accurate jaw relations and denture extension contribute to the success of the prosthesis in terms of stability, retention and ultimately patient acceptance and satisfaction.

References

1. Fiske J, Davis DM, Frances C, Gelbier S. The emotional effects of tooth loss in edentulous people. Br Dent J. 1998;184:90–3.
2. The Glossary of Prosthodontic Terms: Ninth Edition. J Prosthet Dent 2017; https://doi.org/10.1016/j.prosdent.2016.12.001.
3. Ellis JS, Pelekis ND, Thomason JM. Conventional rehabilitation of edentulous patients: the impact on oral health-related quality of life and patient satisfaction. J Prosthodont. 2007;16:37–42.
4. Berg E. Acceptance of full dentures. Int Dent J. 1993;43:299–306.
5. Leyssen W, Jayachandran S, Walmsley AD. Complete denture series part 1: referrals for complete dentures—identifying the reasons. Dent Update. 2019; https://doi.org/10.12968/denu.2019.46.5.466.
6. Shigli K, Awinashe V. Patient-dentist communication: an adjunct to successful complete denture treatment. J Prosthodont. 2010;19:491–3.
7. Bell DH. Provocative diagnosis: a rational approach to the management of problem denture patients. In: Lefkovitz W, editor. Proceedings of the Second International Prosthodontics Congress. CV Mosby; 1979. p. 31–2.
8. Someya S. The anatomical study of the sinew string observed on the buccal mucosa of mandibular second molar and posterior of retromolar pad. J Acad Clin Dent. 2008;28:14–20.
9. Watt DM, MacGregor A R. Designing complete dentures. Chapter 2. WB Saunders, 1976.

Part VII

Paediatric Dentistry

Examination and Treatment Planning 35

David Baldwin, Anne Williams, and Ewen McColl

Learning Points

- Understand the importance of effective communication with paediatric patients.
- Recognise the need for familiarity and acclimatisation to the dental environment as early as possible.
- Appreciate methods in communicating dental procedures to child patients to promote better understanding and compliance.
- Recall the various hard tissue examination techniques for the child patient.
- Understand the role that radiography plays in the early detection of carious lesion.
- Distinguish between the different methods of managing carious lesions in the child patient depending on the progression of disease.

35.1 Introduction

Paediatric dentistry is often seen as a challenging discipline in primary care, considering the management and technical variances when compared to adult patients. The top tips discussed come from years of experience and will optimise care, cognisant of the time challenges that often exist in primary care.

Each interaction we have with our child patients will influence how they feel about and the importance they place upon their oral health in the future. Will they become adults with a positive outlook on oral health, or will they remember a childhood experience that negatively influenced their relationship with dental care for the rest of their lives? [1]

D. Baldwin
London, UK

A. Williams · E. McColl (✉)
Peninsula Dental School, Plymouth, UK
e-mail: ewen.mccoll@plymouth.ac.uk

E. McColl, A. Alani (eds.), *Practical Tips in Clinical Dentistry*, BDJ Clinician's Guides, https://doi.org/10.1007/978-3-031-90355-7_35

35.2 Early Introduction to the Dental Environment

Encourage parents to bring their children at an early age for examination as per Dental Check by One, ChildSmile and Designed to Smile guidance [2–4]. These early visits for children under the age of 3 years are about delivering key preventive messages to parents and enabling the dentist to pick up early on any potential high-risk caries activities and provide appropriate preventative advice as per *Delivering better oral health* guidance [5].

For the patient, these early visits are about acclimatisation to the dental environment and beginning a positive, lifelong relationship with dentistry, even though the examination may be very brief and no clinical intervention may be required.

35.3 Appropriate Behaviour Management

Behaviour management starts even before the child enters the surgery.

Make sure the practice website is up to date with photos of the reception, waiting room and the surgery so that children can become familiar with where they are going. Have photos of the staff that they may see and pictures of the dental chair, mouth mirrors and toothbrushes to further inform them of the reason for their visit. Widgit Health [6] has produced easy-to-read communication support dental information sheets. Consider using, or produce your own versions of, their dental documents to help acclimatise younger children to the dental environment.

35.4 Communication Is Key

Prepare the parents for what will happen when they bring their child for the first visit. A good, trusting relationship with the child, the parents and the dental team is vital so that everyone is aware of the roles they should play. The parents may be able to prepare the child for what will happen at the next visit—as long as they themselves have a positive attitude towards dental care and oral health.

Tailor your communication to the age of the child, using child-friendly language and avoiding technical terms. Use words like 'stroke' or 'touch' rather than 'probe'; use 'picture' rather than 'bitewing radiograph'. Avoid trigger words such as pain, needle or sharp.

Vary the tone of your voice; young children respond to the speed and pitch of the voice often more than the words that are used. Keep talking while you treat a child. Prolonged silences are off-putting and not reassuring. You can distract and soothe if you talk to your patients as you treat them.

Tell them what they are doing well rather than just repeating 'good girl' or 'good boy' over and over. Say 'When you open your mouth really wide I can see all your teeth right at the back of your mouth – so that's great, thank you'.

Children like to please, so telling them what they are doing well is positive reinforcement for them.

Let the children know you care about them; ask if they are okay. Smile behind the mask and glasses; crinkly eyes are more friendly than blank staring ones.

Try not to label a child as uncooperative, which implies they are doing it on purpose. Children under three are usually pre-cooperative—that is, they don't know how to cooperate. All children have the potential to become cooperative; it just takes some longer than others. Some may simply be at an age where they are unable to tolerate what you want from them at that time.

Use one of the many non-pharmacological behaviour management techniques to help a child who needs reassurance, such as 'Tell, show, do', or distraction [7, 8]. Putting a cartoon on the overhead monitor has been shown to calm and soothe a child while you are looking at their teeth. Use positive reinforcement to reward them with stickers or toothbrushes.

35.5 Clinical Examination of the Child

Always start with an extra-oral examination, looking at the child as they come into the surgery and noting any asymmetry, rashes, bruises or cold sores.

Palpate for lymph nodes in the submandibular and cervical areas and check the TMJ, explain you are going to 'tickle' their neck and face.

Intraorally, look at the soft tissues before the hard tissues; check the tongue, gingivae, palate, floor of mouth and labial and buccal mucosa; and note common conditions such as minor aphthous ulceration or geographic tongue.

35.6 Hard Tissue Examination: Common Findings and Points to Remember

35.6.1 Caries

Dental caries is common. The 2019 oral health survey of 5-year-olds 2019 found that 23.4% of 5-year-old children in England had experience of dental decay, with an average number of 3.4 teeth with experience of dental decay [9].

As clinicians, we know that a significant proportion of clinical caries may not be visible in the mouth on clinical examination. Although caries can present on occlusal surfaces of posterior teeth and labial surfaces of upper incisors and canines in severe cases, there will likely also be caries interproximally, especially where there are tight contact points. Check the marginal ridges of primary molars for signs of shadowing or early breakdown. Back up any clinical findings with appropriate radiographic examination.

35.6.2 Dental Development, Eruption Patterns, Infra-occlusion and Orthodontic Assessment

Look at the eruption pattern of the teeth and question whether this fits what you would expect.

Delayed eruption of upper permanent incisors can occur due to the presence of supernumerary teeth or trauma to the primary tooth. If the contralateral incisor has been erupted for more than 6 months or a central incisor remains unerupted and the lateral incisor has erupted, investigate with an upper standard occlusal or periapical radiograph to assess the position of the unerupted tooth. Be aware that supernumerary teeth occur in approximately 1–2% of the population, and approximately 80% will occur in the upper midline often causing delayed eruption of permanent incisors.

First permanent molars can impact into the distal aspect of the second primary molars, thus delaying their eruption or speeding the exfoliation of the primary molar tooth. If mildly impacted, placing an orthodontic separator for a week may be enough to disimpact the first permanent molar to allow it to erupt. Severe impactions where the first permanent molar has resorbed the second primary molar excessively (sometimes involving the pulp) may require primary molar extraction, and once erupted enough, space maintenance of the first permanent molar.

Be aware of deciduous molars that are in infra-occlusion. Monitor them carefully and extract if they continue to 'submerge'; this should be done as soon as the occlusal surface of the infra-occluded tooth passes past the most bulbous part of the contact point of the adjacent teeth, and before they sink below the gingival margin and require a surgical approach.

At the age of nine, assess the overall stage of dental development and palpate the buccal sulcus for the position of the unerupted canine teeth. If it is not obvious where they are, then take radiographs to find them, an OPG if you have one or periapicals if not. Know who your local orthodontic specialists and consultants are and how to refer to them. Refer early to the orthodontist for misplaced/ectopic canines.

35.6.3 Caries Risk Assessment, BEWE and BPE

All children should have caries risk assessment and BEWE undertaken, and those 7 years or older who are cooperative should have a BPE undertaken.

Include these assessments as part of your examination template and complete them each time you see a child for examination. They will help you form your diagnoses and guide treatment planning.

Once you have completed your clinical examination, consider which radiographs you want to take and given the child's caries risk assessment how frequently they should be repeated. The timing of repeat bitewing radiographs for children should follow the FGDP guidelines [10] depending on the caries risk of the child and whether any new decay is present.

35.6.4 Radiographic Examination

Dental radiography is an essential adjunct to patient assessment and a critical part of the treatment planning process. This is just as true in children as it is in adult patients.

If caries is clinically visible in one or more teeth, or if the caries risk assessment indicates that the patient is at increased risk of developing caries, then radiographs should be attempted. Remember not all caries present will be clinically visible.

Figure 35.1 shows a 5-year-old patient with no symptoms.

Clinical presentation:

URE^{o}, ULE^{o}

Radiographic presentation:

Caries URE^{o,m}, URD^{d,m}, URC^{d}, ULC^{d}, ULD^{d}, ULE^{m,o}, LLE^{m}, LLD^{d}, LRD^{d}, LRE^{m}

Many children, however, may find bitewing holders difficult to tolerate. The shape and size of the patient's mouth is the main factor. In a vertical dimension, the depth of the lingual sulcus and height of palate are important; in a horizontal dimension, a longer film may trigger a gag reflex. Various behaviour management techniques such as tell, show, do and distraction can be used to help.

It is important to recognise the different size film/plates available for intraoral imaging. Use paediatric bitewing holders, which are smaller and easier for the child to tolerate, with size 0 recommended for the primary dentition only (22 × 31 mm) or size 1 for mixed dentition (24 × 40 mm) (Fig. 35.2).

From the age of four, start introducing bitewing holders; get the patient to try them in themselves first even without a film/plate in place rather than trying yourself (Fig. 35.3). Detach the bite block from the rest of the film holder/aiming device to make it less obtrusive. As soon as the child can tolerate them and bite down fully, take radiographs to check for interproximal caries.

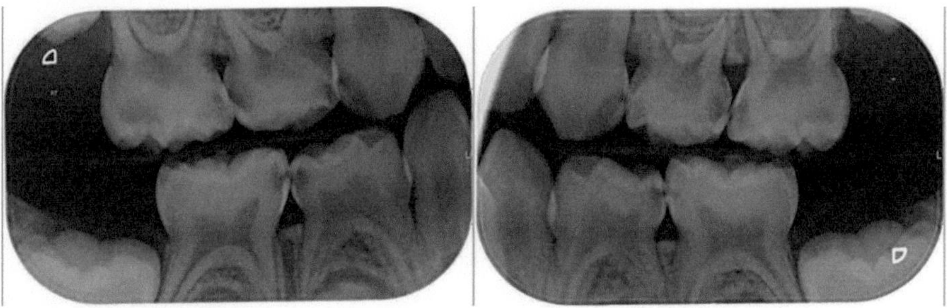

Fig. 35.1 Example of caries in a 5-year-old patient with no symptoms. (Images taken July 2019. Source D. Baldwin)

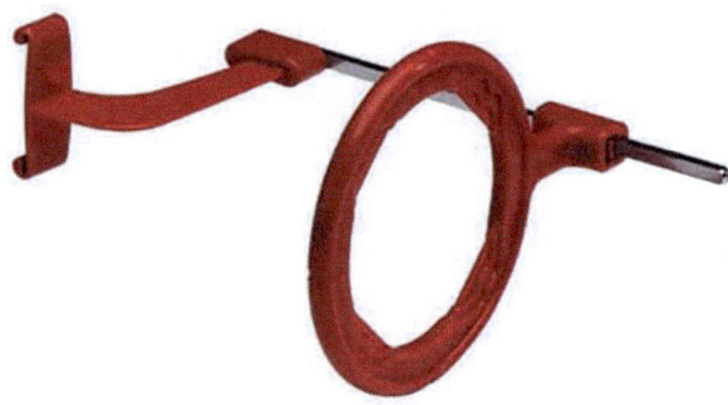

Fig. 35.2 Rinn XCP

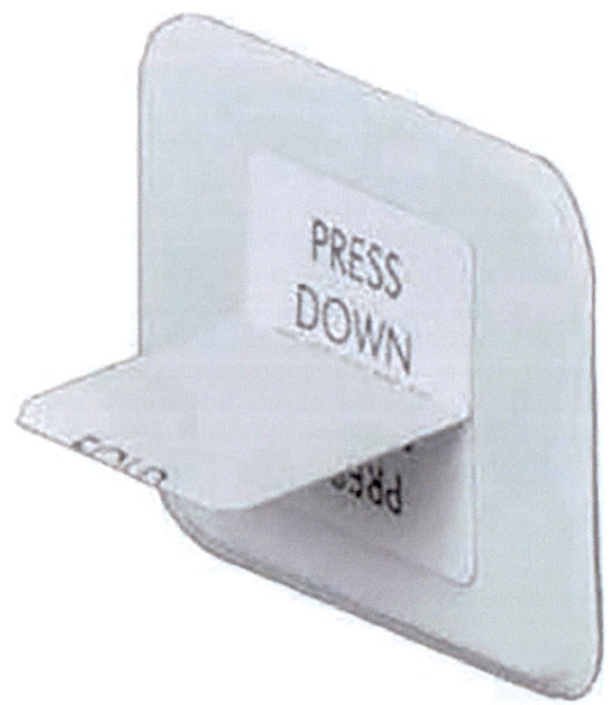

Fig. 35.3 Bitewing sticky tabs

A size 2 film can be used to take an occlusal view in very young children following trauma to the deciduous incisors. They can bite down very gently on the film rather than trying to fit a standard size 4 occlusal film or a periapical holder. See Table 35.1.

Use a system that is tolerable to the patient, that gives reproducible images and that reduces the risk of poor-quality images being taken to adhere to ALARA principles to reduce the need to repeat an image.

Table 35.1 The properties of Rinn XCP and bitewing sticky tabs

Rinn xcp (Fig. 35.2)	Bitewing sticky tabs (Fig. 35.3)
Minimally invasive in oral cavity Size 0/1 specific holder Beam aiming device Good reproducibility Able to position appropriately	Least invasive – only film sits in oral cavity
More bulk for patient to tolerate	No aiming device Difficult to ensure film is in correct position Increased likelihood of overlap on image risk of cone cutting Can produce poorer quality image

When you have gathered all the information from the patient history, caries risk assessment, BEWE, BPE and clinical and radiographic examination, you will be in a position to make a clear diagnosis and use this to guide your treatment plan.

Schedule treatment according to clinical and radiographic findings and prioritise as follows:

1. Urgent treatment.
2. Preventative care based on caries risk assessment and utilising advice from DBOH[5].
3. Operative treatment—based on clinical and radiographic findings.
4. Recall plans—based on caries risk assessment.

35.6.5 Operative Treatment Planning Pathway

Understand what your clinical and radiographic findings mean and develop a whole mouth operative treatment plan based on these findings. Follow a decision-making pathway for deciding what treatment is required for what tooth, which may include:

- Caries into pulp/inter-radicular radiolucency/history of irreversible pulpitis/clinical sinus/infection—extraction.
- Interproximal molar caries in dentine with reversible pulpitis—stainless-steel crown.
- Anterior caries in dentine with reversible pulpitis—composite restoration.
- Single surface molar caries in dentine with reversible pulpitis—intra-coronal composite restoration or stainless-steel crown.
- Enamel-only lesions—increased risk preventative care and reduced recall period monitoring.

35.6.6 Conclusion

This chapter has highlighted the undoubted importance of good communication with the paediatric patient and how this sets the foundations for future care and treatment. A comprehensive systematic approach to examination and treatment planning is important to ensure optimal management of all presenting pathology in the growing patient.

References

1. Benjamin F. Childhood lasts a lifetime. Br Dent J. 2018;224:577–9.
2. Dental Check By One. Available at: https://dentalcheckbyone.co.uk/profession/. Accessed 28 Mar 2022.
3. NHS Scotland. ChildSmile. Available at: http://www.child-smile.org.uk/. Accessed 28 Mar 2022.
4. Public Health Wales. Designed to Smile. Available at: https://phw.nhs.wales/services-and-teams/designed-to-smile/. Accessed 28 Mar 2022.
5. Office for Health Improvement and Disparities, Department of Health and Social Care, NHS England and NHS Improvement. Delivering better oral health: an evidence-based toolkit for prevention. Updated 9 November 2021. Available at: https://www.gov.uk/government/publications/delivering-better-oral-health-an-evidence-based-toolkit-for-prevention. Accessed 28 Mar 2022.
6. Widgit Health. Dental procedures: My visit to the dentist. Available at: https://widgit-health.com/downloads/dental-procedures.htm. Accessed 28 Mar 2022.
7. Campbell C, Soldani F, Busuttil-Naudi A, Chadwick B. Update of non-pharmacological behaviour management guideline. Clinical guidelines in paediatric dentistry. Available at:. https://www.bspd.co.uk/Portals/0/Public/Files/Guidelines/Non-pharmacological%20behaviour%20management%20.pdf. Accessed 28 Apr 2022.
8. Chadwick BL, Hosey MT. Child taming: how to manage children in dental practice. 2nd ed. Quintessence Publishing Co Ltd; 2017.
9. Public Health England. National Dental Epidemiology Programme for England: oral health survey of 5-year-olds 2019. A report on the variations in prevalence and severity of dental decay. Available at: https://assets.publishing.service.gov.uk/government/uploads/system/uploads/attachment_data/file/873492/NDEP_for_England_OH_Survey_5yr_2019_v1.0.pdf. Accessed 28 Mar 2022.
10. Horner K, Eaton KA (eds). Selection criteria for dental radiography. 3rd edn. 2018. Available at: https://cgdent.uk/wp-content/uploads/2021/08/FGDP-SCDR-ALL-Web.pdf. Accessed 28 Mar 2022.

Prevention and the Whole Team Approach to Care

36

David Baldwin, Anne Williams, and Ewen McColl

Learning Points

- Recall the various methods of preventing dental disease at the disposal of dental care professionals.
- Appreciate the need to assess caries risk status of a child and how these effects recall intervals.
- Recognise patients with high sugar intake and instigate advice and preventive regimes to reduce lesion development.
- Recall the various delivery modes for fluoride and how best to incorporate these into a treatment plan for the child patient.
- Understand the need to involve dental team members in the delivery of prevention to best maximise opportunities for patients' benefit.

36.1 Introduction

When considering the management of paediatric dental patients in any dental setting, perhaps the most important component of any management plan, but that which is at greatest risk of being overlooked or given less importance, is prevention.

If the appropriate preventative practices aren't adopted by both the practitioner and most importantly by the patient and their families, then the chance of developing new carious lesions remains high and any operative work provided has increased risk of failure.

D. Baldwin
London, UK

A. Williams · E. McColl (✉)
Peninsula Dental School, Plymouth, UK
e-mail: ewen.mccoll@plymouth.ac.uk

E. McColl, A. Alani (eds.), *Practical Tips in Clinical Dentistry*, BDJ Clinician's Guides, https://doi.org/10.1007/978-3-031-90355-7_36

36.2 Caries Risk Assessment-Dependent Preventative Care

- Will depend on clinical and radiographic findings and caries risk status. Utilise *Delivering better oral health* (DBOH) [1] to help you shape your preventative management plan.
- Set a recall interval based on the caries risk assessment. Children at no increased risk can be seen every 6 months whilst those at increased risk should be seen more than twice a year.
- If the child has enamel defects, such as molar incisor hypomineralisation (MIH), this also increases caries risk; discuss it with the parents and the treatment plan accordingly.

36.3 Diet Analysis and Advice

Often parental compliance and accuracy of diet diaries is poor. Use a 24-h recall technique to ascertain the child's dietary habits over the last 24 h. Tailor dietary advice to this:

- Drink water only between meals.
- Aim for three regular meals per day.
- No more than one snack per day.
- Keep snacks to savoury foods such as cucumber/carrot/celery sticks, cheese and crackers.

36.4 Fluoride Varnish Application

- Should be applied to all at-risk teeth at each examination appointment, based on *DBOH* guidelines depending on caries risk and age.
- Beware of risk of allergy to colophony-containing fluoride varnishes (linked to Elastoplast allergy) and that certain fluoride varnishes (casein containing) are not suitable for individuals with milk protein allergy.
- Dry and isolate the teeth well with cotton wool rolls before applying varnish.
- Remember to advise avoidance of food/drink for approximately 30 min after application.

36.5 Toothpaste

- 1000–1450 ppm toothpaste should be advised depending on patient age and caries risk status.
- Once 10 years of age, if at increased risk of caries, prescribe 2800 ppm toothpaste—use at least twice daily.

- For all toothpastes, encourage all family members to spit out and not to rinse the mouth after use—you will be surprised at how many people simply wash away all the toothpaste after brushing.
- Taste of toothpaste—if you have a patient who has sensory processing problems, is autistic, or simply doesn't like the strong flavours of traditional toothpastes, remember that in addition to the many fluoride-containing 'berry flavour' toothpastes on the market that oraNurse produces a flavourless non-foaming fluoride-containing toothpaste (https://oranurse.co.uk/).
- Fluoride-free alternatives—if parents wish to use a fluoride-free toothpaste, ask them to consider BioMin C (https://biomin.co.uk/products/biominr-c-toothpaste) or Tooth Mousse (https://europe.gc.dental/en-GB/products/toothmousse).
- Remineralisation of teeth—MIH. Consider advising Tooth Mousse, which provides additional calcium and phosphate (CCP-ACP) or BioMin, which utilises glass silicates (ChloroCalciumPhosphoSilicate) to remineralise the teeth. But it is important to remember that CPP-ACP products are contraindicated in children who are allergic to milk protein due to the presence of casein.
- NovaMin-containing toothpaste can also be recommended that will help with the sensitivity.

36.6 Mouthwash

- If over 7 years of age, consider the use of a fluoride mouthwash and advise that this is used at a separate time to brushing—that is, when the child comes home from school.

36.7 Floss

- A 2017 systematic review [2] found only one study showing evidence of an association between the use of dental floss and proximal caries reduction in the primary dentition. However, they concluded the use of dental floss should never be discouraged, as habits acquired in childhood continue throughout adult life, with numerous oral- and general-health benefits.

36.8 Fissure Sealants

- If at increased risk of caries.
- Once first permanent molars have erupted sufficiently, they should be fissure sealed to prevent caries development.
- Until effective moisture control become possible or if molars are only partially erupted, fluoride varnish can be applied to them.
- Key areas to remember are the buccal grooves of lower molars and the occlusal palatal fissure and around the cusp of Carabelli on upper molars.

- To allow full access to these areas, you may wish to use a flat plastic to gently reflect gingival margin. Ineffective moisture control is the most likely cause of sealant restoration failure. Use a cotton wool roll on either side of lower molars held with non-dominant thumb and index finger. Use dry tips/dry guards to reflect buccal mucosa for upper molars.
- Fissure sealants could and should be applied to any at-risk areas in individuals of increased caries risk, including fissures on primary molar teeth, premolars and second permanent molars.

36.9 Silver Diamine Fluoride

- Has been available since the 1960s but not used regularly in the United Kingdom until recently.
- Rapidly being adopted into dental undergraduate teaching programmes across the United Kingdom.
- Fluoride content is twice that of regular high-strength fluoride (44,800 ppm); silver compounds are antibacterial.
- The British Society of Paediatric Dentistry has produced some important and useful guidance on its use: https://www.bspd.co.uk/Professionals/Resources.
- Benefits:
  - Can help to arrest/slow progression of caries in combination with other preventative practices.
  - Can potentially avoid further operative/interventive care or be used as part of a stabilisation phase of treatment prior to definitive treatment.
  - Good minimally invasive technique.
- Considerations:
  - Requires continued observation and monitoring if adopting a preventative only approach.
  - Not a suitable treatment option for pulpally involved teeth.
  - Can be difficult to place on minimally cavitated interproximal lesions.
  - Stains the carious lesions a dark black colour—potential parental compliance issues regarding post-treatment aesthetics.
  - In the United Kingdom, it is licensed for treating sensitivity only. It is fully licensed for caries management in many countries around the world where it has been safely used for many years.

36.10 Involving Your Whole Dental Team in Paediatric Dentistry

Treating children can sometimes be quite daunting; it may be more suited to certain individuals within a practice and it is beneficial to recognise which team members are best placed to treat paediatric patients. Having child-friendly reception staff and a portion of the waiting room being child friendly and dentally interactive can help to further acclimatise patients.

The recent publication of Health Education England's (HEE) Advancing Dental Care Review [3] highlighted the underutilisation of dental therapists in general dental practice. Optimising the full scope of practice [4, 5] of not only dental therapists but also dental hygienists and dental nurses would allow dentists to focus on more complex treatments unique to their scope whilst allowing the practice to be child friendly.

Dental nurses can apply fluoride varnish either on prescription from a dentist or direct as part of a structured dental health programme.

Dental therapists working in NHS dental practices are able to carry out direct restorations on primary and secondary teeth, carry out pulpotomies on primary teeth, extract primary teeth and place pre-formed crowns on primary teeth.

Dental therapists and hygienists working in NHS practices are able to obtain a detailed dental history from patients and evaluate their medical history; carry out a clinical examination within their competence; diagnose and prepare treatment plan within their competence; prescribe radiographs; take, process and interpret various film views used in general dental practice; plan the delivery of care for patients; apply fluoride varnish; and place fissure sealants. Additionally, dental therapists can develop skills to administer inhalation sedation.

The time saved by involving the entire dental team in paediatric dental care makes sense not just from a financial point of view but in also allowing individual team members to excel at what they do best.

36.11 Conclusion

This chapter has highlighted the important role that fully integrated prevention has in the holistic management of the paediatric patient. A team approach to prevention underpins dental care for the young patient by nurturing a culture of self-care and maintenance with behaviours and routines for lifelong oral health.

References

1. Office for Health Improvement and Disparities, Department of Health and Social Care, NHS England and NHS Improvement. Delivering better oral health: an evidence-based toolkit for prevention. Updated 9 November 2021. Available at: https://www.gov.uk/government/publications/delivering-better-oral-health-an-evidence-based-toolkit-for-prevention. Accessed 28 Mar 2022.
2. de Oliveira KMH, Nemezio MA, Romualdo PC, da Silva RAB, de Paula E, Silva FWG, Küchler EC. Dental flossing and proximal caries in the primary dentition: a systematic review. Oral Health Prev Dent. 2017;15:427–34.
3. Health Education England. HEE's Advancing Dental Care Review: Final report. Available at: https://www.hee.nhs.uk/sites/default/files/documents/Advancing%20Dental%20Care%20Report%20Sept%2021.pdf. Accessed 28 Mar 2022.

4. General Dental Council. Scope of practice. 30 Sept 2013. Available at: https://www.gdc-uk.org/docs/default-source/scope-of-practice/scope-of-practice.pdf?sfvrsn=8f417ca8_4. Accessed 28 Mar 2022.
5. Pivoda L, McColl E. Advancing dental care—Utilising the dental therapist workforce to optimise patient outcomes. BDJ Team 2022; 9: 16–18.

37 Operative Care, Stainless Steel Crowns and Management of Molar Incisor Hypomineralisation

David Baldwin, Anne Williams, and Ewen McColl

Learning Points

- Understand the importance of communication when delivering local anaesthesia.
- Appreciate how the variety of dental procedures in the child patient require different methods of delivering anaesthesia.
- Recall how stylising language when describing operative dentistry allows better understanding and so compliance.
- Understand the indications for use of preformed metal crowns and spacers.
- Recognise the various challenges MIH provides the clinician and how these can be overcome.
- Understand how management differs between posterior and anterior teeth affected by MIH.
- Appreciate how local secondary care services can aid in the treatment of the child patient and how best to liaise with managed clinical networks in their management.

37.1 Introduction

In patients presenting with established carious lesions or enamel breakdown secondary to MIH, the provision of operative dentistry needs to be planned and delivered as efficiently as possible to maximise the opportunity to definitively restore. Various tips and techniques are presented that aid the clinician in ensuring

D. Baldwin
London, UK

A. Williams · E. McColl (✉)
Peninsula Dental School, Plymouth, UK
e-mail: ewen.mccoll@plymouth.ac.uk

E. McColl, A. Alani (eds.), *Practical Tips in Clinical Dentistry*, BDJ Clinician's Guides, https://doi.org/10.1007/978-3-031-90355-7_37

restorative procedures are predictable without compromising residual tooth tissue with the aim of maintaining deciduous units until they naturally exfoliate or retain adult units definitively.

37.2 How to Give Effective LA

Effective anaesthesia is essential to ensure successful operative treatment when considering intra-coronal restorations or tooth extraction.

Use age-appropriate explanations and continually talk through sensations being felt whilst administering both topical and local anaesthetic. Reassure the patient that the sensations they feel are what is expected and are entirely normal. Develop your own specific script for this kind of scenario that you can become comfortable with repeating each time you give topical/local anaesthetic to a child. Remember as previously mentioned to vary the tone and speed of your voice as you give this information; young children respond to the speed and pitch of the voice often more than the words that are used.

Always use topical anaesthetic before giving local anaesthetic.

You need to apply topical anaesthetic to dry mucosa for at least 3 min for it to be effective. By doing this, even keratinised mucosa on the palate can be anaesthetised at least enough to help reduce the sensation when administering local anaesthetic.

37.3 Other Local Anaesthetic Considerations

- For the majority of infiltration anaesthesia, an ultrashort purple needle is all that is required.
- Restoration of a single tooth—Buccal infiltration can be effective. For lower teeth, articaine is more effective than lidocaine.
- Quadrant dentistry—Consider if attempting to treat lower canine and both primary molars in one visit that block anaesthesia may be a more effective approach than infiltration anaesthesia.
- Extraction of a tooth—a painless infiltration technique—takes time:
  - Apply topical anaesthetic for a minimum of 3 min, administer buccal infiltration, wait, administer intra-papillary infiltration from buccal aspect through already anaesthetised mucosa chasing anaesthetic through to palatal/lingual aspect of tooth, wait and perform direct lingual/palatal infiltration through already anaesthetised mucosa to complete anaesthesia.

37.4 The Use of Dental Handpieces

When considering handpieces, use relevant child-friendly terms to describe them such as 'fast and slow electric toothbrushes'; remember a child is unlikely to have ever experienced anything like this before. Therefore, it is important to first show them and explain their use using the tell-show-do approach [1]. Explain the different noises they produce, get the child to hold out their hand to feel air (and water) coming out of the handpieces, allow them to feel the roughness of a diamond bur (to polish and clean the teeth) and explain the 'bumping' sensation of the slow speed handpiece, all before even starting work in the mouth. Before touching a tooth, switch on thc fast handpiece and hold it in the mouth with suction so the child is aware of the sensation of water cooling and suction. When working on a particular tooth, give regular breaks or use a countdown technique from 10–15 s to zero; give stop signals 'hand up' to patient; make them feel like they are in control of the appointment; always explain what is happening and how well the patient is doing.

37.5 Composite Restorations

Use the same principles you do when restoring permanent teeth. Consider how you will achieve effective moisture control. However, primary tooth enamel is thinner and has a lower mineralised content than permanent teeth—composite bond strengths will be reduced.

37.6 Preformed Metal Crowns

With the advent of the Hall Technique [2], fitting stainless steel crowns to deciduous molars has become technically much easier than the alternative multisurface composite restoration.

Glass ionomer cement restorations should only ever be considered as stabilising or temporary restorations, and thus, a 5-year-old child presenting for definitive treatment of a decayed primary molar tooth does not need a temporary restoration but one that will last until the tooth exfoliates, 5–7 years later, such as a stainless steel crown.

Placing crowns using the Hall Technique usually involves no local anaesthetic and no tooth preparation so is better tolerated by the children.

The Hall Technique guide [2] is highly recommended as additional reading: https://upload.wikimedia.org/wikipedia/commons/9/91/HallTechGuide_V4.pdf.

There are three ways to fit a Hall Technique stainless steel crown:

- Using orthodontic separators to create space for a few days before the crown is fitted. This is the best way as it avoids any tooth preparation.
- By slicing through the contact points mesially and distally to create space.
- By getting the child to bite the crown into place if there is enough space naturally.

Placing crowns by fitting spacers first is often the preferred method—this will however require two short visits, one to fit the spacers and another to remove the spacers and place the crown. Explain the technique to the parents and the child; it

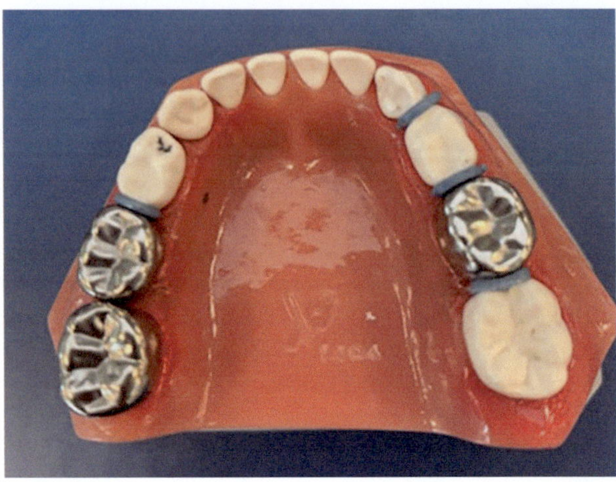

Fig. 37.1 Model showing both separators and crowns on primary and permanent molars

helps to have a model to show them so there is no misunderstanding as to what the spacers are and what the crown will look like once placed (Fig. 37.1).

37.7 Spacer Placement

Placing spacers is best done using two pieces of non-waxed floss threaded through to stretch the spacer. Waxed floss can be too slippy. Wind the floss round your middle fingers and use your index fingers and thumbs to apply pressure to literally floss the spacer through the contact point. It's often easier to start on the buccal side rather than trying to go straight down from the occlusal surface. When correctly seated, the spacer should fit around the contact point, not completely below it.

It's fine to crown more than one tooth in each appointment, although it is preferable to avoid placing crowns on opposing or adjacent teeth at the same time as this opens the bite too much or risks not having enough anterior-posterior space.

Leave the spacer in for a few days, up to a week is fine, and explain that initially there will be some tightness as if a piece of food is stuck between the teeth—simple analgesia can be given if required. At the fit appointment, size up the crown before removing the bands, which should only be removed at the last minute to prevent loss of space. The crowns are very small and slippery, so positioning the patient in a sitting up position protects the airway should you drop the crown. Using Pic-n-Stics (Pulpdent) or other adjuncts can help when trying in the crown (Fig. 37.2).

The crown should fit both mesio-distally and bucco-palatally. If it feels very loose, try a smaller size. If fitting crowns on second deciduous molars, or when planning to place stainless steel crowns on adjacent teeth, it's a good idea to flatten the mesial and distal surfaces with crimping forceps to reduce bulbosity and shorten the length of the crown. You may also need to reshape the crown buccolingually if interproximal caries has resulted in tooth surface loss and a shortening of the anterior-posterior length of the tooth (Figs. 37.3, 37.4 and 37.5).

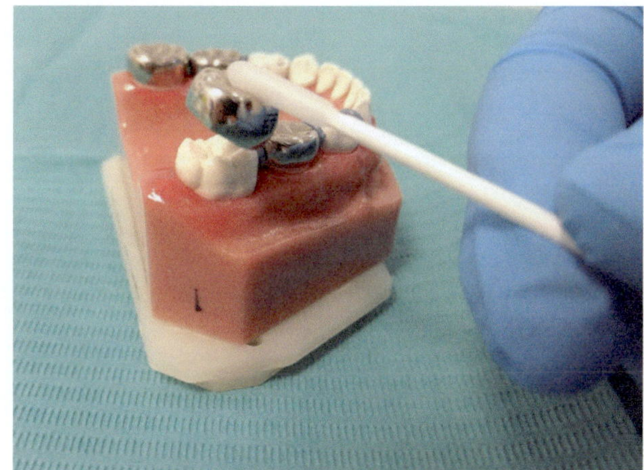

Fig. 37.2 Model showing the use of Pic-n-Stics (Pulpdent) to help when trying in the crown

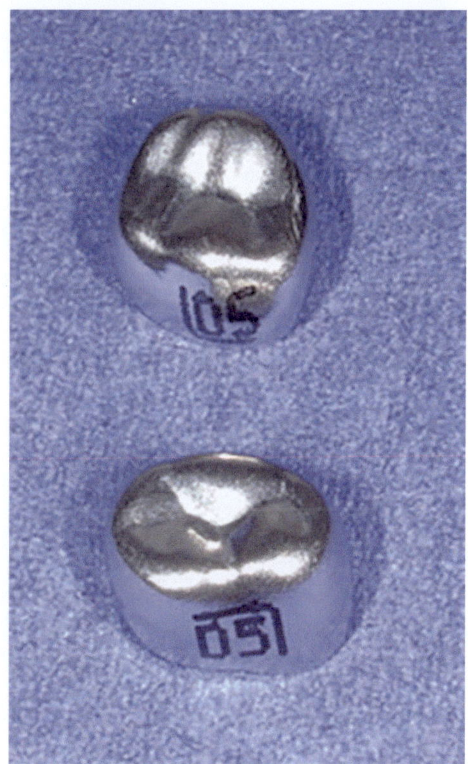

Fig. 37.3 Using an upper left (shorter and fatter) for a lower right crown (longer and thinner) when there has been space loss on a lower first molar due to caries

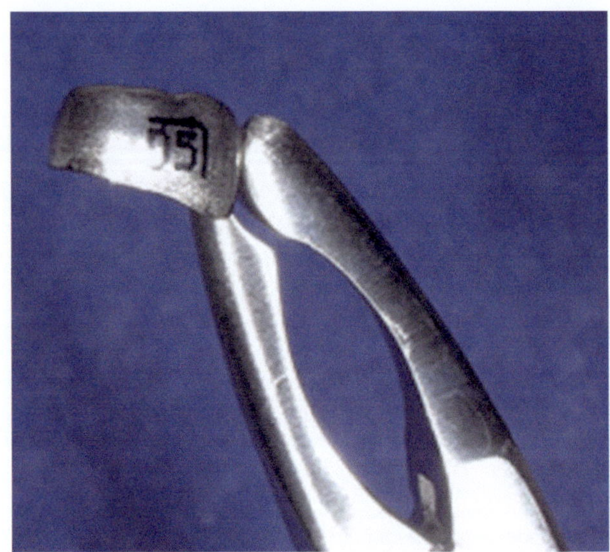

Fig. 37.4 Using the crown crimping pliers in reverse to flatten the bulbosity of the crown to manage reduced space requirements. 'HS Pliers No 114 Johnson Contouring'

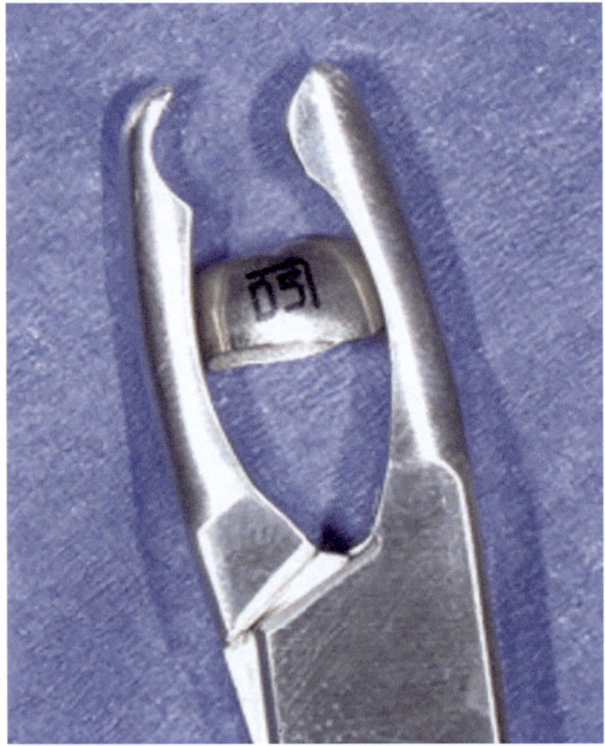

Fig. 37.5 Reducing the anterior-posterior length by applying pressure to the crown between the beaks of the crown crimping pliers

When you're happy that you have the correct size, remove the bands, try the crown one more time and then cement into place with a glass ionomer-luting cement. Seat firmly and ask the child to bite on a cotton wool roll and check the gingival margins are blanched. Remove any extra cement and reassure the child and the parent that their crown will feel big to begin with but that the bite will quickly settle.

37.8 Common Problems

We would encourage you to practise modifying the circumference of the crown to adjust the fit to teeth where there has been space loss due to interproximal caries. Stainless steel crowns can be quite forgiving, and with practice and the careful use of crimping pliers, the mesio-distal length and buccolingual width can be adjusted.

Lower first primary molar crowns are commonly the most difficult crown to fit, especially when there has been space loss due to caries. In addition to advice given in the Hall Technique [2] regarding crown modification, we recommend using a contralateral upper crown (i.e., ULD to fit LRD) that are often shorter and fatter than the lower first molar crowns and will fit the affected tooth better.

37.9 Molar Incisor Hypomineralisation

Hypomineralisation occurs commonly; the 2013 Children's Dental Health Survey [3] found that 19% of 12-year-olds had one or more teeth with a well-demarcated opacity. In many cases, this is likely to be molar incisor hypomineralisation (MIH).

Hypomineralisation and hypoplasia are commonly confused. Enamel hypomineralisation is a qualitative defect, with reduced mineralisation resulting in discoloured enamel in a tooth of normal shape and size. Because the enamel is weaker, teeth can undergo post-eruptive breakdown, resulting in missing enamel, which is rough, discoloured and often sensitive. Enamel hypoplasia is a quantitative defect of the enamel, where less enamel forms initially, presenting as pits, grooves, missing enamel or smaller teeth, but often with normal levels of mineral content [4].

Common presentation in younger children can be post-eruptive breakdown (possibly also with caries) of the second primary molar teeth. Often, this can present in an otherwise healthy mouth with abnormal caries pattern, as second primary molars do not normally become the first carious teeth.

Permanent teeth affected by molar incisor hypomineralisation can include first permanent molars, permanent incisors and, in severe cases, permanent canines. Opacites are often well defined and can present as white/cream/yellow or brown in colour with increasingly less mineral content (Figs. 37.6 and 37.7).

Teeth can be more sensitive (hot and cold, as well as touch—even from tooth brushing). Patients are less likely to want to brush them. As a result, they are more likely to breakdown; more likely to develop caries, which can pass more rapidly through the tooth; more difficult to anaesthetise; and more difficult to bond to due

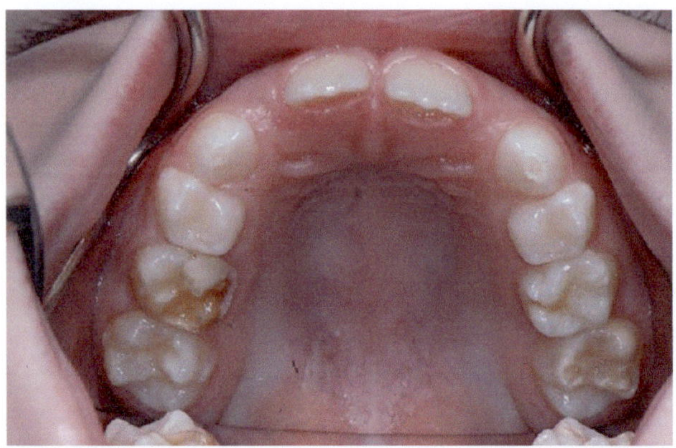

Fig. 37.6 Opacities due to MIH are often well defined and can present as white/cream/yellow or brown in colour with increasingly less mineral content

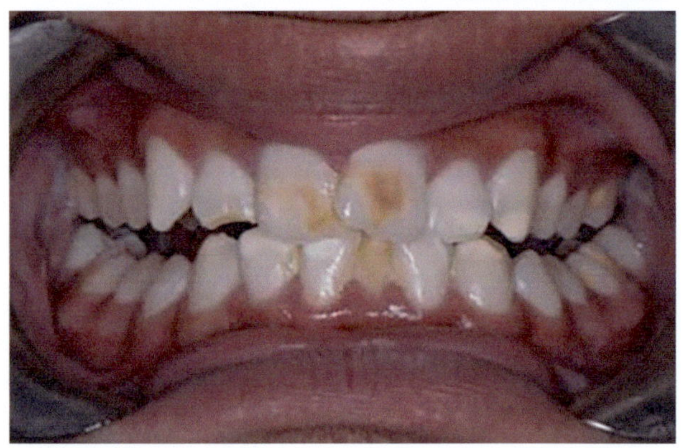

Fig. 37.7 Opacities that present anteriorly with MIH are likely to coincide with aesthetic concerns from the patient or guardian

to reduced mineral content, and affected anterior teeth can be unsightly and patients will often complain of teasing at school due to appearance of teeth.

37.10 Management Tips

As soon as the teeth erupt and MIH is recognised, it is important to start enhanced preventive measures as advised by *Delivering better oral health* [5] but also to include:

- Encouraging parents to help younger children brush effectively around affected first permanent molar teeth on a daily basis—if sensitive, these may be being missed.
- Apply 22,600 ppm fluoride varnish to affected teeth more than twice a year in the surgery.
- When they are able to rinse, prescribe a fluoride mouthwash.
- Prescribe 2800 ppm NaF toothpaste from the age of 10.

- Consider brushing a third time during the day or rubbing toothpaste directly over the affected teeth with a finger last thing at night before bed.

37.11 Posterior Teeth

Minimally affected first permanent molars (and second primary molars) should be fissure sealed. The strength of the bond may be increased by using an etch, bond, seal technique [6, 7] rather than the usual etch, seal.

If moisture control cannot be achieved, then use glass ionomer sealant (GC Fuji TRIAGE) placed over the affected occlusal or buccal surfaces to temporarily stop the sensitivity and protect the tooth.

When local anaesthetic is required for restoration, infiltration of 4% articaine HCL is more effective than 2% lidocaine HCL in achieving the depth of anaesthesia needed for restoration. Lidocaine block anaesthesia in the mandible can be supplemented with articaine as an infiltration buccally.

Small areas of post-eruptive breakdown on molars can be restored with composite. It is usually better to remove all of the hypomineralised enamel and dentine, cutting back to unaffected tooth tissue, prior to restoration, rather than merely attempting to fill the area of breakdown.

Where posterior teeth exhibit extensive post-eruptive breakdown, long-term prognosis is often poor. Early intervention to extract them is better than attempting to maintain a heavily restored tooth in the longer term. The ideal age to consider loss is around 9½ years old. Glass ionomer sealants or stainless steel crowns can be used to maintain teeth until this time. At this age, paediatric dental specialist and orthodontic opinion should be sought to consider compensating extractions [8].

37.12 Anterior Teeth

Opacities associated with molar incisor hypomineralisation on anterior teeth can often be a source of embarrassment for the patient with regard to their appearance. They can sometimes be sensitive, but only in the most severe cases is there any breakdown that requires management.

Know the options available for aesthetic management in children; this includes direct composite restoration to mask the opacity and minimally invasive techniques such as acid pumice microabrasion Opalustre (Ultradent Products, Inc) and Icon resin infiltrant (DMG), which are useful adjuncts to remove mild to moderate opacities.

The aesthetic improvement of the front teeth can be approached in different ways. It's important to take photographs of the teeth before any treatment is commenced.

With younger children (under 10 years old), if they are being teased at school regarding the opacity, the simplest option may be to place composite directly over the top of the opacity without doing any treatment of the opacity. This leaves all options open for the future whilst hiding the opacity for the time being. This type of treatment will require maintenance.

There is no one technique that will cover all eventualities and often, a combination of methods is required. Be honest with the parents and child about the limitations of treatment from the beginning as it is unlikely you will ever resolve 100% of aesthetic concerns.

37.13 Local Referral Pathways and How You Can Achieve Shared Care with Specialist Services

Paediatric Dental Managed Clinical Networks are either already established or are currently being established around England [9]. Know who your local secondary and tertiary paediatric dental services are and how to refer to them. Many of these services will be happy to help out with treatment planning advice if you are keen to attempt to treat the patient and will want to act in a shared care approach. These services may have access to inhalation sedation (possibly intravenous sedation) and general anaesthetic.

Think what you can do to benefit your patients as part of shared care in the referral process. If your patient won't tolerate local anaesthetic and has grossly carious primary first molars and minimally carious primary second molars, consider what you may be able to achieve before referring for tooth extraction, such as placing Hall crowns on the second primary molars. There is great benefit in maintaining the second primary molars that would otherwise be extracted if no treatment was attempted before referring for GA extractions including:

- Maintaining posterior occlusion.
- Stopping first permanent molars from mesially migrating.
- Holding some space for premolars.
- Reducing potential future crowding.

We hope these tips will be useful in managing paediatric patients presenting in your practice. As with other dental specialties, there are unique challenges, but the rewards of establishing behaviours and attitudes that will set a child on a path to dental health is extremely rewarding if managed appropriately.

37.14 Conclusion

There are numerous options for the operative management of established pathology in the paediatric patient. Spacer placement in combination with preformed metal crowns can aid the clinician in managing established carious multisurface lesions efficiently. MIH present a significant challenge to the clinician from both an aesthetic and functional aspect due to the compromised structural nature of the enamel.

References

1. Campbell C, Soldani F, Busuttil-Naudi A, Chadwick B. Clinical guidelines in Paediatric dentistry. Update of non-pharmacological behaviour management. Revised 2011. Available at: https://www.bspd.co.uk/Professionals/Resources/Clinical-Guidelines-and-Evidence-Reviews/BSPD-Guidelines. Accessed 28 Mar 2022.
2. Innes N, Evans D, Stewart M, Keightley A. The Hall Technique: a minimal intervention, child centred approach to managing the carious primary molar. A users manual, version 4. Dundee: University of Dundee; 2015. Available at: https://upload.wikimedia.org/wikipedia/commons/9/91/HallTechGuide_V4.pdf. Accessed 28 Mar 2022
3. NHS Digital. Child Dental Health Survey 2013, England, Wales and Northern Ireland. 19 March 2015. Available at: https://digital.nhs.uk/data-and-information/publications/statistical/children-s-dental-health-survey/child-dental-health-survey-2013-england-wales-and-northern-ireland#highlights. Accessed 28 Mar 2022.
4. Parekh S. Hypomineralisation or hypoplasia? UCL discovery. Available at: https://discovery.ucl.ac.uk/id/eprint/10086728/3/Parekh_Hypomineralisation%20or%20hypoplasis_AAM.pdf. Accessed 28 Mar 2022.
5. Office for Health Improvement and Disparities, Department of Health and Social Care, NHS England, NHS Improvement. Delivering better oral health: an evidence-based toolkit for prevention. Last updated 9 November 2021. Available from: https://www.gov.uk/government/publications/delivering-better-oral-health-an-evidence-based-toolkit-for-prevention. Accessed 28 Mar 2022.
6. Almuallem Z, Busuttil-Naudi A. Molar incisor hypomineralisation (MIH)—an overview. Br Dent J. 2018;225:601–9.
7. Lygidakis NA, Garot E, Somani C, Taylor GD, Rouas P, Wong FSL. Best clinical practice guidance for clinicians dealing with children presenting with molar-incisor-hypomineralisation (MIH): an updated European Academy of Paediatric Dentistry policy document. Eur Arch Paediatr Dent. 2022;23:3–21.
8. Cobourne MT, Williams A, Harrison M. National clinical guidelines for the extraction of first permanent molars in children. Br Dent J. 2014;217:643–8.
9. Gallagher J. The future oral and dental workforce for England. Liberating human resources to serve the population across the life-course. 7 March 2019. Available at: https://www.hee.nhs.uk/sites/default/files/documents/FDWF%20Report%20-%207th%20March%202019.pdf. Accessed 28 Mar 2022.

Part VIII

Orthodontics

Five Tips for Orthodontic Practitioners

38

Padhraig S. Fleming

Learning Points

- Appreciate the importance of diagnosis in the treatment planning of orthodontic treatment.
- Understand the importance of post-treatment stability in the maintenance of the desired outcome.
- Recognise and apply the various strategies to anchorage management.

38.1 Introduction

Orthodontics has witnessed meaningful progress in recent decades with renewed interest in self-ligation; the advent, wider adoption and continued growth of aligner therapy; and the dawn of a range of surgical and non-surgical adjuncts just some of the more salient developments. While progress challenges us to adapt, to update our knowledge and understanding and to embrace new technologies, the primacy of fundamental knowledge, careful planning and diligent oversight and the centrality of the orthodontist rather than the tools we use remains unchallenged. As such, the requirement for guiding principles remains pivotal and the challenge of condensing these into digestible tips is considerable. We emphasise the importance of fundamental keys embracing orthodontic diagnosis including the relationship between planning and prospective stability, principles of treatment planning and objective setting and anchorage management. These aspects represent a cornerstone of planning irrespective of the force delivery system.

P. S. Fleming (✉)
School of Dental Science, Dublin Dental University Hospital, The University of Dublin, Trinity College Dublin, Dublin, Ireland

Barts and The London School of Medicine and Dentistry, Queen Mary University of London, London, UK
e-mail: padhraig.fleming@dental.tcd.ie

E. McColl, A. Alani (eds.), *Practical Tips in Clinical Dentistry*, BDJ Clinician's Guides, https://doi.org/10.1007/978-3-031-90355-7_38

1. *Diagnosis is key.* As with any other area of dentistry or medicine, safe, effective and predictable outcomes are predicated on careful diagnosis. Orthodontic diagnosis involves the distillation of a range of factors spanning patient concerns, dental health, facial pattern (including skeletal and soft tissue factors and likely growth patterns) and occlusal features. Clear objectives should be formulated on the basis of thorough diagnosis. The quality of outcome, the prospective stability of treatment, optimal function and dental health all hinge on these pivotal considerations.

   The advent of three-dimensional technologies and digital planning do not obviate the need for this cornerstone of planning. Similarly, while technological advances have helped to simplify the process of treatment for adult patients in particular, none have been shown to enhance treatment outcomes, in isolation. There are also accepted weaknesses inherent in certain systems [1]. It is important, therefore, that the emphasis remains on the provision of quality care with a range of possible systems founded upon careful consideration, knowledge and planning.
2. *Key considerations when planning antero-posterior, vertical or transverse correction.* Meaningful orthodontic change should be based on the likely implications of treatment on health, aesthetics and stability. This should further be balanced with the potential unwanted effects of any proposed (non-surgical or surgical) intervention. In particular, significant arch lengthening may risk advancement of the incisors, which may lead to reduced periodontal support, while also destabilising the lower incisor position [2]. Moreover, the advancement of the incisors may also have aesthetic implications. Similarly, in the transverse plane, crossbite correction can be achieved by maxillary arch expansion, mandibular arch constriction or a combination of these movements. The scope for lower arch constriction is more limited. However, it can be helpful and may serve to limit the amount of required upper arch expansion, which is accepted to be particularly unstable with excessive dental expansion also risking periodontal compromise.
3. *Consideration of prospective stability from the outset.* There is an appreciation that tooth movement is an insidious and ongoing process with natural change unmitigated by orthodontics and genuine relapse following treatment also a potential risk. Diligent retention has proven effective in limiting both types of change in the longer term. [3, 4] However, there is also a recognition that specific treatment-related changes and features of malocclusion, for example, anterior open bite correction due to extrusion of the anterior dentition in the presence of skeletal discrepancy, may be particularly unstable. As such, treatment planning decisions and informed consent processes should involve due consideration of the prospective stability of treatment. [5]
4. *Detailed inter- and intra-arch treatment objectives.* Typically, full occlusal correction will be planned with Class I relationships targeted. However, it is also important that bespoke planning is undertaken for each dental arch concerning the intended position for both the upper and lower anteriors. Specifically, in a Class III case, for example, correction of the incisor relationship may be achieved by retracting the lower anteriors, in isolation; by advancing the maxillary incisors alone; or with a combination of these movements (Fig. 38.1). This logic can all be applied to the reduction of an increased overjet with retraction of the

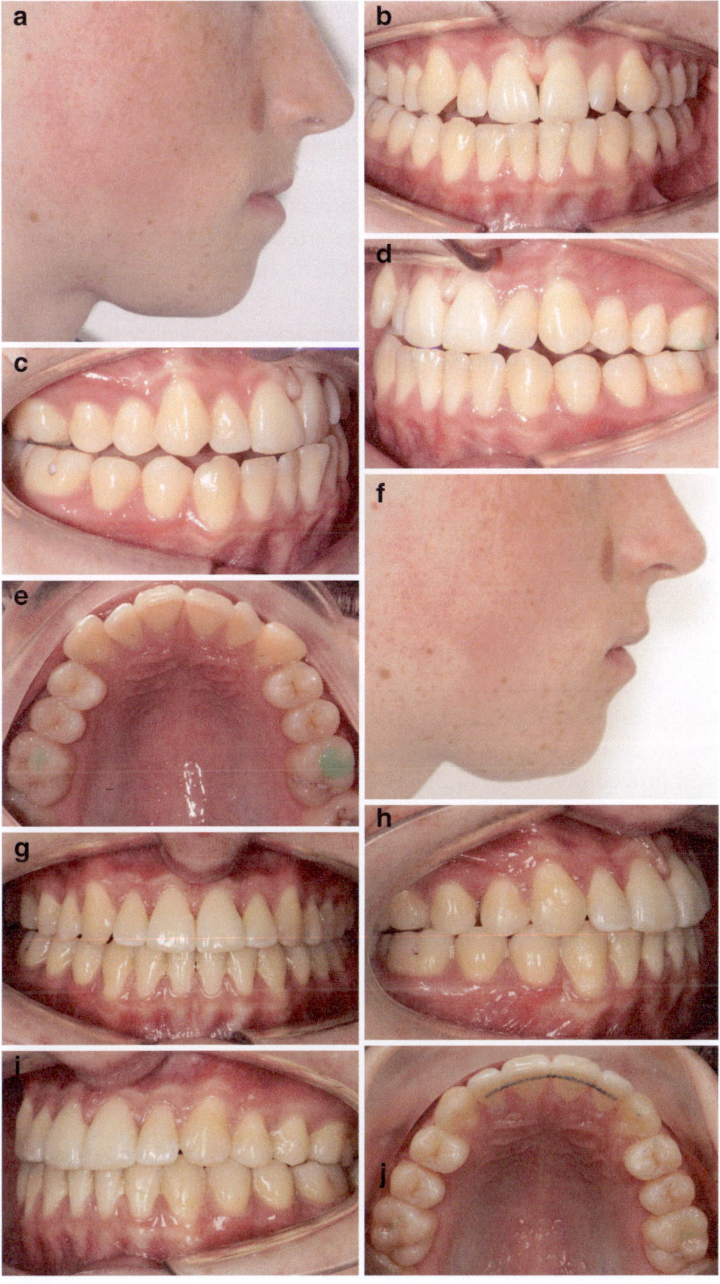

Fig. 38.1 A 15-year-old male presented with a Class III incisor relationship on a mild skeletal III pattern with a procumbent lower lip (**a**). The overjet was reduced with a reduced overbite and the presence of dual-arch crowding (**b–e**). From an aesthetic perspective, it was felt that scope existed to advance the maxillary incisors. A decision was made to treat this patient with fixed appliances to correct the occlusion both by retraction of the mandibular incisors and minimal advancement of the maxillary incisors. This approach lent itself to enhanced dental aesthetics by advancing the maxillary incisors, while retraction of the lower incisors promoted lower lip retraction (**f**). The retraction of the mandibular incisors also assisted with increase in the overbite (**g–j**)

maxillary incisors, advancement of the mandibular incisors or a combination of these movements representing possible options. In the presence of particularly prominent maxillary incisors and a protrusive upper lip and soft tissue pattern, retraction of the maxillary incisors is likely to maximise the aesthetic benefit of treatment. In addition, posterior movement of the maxillary incisors may promote the achievement of lip competence, which may decrease the tendency for overjet relapse. Similarly, by limiting advancement of the mandibular incisors, the risk of recurrence of lower anterior irregularity of overjet relapse may be offset. On the other hand, a retrusive soft tissue profile with relatively thin soft tissues and little upper lip support may preclude retraction of the maxillary incisors due to the aesthetic implications [6]. The overjet may be corrected, therefore, by advancement of the mandibular incisors, in isolation or in conjunction with limited retraction of the maxillary incisors. This plan will help to optimise both facial and dental aesthetics but does increase the risk of relapse associated with uprighting of the mandibular incisors in the post-treatment phase. This may lead to mandibular incisor irregularity and increased overjet. Alternatively, a residual overjet may be accepted in the presence of a skeletal II discrepancy or retrusive soft tissue profile, where orthognathic surgery is not considered appropriate. Permanent bonded retention may be mandatory in these cases.

5. *A hierarchy of intervention for anchorage management.* Optimal anchorage management is key to the fulfilment of intra- and inter-arch objectives. While space creation may well be required in order to achieve objectives, five further key strategies exist. These range from simple and predictable interventions that involve no additional risk or burden with wide potential application to more involved procedures (Fig. 38.2). The more invasive options may be required in cases or isolated arches with higher anchorage demands. However, by carefully considering objectives and planning, allied to careful use of the less invasive options, it may be possible to limit or obviate the need for these approaches. The range of possible options include:

Fig. 38.2 A hierarchy of approaches to anchorage management including conservative approaches (green font) such as appropriate selection of fixed appliance prescription and local bracket variations. More positive approaches (red font) do exist; however, these generally require additional invasiveness, risks and costs. A distinction can also be drawn between these approaches in respect of mode of action with elastics and springs exerting an inter-arch effect, while the impact of other approaches can be isolated to one arch. It is therefore possible to select appropriate means of anchorage management based on clear intra- as well as inter-arch objectives

(a) *Choice of bracket prescription:* A system appropriate for the arch should be selected. In particular, ample palatal root torque on the maxillary incisors may be helpful in withstanding the risk of unwanted retroclination during retraction of the maxillary incisors during overjet reduction. However, palatal root torque may be unhelpful in certain Class II cases and may also increase posterior anchorage demands in the maxillary arch.
(b) *Local bracket variations:* The alteration of tip on canine brackets may be useful. In particular, reversal or artistic placement of canine brackets may help to neutralise the bracket prescription limiting mesial tip expression as this can be anchorage demanding. Mesial crown tip expression induces an anchorage demand to position the root distally. This may accentuate anchorage-related challenges in the maxillary arch in Class II and in the mandibular arch in Class III scenarios, in particular.
(c) *Intra-arch considerations:* Wire gauge can be varied particularly to titrate the amount of bucco-palatal torque expression. Classically, full torque expression of the mandibular incisors may be unwanted in Class III cases especially where camouflage involving retraction or retroclination of the mandibular incisors is planned.
(d) *Inter-arch auxiliaries:* The use of inter-maxillary elastics and springs may be very effective in altering inter-arch relationships [7]. Clearly, however, it is important to appreciate that these mechanics either require compliance, have associated patient impacts or both. These mechanics also have reciprocal effects, for example, maxillary incisor retraction and lower incisor proclination with Class II elastics or flexible Class II correctors. Unwanted effects may of course be mitigated with adjunctive use of mini-implants or other compensations. However, the relative benefits of these auxiliaries in the antero-posterior plane should be balanced against these potential side effects.
(e) *Other fixed auxiliaries:* These include temporary anchorage devices (TADs) as well as palatal arches. There is equivocal evidence of benefit associated with trans-palatal arches; therefore, TADs may well afford a more predictable means of maximal anchorage provision [8]. However, failure with TADs does occur with associated risks including root contact and fracture of the screw.

38.2 Conclusion

As educated practitioners, we should be at the cutting edge being fully apprised of the contemporary options and trained in the use of any of these options in the correct scenario. However, with diagnostic skills and understanding, perhaps we should err on the side of keeping things as simple as possible. By exploring the least invasive options routinely, we may limit the need for more complex procedures with higher risk of failure or suboptimal compliance potentially leading to more predictable outcomes.

Predictability—that's a goal that we can all reasonably aim for, irrespective of the presenting malocclusion or the tool used to satisfy our clear and considered objectives.

References

1. Haouili N, Kravitz ND, Vaid NR, Ferguson DJ, Makki L. Has Invisalign improved? A prospective follow-up study on the efficacy of tooth movement with Invisalign. Am J Orthod Dentofacial Orthop. 2020 Sep;158(3):420–5. https://doi.org/10.1016/j.ajodo.2019.12.015.
2. Mills JR. The stability of the lower labial segment. A cephalometric survey. Dent Pract Dent Rec. 1968;18(8):293–306.
3. Al-Moghrabi D, Johal A, O'Rourke N, Donos N, Pandis N, Gonzales-Marin C, Fleming PS. Effects of fixed vs removable orthodontic retainers on stability and periodontal health: 4-year follow-up of a randomized controlled trial. Am J Orthod Dentofacial Orthop. 2018 Aug;154(2):167–174.e1. https://doi.org/10.1016/j.ajodo.2018.01.007.
4. Kocher KE, Gebistorf MC, Pandis N, Fudalej PS, Katsaros C. Survival of maxillary and mandibular bonded retainers 10 to 15 years after orthodontic treatment: a retrospective observational study. Prog Orthod. 2019;20(1):28. https://doi.org/10.1186/s40510-019-0279-8.
5. Fleming PS. Orthodontic treatment planning: can we plan for stability? Br Dent J. 2021 Jun;230(11):717–21. https://doi.org/10.1038/s41415-021-2891-5.
6. Alkadhi RM, Finkelman MD, Trotman CA, Kanavakis G. The role of lip thickness in upper lip response to sagittal change of incisor position. Orthod Craniofac Res. 2019;22:53–7.
7. McNamara JA, Franchi L, McClatchey LM, Kowalski SE, Cheeseman CC. Evaluation of adolescent and adult patients treated with the Carriere motion class III appliance followed by fixed appliances. Angle Orthod. 2021;91(2):149–56. https://doi.org/10.2319/073120-669.1.
8. Sandler J, Murray A, Thiruvenkatachari B, Gutierrez R, Speight P, O'Brien K. Effectiveness of 3 methods of anchorage reinforcement for maximum anchorage in adolescents: a 3-arm multicenter randomized clinical trial. Am J Orthod Dentofacial Orthop. 2014 Jul;146(1):10–20. https://doi.org/10.1016/j.ajodo.2014.03.020.

Managing Orthodontic Emergencies in Primary Care

39

Jamie Deans, Ewen McColl, and Sean Hamilton

Learning Points

- Recall the various presentations of orthodontic emergencies.
- Understand the principles in managing orthodontic emergencies.
- Appreciate the need to minimise disruption to the orthodontic treatment through efficient and timely management of orthodontic emergencies.

39.1 Introduction

The General Dental Council (GDC) in *Preparing for practice* [1] states the following learning objectives should have been achieved by dentists upon qualification, in relation to supporting patients undergoing orthodontic treatment. These objectives include explaining to patients the risks of orthodontic treatment and being able to undertake limited orthodontic appliance emergency procedures.

Whilst most orthodontic appliance emergencies are dealt with by specialist practices, there are occasions where the general dental practitioner (GDP) is faced with an anxious parent or patient with an emergency they may not be so familiar with. Dentists report seeing an average of one orthodontic emergency every 6 months and reassuringly most are confident in how to deal with the majority of common problems [2].

J. Deans
Borders General Hospital, Melrose, UK

E. McColl (✉)
Peninsula Dental School, Plymouth, UK
e-mail: ewen.mccoll@plymouth.ac.uk

S. Hamilton
Peninsula Dental School (University of Plymouth), Derriford Dental Education Facility, Plymouth, UK

E. McColl, A. Alani (eds.), *Practical Tips in Clinical Dentistry*, BDJ Clinician's Guides, https://doi.org/10.1007/978-3-031-90355-7_39

That said, there are times when patients can't access specialist practice facilities to deal with the problem for geographical or financial reasons, and problems relating to retention can occur long after discharge from their orthodontic practitioner.

Detailed guidance has previously been published on the management of orthodontic emergencies in a general practice [3–5] but in this short paper, we discuss five likely presentations of orthodontic emergencies and share our pragmatic tips on how the GDP can manage them.

39.2 Trauma from a Broken Fixed Appliance

This is documented as the most common cause of an orthodontic emergency [6] and is usually a lost bracket or a protruding archwire. We do not recommend that GDPs replace lost brackets but may be called upon to manage a problematic archwire. When faced with this, we recommend that the practitioner considers why the archwire has become traumatic. These problematic archwires can cause trauma to the oral mucosa (Fig. 39.1) and this is often due to the following:

1. Tooth movement. When spaces are closed due to sliding mechanics on a straight wire appliance, wire begins to protrude out of the distal tube or band slot. *Consider*—wax and reassurance if mild (Fig. 39.2) or cut the offending distal end of the wire with distal end cutters (Fig. 39.3).
2. Swivelled or rotated archwire. This normally happens to patients in flexible aligning archwires due to occlusal forces directly or indirectly flexing the archwire between the brackets or tubes, causing it to move round. It is not dissimilar to losing one end of the cord in your swimming trunks! Archwire swivelling can also occur when an aligning archwire has been asymmetrically cut and placed into a symmetrical arch form (Fig. 39.4). The asymmetric archwire rotates over time to fit the arch form and protrudes out one end. To diagnose a swivelled wire, look at the contralateral side to see if it is short. *Consider*—wax and reassurance

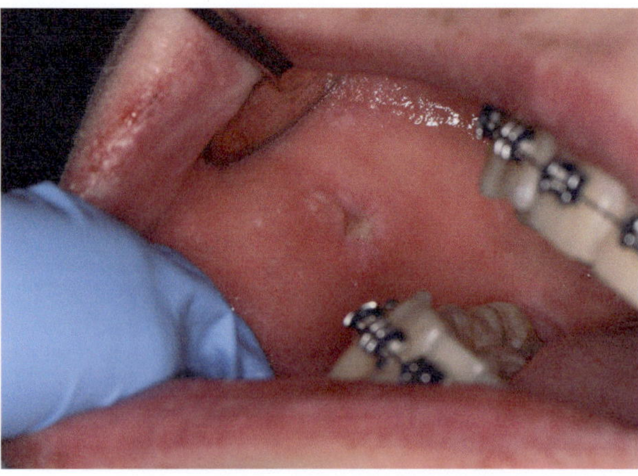

Fig. 39.1 Trauma to the oral mucosa from an archwire

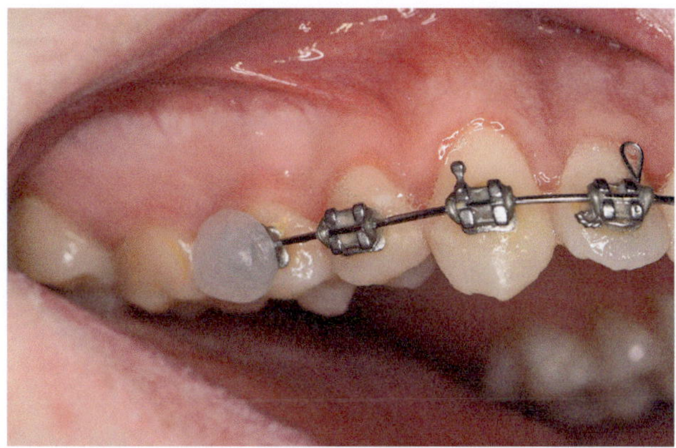

Fig. 39.2 Wax on a protruding archwire end

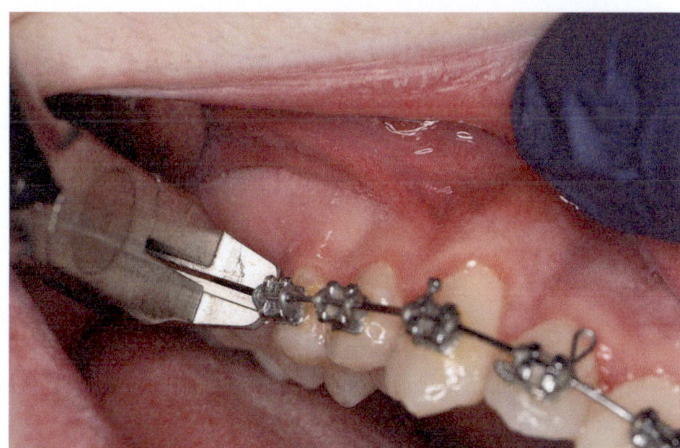

Fig. 39.3 Cutting the distal end of an archwire

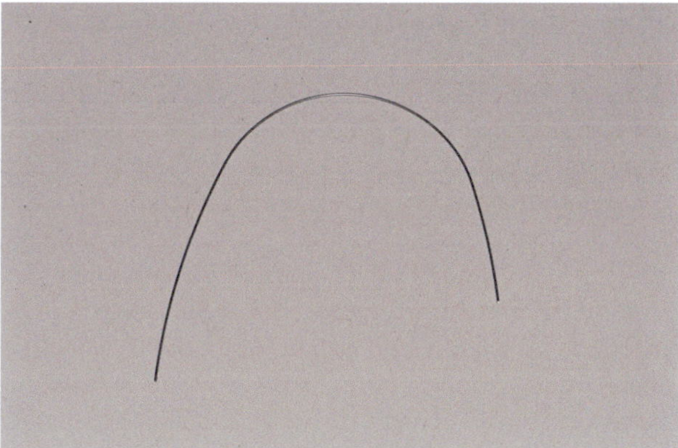

Fig. 39.4 An asymmetrically cut archwire

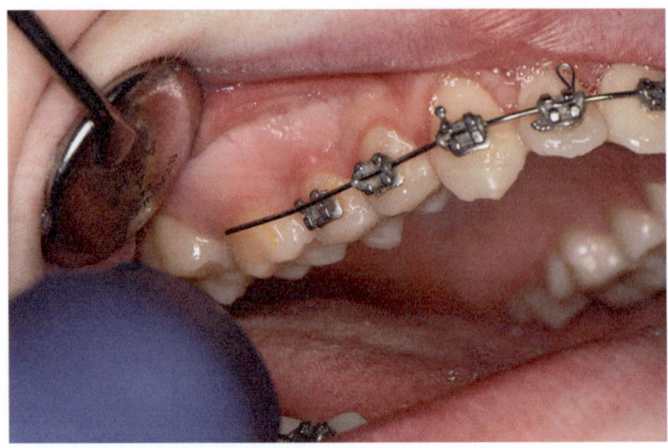

Fig. 39.5 Loss of a terminal molar band or tube

if mild, cut the distal end with distal end cutters or (if confident) grip and reposition the swivelled wire with a pair of utility pliers.

3. Loss of distal band or tube. Sometimes, the distal tube or band becomes detached from the tooth, leaving a long length of wire protruding (Fig. 39.5). *Consider*—cut the distal end of the wire with distal end cutters.
4. Wire displaced from distal tube or band slot. When the orthodontist has included the second molars on the appliance in addition to first molars, the wide inter-slot length can result in a flexible wire being displaced out of the tube slot due to occlusal forces. The wire can also come out of the first molar tube slot when unsupported in extraction or hypodontia cases. *Consider*—replace the archwire in the slot with a pair of utility pliers or cut the archwire distal to the terminal bracket with distal end cutters.

39.3 Pain from Orthodontic Tooth Movement

Orofacial pain is a common side effect of orthodontic treatment occurring in 72–100% of patients [7]. The pain usually starts 12 h after orthodontic force application, peaks after 24 h and lasts for 3–7 days. In a minority of cases, it can take up to 1 month to return to pre-treatment levels.

Orthodontic pain is caused by ischaemic changes in the PDL [periodontal ligament] and a resulting cascade of inflammatory responses that form part of the biology of tooth movement. The pain is ultimately controlled by endogenous analgesic mechanisms, but some patients benefit from intervention. Despite many interventions claiming to regulate orthodontic pain, the only approach based on robust evidence is a pharmacological one. *Consider*—reassurance in the form of demonstrating an understanding of what is happening to the patient and the appropriate prescription of non-opioid analgesics or non-steroidal anti-inflammatory drugs.

39.4 Lost or Broken Retainers

Most orthodontic patients require indefinite retention to prevent long-term post-treatment changes to their occlusions [8]. Therefore, the breakage or loss of a retainer must be addressed with urgency. We have identified the following as retainer emergencies and recommend some basic interventions to those practitioners with limited orthodontic experience, equipment and materials:

1. Loss of a removable retainer. *Consider*—an impression or intra-oral scan followed by provision of a replacement retainer to be worn as recommended by the patient's orthodontist.
2. Complete loss of a bonded retainer. *Consider*—removal of the residual composite with a composite-removing bur followed by an impression or intra-oral scan to provide a removable pressure-formed retainer. This will buy the patient time to find a practitioner to consider having the bonded retainer replaced if appropriate.
3. Partial fracture of a bonded retainer. *Consider*—removal of redundant residual composite with a composite-removing bur and smoothing down of potentially traumatic wire ends with an abrasive disc. This can then be followed by an impression or intra-oral scan to provide a removable pressure-formed retainer.
4. Partial debond of a bonded retainer. *Consider*—removal of redundant residual composite from the tooth (fluted tungsten carbide bur and a slow handpiece) and retainer wire (utility pliers) followed by careful repair with new composite resin bonded by the practitioner's choice of system. Care must be taken to ensure the retainer wire is recemented correctly, ensuring that it is passive so as not to cause any unwanted tooth movement.

In the absence of any pre-existing instructions for the wear of removable retainers, we recommend overnight wear until the patient can return to the orthodontist supervising their retention.

39.5 Demineralisation

Demineralised lesions are caused by poor appliance cleaning and cariogenic diet (Fig. 39.6). They can take only 4 weeks to occur during orthodontic treatment [9] and are prevalent in a significant percentage of orthodontic patients [10]. The reinforcement of oral hygiene instructions to clean an orthodontic appliance and diet advice to reduce the frequency of sugars are paramount. The professional application of fluoride every 6–8 weeks during appliance therapy is associated with a reduction in the development of demineralised lesions [11].

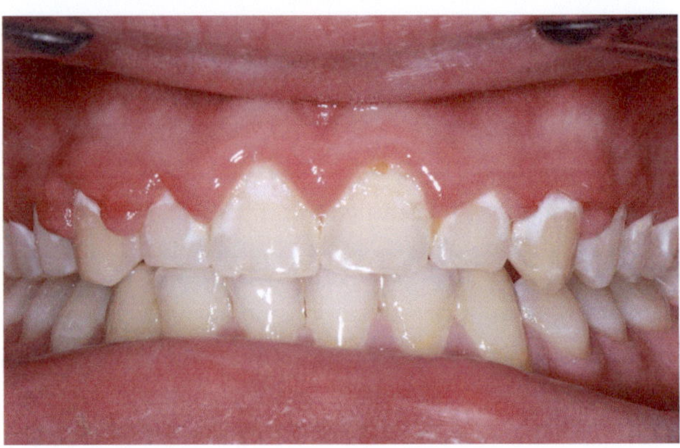

Fig. 39.6 Orthodontic appliance-related demineralisation

With demineralisation in mind, it is imperative to have effective communication between dental colleagues when orthodontic treatment is planned. This allows the general dental practitioner to contribute to the risk assessment before treatment begins and develops a shared responsibility between all parties in the prevention of damage to the oral tissues.

Should the dental practitioner have concerns about the patient's oral hygiene or suspect that demineralisation has already occurred and the patient cannot immediately return to the orthodontic specialist, we recommend the following *action*:

1. Clean the teeth and appliance with a combination of prophylactic paste and rubber cup, ultrasonic scaler to remove calculus deposits and interproximal brushes to clean under the archwire adjacent to brackets.
2. Rinse and dry the dentition and examine all teeth for demineralisation.
3. Consider intra-oral photographs, document findings and inform the patient.

If demineralisation has NOT occurred, then we recommend the following immediate *action*:

1. Reinforce diet advice and appliance cleaning instructions.
2. Consider professional application of high-dose fluoride [12].
3. Strongly advise the patient to seek a timely review with their orthodontic specialist.
4. Communicate to the orthodontic specialist your findings and management actions.

If demineralisation HAS occurred and the patient has no timely access to an orthodontic practitioner, then we recommend the following immediate *action*:

1. Reinforce diet advice and appliance cleaning instructions.
2. Remove the brackets and leave the residual composite resin on the tooth surface. DO NOT use a composite-removing bur and handpiece as this may cause damage to the enamel.

3. Take an impression or intra-oral scan and provide removable pressure-formed retainers for part-time wear.
4. Consider prescription of products containing casein phosphopeptide amorphous calcium phosphate (CPPACP) [13].
5. Strongly advise the patient to seek a timely review with their orthodontic specialist.
6. Communicate to the orthodontic specialist your findings and management actions.

The removal of orthodontic brackets and composite can result in minor enamel loss for all orthodontic patients [14] but is worse in patients with evidence of enamel demineralisation [15]. As this iatrogenic enamel damage is mainly associated with the composite removal stage of appliance removal, we recommend that careful composite removal is carried out by the orthodontic specialist after attempting to remineralise the tooth surface.

Demineralisation can improve in the first 6 months following cessation of orthodontic treatment with improved diet and toothbrushing [16]. High-dose fluoride applications are effective in preventing demineralisation but should be avoided in the immediate management of orthodontic demineralisation. The use CPPACP (tooth mousse) could be considered.

39.6 Acute Gingival Conditions

Plaque-related gingivitis is common in orthodontic patients and, although important to diagnose, inform and manage, in isolation is not an orthodontic emergency.

However, there are gingival conditions that present during orthodontic treatment that either require urgent management such as necrotising gingivitis/necrotising periodontitis (NG/NP) or cause great concern to patients due to the appearance, such as severe gingival enlargement (SGE).

NG/NP classically presents with pain, loss of inter-dental papilla, bleeding, halitosis, fever, malaise and lymphadenopathy. The incidence of NG/NP in orthodontic patients is unknown [17], but it may be more common in orthodontic patients due to the plaque-retentive nature of fixed appliances.

It can present in a variety of forms with varied severity [18], and as NUG [necrotising ulcerative gingivitis] can cause irreversible damage to the gingiva, we recommend the following:

1. Cessation of modifying factors such as smoking.
2. Oral hygiene instruction.
3. Debridement of areas affected.
4. If the patient is pyrexic, prescription of metronidazole 400 mg three times daily for 3 days with chlorhexidine mouthwash to be used twice a day for 7 days.
5. Review.

Unless the orthodontic appliance is preventing access for debridement or is associated with enamel demineralisation, an immediate debond for NG/NP may not be indicated. A debond of the appliance followed by provision of removable retention could be considered if:

1. This is requested by a specialist periodontologist.
2. The oral hygiene is extremely poor.
3. The gingival condition fails to resolve after standard intervention.
4. Loss of attachment is severe.

Gingival enlargement is positively associated with fixed appliance orthodontic treatment and, when it occurs anteriorly, has a negative effect on oral health-related quality of life [19]. It is believed to be caused by plaque accumulation or local irritation from the appliances but can also be hereditary, allergic response or drug induced. Interestingly, the amount of plaque present is not directly related to the severity of gingival enlargement but appears to be due to the make-up of the plaque and the host response [20].

Severe gingival enlargement is a chronic condition that is not normally associated with pain or loss of attachment but can be a cause of severe concern to a parent or patient. Although it is generally agreed that gingival enlargement resolves after completion/cessation of orthodontic treatment, some cases persist and may need gingival surgical procedures [21].

If the dental practitioner is presented with a patient deeply upset by severe orthodontic-associated gingival enlargement, *consider* either:

1. Reinforcement of appliance cleaning and reassurance that 'most' cases resolve after completion of orthodontic treatment. Advise orthodontic review when next possible.
2. If no foreseeable orthodontic review possible, gain consent for cessation of orthodontic treatment and provision of part-time removable retainers if patient wishes to retain significant tooth movements. As above, reassure patient that 'most' cases resolve after completion of orthodontic treatment.

We have described some simple interventions and equipment required (Box 39.1) to manage some common orthodontic emergencies. We encourage undergraduate dental students and general dental practitioners to work with their orthodontic colleagues to develop competencies (Box 39.2) to confidently deal with these situations.

Box 39.1 Orthodontic Equipment for Managing Orthodontic Emergencies

Distal end cutters
Bracket removal pliers
Utility orthodontic pliers (Weingarts)
Composite-removing bur
Orthodontic wax
Band removing pliers

Box 39.2 Simple Skills to Develop for Managing Orthodontic Emergencies

Cutting a distal end
Placing orthodontic wax
Removing and placing elastomeric modules
Removing an archwire
Repositioning a swivelled archwire
Repair of a partially debonded fixed retainer
Removing orthodontic brackets and bands

39.7 Conclusions

Orthodontic emergencies, whilst relatively rare, can present at inopportune moments. The tips presented in this paper allow guidance on how some frequently presenting acute orthodontic problems may best be managed in primary care when timely access to a specialist orthodontist may not be feasible.

References

1. General Dental Council. Preparing for practice. Dental team learning outcomes for registration (2015 revised edition). Available at: https://www.gdc-uk.org/docs/default-source/quality-assurance/preparing-for-practice-%28revised-2015%29.pdf. Accessed February 2023.
2. Popat H, Thomas K, Farnell DJJ. Management of orthodontic emergencies in primary care—self-reported confidence of general dental practitioners. Br Dent J. 2016;221:21–4.
3. Sodipo I, Birdsall J. Orthodontic first aid for general dental practitioners. Dent Update. 2016;43:461–71.
4. Dowsing P, Murray A, Sandler J. Emergencies in orthodontic practice part 1: management of general orthodontic problems as well as common problems with fixed appliances. Dent Update. 2015;42:131–40.

5. Dowsing P, Murray A, Sandler J. Emergencies in orthodontic practice part 2: management of removable appliances, functional appliances and other adjuncts to orthodontic treatment. Dent Update. 2015;42:221–8.
6. Kwon O, Sivamurthy G, McIntyre G. Patient experience and usage of orthodontic emergency clinics: a local re-audit. BOS Clinical Effectiveness Bulletin, November 2019.
7. Long H, Wang Y, Jian F, Liao L, Yang X, Lai W. Current advances in orthodontic pain. Int J Oral Sci. 2016;8:67–75.
8. Littlewood S, Dalci O, Dolce C, Holliday S, Naraghi S. Orthodontic retention: what's on the horizon? Br Dent J. 2021;230:760–4.
9. Reilly MM, Featherstone JD. Decalcification and remineralization around orthodontic appliances: an in vivo study. Am J Orthod Dentofacial Orthop. 1987;92:33–40.
10. Ogaard B. Prevalence of white spot lesions in 19 year olds: a study on untreated and orthodontically treated persons 5 years after treatment. Am J Orthod Dentofacial Orthop. 1989;96:423–7.
11. Benson PE, Parkin N, Dyer F, Millett DT, Germain P. Fluorides for preventing early tooth decay (demineralised lesions) during fixed brace treatment. Cochrane Database Syst Rev. 2019; https://doi.org/10.1002/14651858.CD003809.pub4.
12. NHS Education for Scotland. Prevention and management of dental caries in children. Dental Clinical Guidance. Scottish Dental Clinical Effectiveness Programme, 2018. Available at: https://www.sdcep.org.uk/published-guidance/caries-in-children/. Accessed August 2023.
13. Sampson V, Sampson A. Diagnosis and treatment options for anterior white spot lesions. Br Dent J. 2020;229:348–52.
14. Ryf S, Flury S, Palaniappan S, Lussi A, van Meerbak B, Zimmerli B. Enamel loss and adhesive remnants following bracket removal and various clean up procedures in vitro. Eur J Orthod. 2012;34:25–32.
15. Cochrane N, Ratneser S, Reynolds E. Effect of different orthodontic adhesive removal techniques on sound, demineralized and remineralized enamel. Aust Dent J. 2012;57:365–72.
16. Khoroushi M, Kachuie M. Prevention and treatment of white spot lesions in orthodontic patients. Contemp Clin Dent. 2017;8:11–9.
17. Sangani I, Watt E, Cross D. Necrotizing ulcerative gingivitis and the orthodontic patient: a case series. J Orthod. 2013;40:77–80.
18. Rodríguez-Pulido J, Quiroga-Zúñiga N, Martínez-Sandoval G. Clinical diagnosis and treatment of necrotizing ulcerative gingivitis in the orthodontic patient. A case report. J Oral Res. 2016;5:119–23.
19. Pinto A, Alves L, Eduardo J, Zenkner A, Zanatta F, Maltz M. Gingival enlargement in orthodontic patients: effects of treatment duration. Am J Orthod Dentofacial Orthop. 2017;152:477–82.
20. Vincent-Bugnas S, Borsa L, Gruss A, Lupi L. Prioritisation of predisposing factors of gingival hyperplasia during orthodontic treatment: the role of the amount of biofilm. BMC Oral Health. 2021;21:84. https://doi.org/10.1186/s12903-021-01433-2.
21. Kouraki E, Bissada N, Paloma J, Ficara A. Gingival enlargement and resolution during and after resolution. N Y State Dent J. 2005;71:34–7.

Part IX

Practice Management, Governance and Wellbeing

Keeping Dentistry Stimulating

40

R. J. R. Smith, Ewen McColl, and G. E. Bryce

Learning Points

- Recognise that self-reflection can help with maintaining career stimulation.
- Identify opportunities during the week for improving your clinical skills or enhancing the clinical environment to make work easier to manage.
- Appreciate areas of development that can aid self-fulfilment and career satisfaction.

40.1 Introduction

The average career of a dentist may be 40 years [1] and proactivity is needed to ensure that the professional does not stagnate. This can be challenging especially as the demands of dental service provision often necessitate a steadfast routine that, whilst efficient, may lead to 'rust out' or 'burn out' (Table 40.1). In this article, we provide top tips for keeping dentistry stimulating.

Table 40.1 Symptoms and causes of 'rust out' and 'burn out'

	Symptoms	Examples of contributory factors
Rust out [2]	Day-to-day feels mundane Feeling unstimulated and uninspired Day goes 'slowly'	Insufficient variety and challenge Skill set is not being stretched (and developed)
Burn out [3]	Feeling tired, helpless, trapped, detached, cynical or overwhelmed Procrastinating over decisions	Sustained excessive workload Poor work-life balance Real (or perceived) lack of control

R. J. R. Smith
Defence Centre for Rehabilitative Dentistry, Aldershot, UK

E. McColl (✉)
Peninsula Dental School, Plymouth, UK
e-mail: ewen.mccoll@plymouth.ac.uk

G. E. Bryce
Restorative Dentistry, Defence Centre for Rehabilitative Dentistry, Aldershot, UK

E. McColl, A. Alani (eds.), *Practical Tips in Clinical Dentistry*, BDJ Clinician's Guides, https://doi.org/10.1007/978-3-031-90355-7_40

40.2 Reflect and Refine Your Working Practice

40.2.1 Identify Good and Bad Habits

A habit can be defined as a 'fixed way of thinking, willing, or feeling acquired through previous repetition of a mental experience' [4] and is central to developing routine, a core component of working life. Self-reflection with adjustments to habits or routine are essential to the reinforcement of good and reduction of bad practices. Crucially, this can help check negative thoughts such as 'what's the point; I am going have a bad day; nobody understands the difficulties we face' and reduce the risk of falling into spirals of self-doubt.

40.2.2 Pause and Take Time

Consider:

(i) Am I happy in what I do?
(ii) What do I like about my job/profession?
(iii) What don't I like about my job?
(iv) How can I build upon what I like?
(v) How can I change what I don't like?

40.2.3 Plan

A professional development plan (PDP) is great for specifying short, medium and long-term goals, not least because it requires the individual to consider what they want to achieve. Once you know *what* you want to achieve, turning these aspirations into a Specific/Measurable/Achievable/Relevant/Time-bound (SMART) objectives can help formulate a pathway for *how* you will attain them [5].

40.3 Keep Challenging Yourself—Avoid 'Rust Out'

40.3.1 Vary Your Routine

It can be really easy to fall into a working pattern where the complexity of the clinical work becomes less challenging and requiring reduced proactive thought for the planning and execution. Subsequently, clinicians run the risk of becoming 'stale' and, without change, may exacerbate the feeling of being 'imprisoned' within the four walls of their surgeries.

40.3.2 Identify a 'Problem of the Week'

Find an area for improvement within your practice environment and work collaboratively with the team to solve this. This can lead to a sense of satisfaction, enhance team cohesion as well as improving the overall operating environment for staff and patients (see Sect. 40.4—Leading Change).

40.3.3 Advance Your Clinical Skills

Clinical practice is a process and not a discrete or 'achieved' event. Dentistry (like medicine) is in a constant state of progression. Failure to consistently strive for clinical advancement leads to stagnation, which risks leaving the individual ever further from the 'gold standard'. Top tips for clinical advancement:

(i) Be humble and constantly willing to enhance your skills.
(ii) Combine innovation, evidence-based dentistry and audit of practice-based outcomes to drive forward improvements to clinical delivery.
(iii) Seek mentorship from a more experienced colleague within your area of interest.
(iv) When identifying cases suitable for safe clinical advancement, look for those which offer one or two aspects for development. Build gradually. Try not to overload on the most difficult cases.
(v) Maintain a logbook of clinical cases with critical reflection on outcomes, assessing both positive aspects (for incorporation into practice) as well as areas for development.

40.3.4 Develop Your Skills with Postgraduate Study

When choosing a course or programme, consider:

(i) Prioritising your learning needs and how these fit with your aspirations for current and future clinical practice.
(ii) What type of educational format will most appropriately meet your learning needs and personal circumstances:
    1. Fully remote online learning.
    2. Blended online/face-to-face learning.
    3. Full-time residential programme.
(iii) Arrangements for funding—whether this needs to be personally funded or whether an employer can partly or fully fund the training.
(iv) Time commitment for travel, attendance and studying.

Table 40.2 The commonest routes to GDC Specialist accreditation

Route	Key features
Three-year formalised training pathway (full or part-time)	Training via an accredited provider, leading to the award of completion of certificate of specialist training (CSST)
'Assessed' application	For those who have not completed a formalised 3-year training pathway but can demonstrate that they have undertaken training equivalent to this

40.3.5 Develop Your Special Interest

The primary care (Tier-1) environment provides an array of opportunities (and challenges) for provision of quality dental care to a broad patient demographic. However, many GDPs (if not all?) will naturally develop a special interest in one or more specific areas of practice. Clinical advancement within an area of 'special interest' may be informal or part of a formalised pathway* leading to accreditation as a:

(i) *Dentist with Enhanced Skills (DES)* [previously known as a Dentist with Special Interest (DwSI)]. This is an NHS appointment that enables practitioners to take referrals of Tier-2 complexity [6]. Currently, DES opportunities are mostly confined to NHS dentists offering Tier-2 oral surgery and orthodontic services.
(ii) *General Dental Council (GDC)-Accredited Specialist*. The GDC maintains lists of dentists who have demonstrated satisfactory completion of training in one of 13 recognised dental specialities [7]. Specialist dental care involves the management of cases of up to Tier-3 complexity. The commonest pathways to specialist accreditation are shown in Table 40.2.

If you wish to become a DES or Specialist, ensure that you familiarise yourself with the regulations for accreditation in these roles (noting that regulations change over time).

40.4 Develop with Your Peers

Engagement with a group of peers who are professionally engaged provides contacts and context to discuss professional challenges and problem solve. Forums include:

40.4.1 Morning Case Discussions

Timetable 10 min before the start of your clinical day to identify the case/s that you are either looking forward to, or concerned about, and present them to your colleagues. This not only provides an immediate and easy forum for success/problem-sharing but also facilitates the opportunity to mentally prepare for the day ahead.

40.4.2 Dental Study Clubs

There are a multitude of dental study groups across the United Kingdom, organised by a range of providers, including GDPs or Specialists, with or without affiliation to public or private organisations. Meetings provide the opportunity to:

(i) Network and make friends with a group of fellow dental professionals.
(ii) Share experiences of challenges encountered (and overcome) in practice, including group case discussions.
(iii) Undertake +/− lead in the delivery of a continuing professional development (CPD) serial.

40.4.3 Professional Associations

There are many UK-based professional dental associations, which seek to develop, promote and educate within their area of interest. Benefits of membership include the opportunity to:

(i) Enhance situational awareness and insight into pathways for career development. For example, the College of General Dentistry has a range of structured career pathways for the whole dental team including the Certified Membership scheme [8].
(ii) Attend regional and national meetings, discuss specific subjects and controversies, whilst gaining CPD.
(iii) Present a poster (either a clinical case report or research project), which can help hone scientific writing and presentational skills.
(iv) Apply to become a member of a board or committee, which provides the opportunity to gain insight into, and contribute to, higher-level leadership.
(v) Participate in or facilitate 'Young Practitioner' groups, to engage and support development of junior dentists.

40.5 Stay with the Vanguard

40.5.1 Keep up to Date with Advances in Healthcare

Change is continuous and, within healthcare, techniques and materials quickly become obsolete as innovations emerge, for instance, the current transformation to digital impression taking. Maintaining awareness of emerging technologies is key to ensuring that you (and your practice) are optimally positioned to adopt change when the timing or environment is correct.

40.5.2 Lead Change

Top tips for leading a change project include:

(i) Not all change has to be revolutionary. Set change targets that are realistic, with outcomes that are easily accessible.
(ii) Get experience with small projects before tackling bigger ones.
(iii) Choose a project that will bring tangible benefits for the clinical team, and ultimately patient care.
(iv) Ask your team what they find challenging/inefficient and offer them the opportunity to come up with the solution. Empowerment is likely to result in greater engagement and superior outputs.
(v) Focus on the outcome rather than (real or perceived) obstacles to change. Believe that within the pursuit of the ultimate goal, as problems are encountered, these issues can be overcome.
(vi) Stick with it! Establishing a new way of working takes times, and the draw of reverting back to the comfort of pre-existing practices is strong. Leading change requires you to energise those around you, patience and fortitude. Use audit to assess the effectiveness of the change project.

40.6 Be an Educator

40.6.1 Learn Whilst You Teach

Teaching often encourages self-reflection where you really probe how much you know or don't know about your subject. Whilst this undoubtedly has benefits for your own professional development, the sharing of knowledge and acquired experience can also be incredibly rewarding.

40.6.2 Develop Your Educational Skills

Ideas for incremental development as an educator include:

(i) Developing and delivering:
   1. In-practice one-to-one training serial.
   2. In-practice training serial to multiple learners.
   3. Presentation at a regional study day.
   4. Presentation or webinar to a national audience.
(ii) Applying to work as an:

1. Educational supervisor.
2. Undergraduate tutor at a dental school.
3. Postgraduate tutor.

(iii) Formalised training and development as a medical educator. For example, a postgraduate certificate in medical (or dental) education, with the option to extend this to diploma or masters level.
(iv) Join and engage with the Faculty of Dental Trainers (Royal College of Surgeons of Edinburgh) or similar organisation.

40.7 Seek to Balance Life and Work—Avoiding 'Burn Out'

40.7.1 Consider What Your Priorities Are in Life

Seek to organise your schedule to flex time towards those things that matter most.

40.7.2 Consider a Change of Scene

Personal and family circumstances vary, but if possible, relocating to a new role or geographical location presents an exciting opportunity to reorientate your outlook and explore new opportunities.

40.7.3 Volunteer Your Time and Skills

Offering your time and skills for the benefit of others, without the expectation of renumeration, often provides a holistic reward to the volunteer whilst also benefitting wider society.

40.8 Conclusions

Maintaining a stimulating career in dentistry improves well-being and job satisfaction. Reflecting on everyday treatment decisions and pathways, potentially making changes to these, promotes variety and challenge that can enthuse clinicians to find new vigour where previous aspects of work may have felt mundane. Advancing your own skills through further postgraduate studying or passing on knowledge and experiences to others through teaching is hugely rewarding and can bring a new aspect to your career and work schedule.

References

1. American Dental Association. Health Policy Institute. Dentist retirements increase. 2022. Available at: https://www.ada.org/resources/research/health-policy-institute/all-hpi-publications. Accessed June 2023.
2. Fox H. Rust-out is the workplace phenomenon making us all feel flat. Harpers Bazaar. 11 May 2023. Available at: https://www.harpersbazaar.com/uk/beauty/mind-body/a43695947/rust-out/. Accessed June 2023.

3. Mental Health UK. Burnout. Available at: https://mentalhealth-uk.org/burnout/. Accessed June 2023.
4. Andrews BR. Habit. Am J Psychol. 1908;14:121–49.
5. Maguire W, Blaylock P. Preparing a personal development plan for all members of the dental team. Br Dent J. 2017;223:402–4.
6. British Dental Association. Dentists with special interests in practice. 2023. Available at: https://bda.org/careers/Generalpractice/Pages/dwsiip.aspx. Accessed June 2023.
7. General Dental Council. Specialist lists. 2023. Available at: https://www.gdc-uk.org/registration/your-registration/specialist-lists. Accessed June 2023.
8. College of General Dentistry. Certified Membership Scheme. 2023. Online information available at https://cgdent.uk/certified-membership/. Accessed June 2023.

Practical Tips on Wellbeing for Dental Professionals

41

Linda Fisher, Jennifer Hare, and Ewen McColl

Learning Points

- Understand that dentistry can be draining mentally and that identifying areas of pressure and stress is beneficial as it is the start of managing these aspects of work
- Appreciate how to apply aspects of cognitive behavioural therapy to the dental environment
- Identify instances of negative thinking and how to manage them
- Appreciate how making connections with colleagues and friends fosters better mental health and wellbeing
- Recognise how exercise and maintenance of good sleep patterns support mental health

41.1 Introduction

Members of the dental team are often so focused on looking after their patients that they neglect to look after themselves. Unfortunately, time pressures and managing patient expectations on a daily basis can be depleting. Looking after your own and your team members' wellbeing is crucial not only for us as individuals; it also ensures optimal patient care is facilitated. This chapter will provide tips for staying well in the context of a busy, often stressful and demanding workplace.

Most people are familiar with the idea of taking exercise and eating well to keep fit and physically healthy, but it is less well known that there are effective strategies that can be used to help to deal with the inevitable work challenges, to promote 'mind-fitness'. It is well known that when we begin to feel 'stressed' or depleted in

L. Fisher · J. Hare
Dental Psychology Service, Guy's and St Thomas' NHS Foundation Trust, London, UK

E. McColl (✉)
Peninsula Dental School, Plymouth, UK
e-mail: ewen.mccoll@plymouth.ac.uk

E. McColl, A. Alani (eds.), *Practical Tips in Clinical Dentistry*, BDJ Clinician's Guides, https://doi.org/10.1007/978-3-031-90355-7_41

some way, we begin to *think* and *feel* and *behave* in particular ways, many of which can be unhelpful.

Whilst this article is written for dental professionals, it is also true to say that each of us only ever works in the context of the wider fabric of our life. Combining a professional life with various challenges across the lifespan, for example, bringing up a young family, caring for elderly relatives and, for women, the menopause, not to mention financial difficulties or problems in our personal relationships, is not to be underplayed.

Increasingly, it is recognised that both self-awareness and the capacity to draw on a range of coping skills make an important contribution to our psychological flexibility and emotional agility and thus our capacity to flourish in both our personal and professional lives. This is not to say that these strategies should be used to put up with intolerable work conditions, rather that they can be applied appropriately, systematically and usefully to support the challenges involved in everyday life.

We have chosen to focus on six key tips for wellbeing and very much hope that you will find something in what follows that adds to your repertoire of coping skills and contributes to your wellbeing in all areas of your life! We have also added links for faith and community-based resources for health and wellbeing for ease of access and completeness at the end of this article.

41.2 Cultivate Self-Awareness

41.2.1 Using a CBT Framework to Pick Up Early Signs of Being Under Pressure

Using a simple cognitive behavioural therapy (CBT) framework on a regular basis to break down experience into *thoughts*, *feelings* (mood and physiology) and *behaviours* can provide a structure around which to usefully 'check-in' with yourself. Recognising early on if you are beginning to feel depleted and need to think about 'resourcing' yourself more fully, or indeed, if you need to change something about the way that you are working, is easier than allowing difficulties to build up and trying to make changes when you are already becoming overwhelmed.

Signs of 'stressed' thinking might be focused on not wanting to go to work or how little you are enjoying your work, or you may begin to think in a repetitive, unproductive and uncontrollable way (ruminate) on problems at work or at home.

Emotions may include beginning to feel low or anxious or indecisive on a persistent basis, and behavioural change might include disruption to your sleep, being irritable, drinking too much alcohol and no longer doing enjoyable things, for example, seeing friends or family or going to the gym. It is not uncommon for people who feel low and anxious to lack energy and experience other minor physical symptoms. In the worst-case scenario, you may begin to have thoughts about wanting to harm yourself in some way, not wanting to wake up in the morning or just not wanting to go on. When things get this bad, it is not unusual for people to feel an increasing sense of shame about what is happening to them and to feel isolated from others whom they would normally turn to for support. If you ever begin to feel this way, it is essential that you seek professional help as a matter of urgency (please see links to suggested sources of help at the end of this article).

If you are feeling very anxious or quite low (both of which can be a strong trigger for the so-called 'negative bias' in human thinking), in order to gain some perspective on whatever it is you are thinking about, it may be helpful to ask yourself:

- What is the worst thing that can happen?
- What is the best thing that could happen?
- What is the most likely thing to happen?

41.3 Focus on the 'Now' in Your Life

Mindfulness strategies are increasingly recognised as useful in helping people to restore balance and a sense of steadiness in challenging situations. Put simply, developing the capacity to notice when you are getting lost in unhelpful thinking (perhaps overly anxious or pessimistic thinking, or just repeatedly 'going around in circles') is the first step in this process. Thinking in unhelpful ways can lower mood or feed into other unpleasant mood states and make you miss what is enjoyable and uplifting in life. Is there really anyone reading this who has not ever been preoccupied with a work problem when out with a loved one or friend, and simply 'missed out' on some of the joy and fun and sense of closeness that has been available to us if only we had not been so wrapped up in our thinking? We think it unlikely!

The idea here is that by noticing these unhelpful thinking styles, you 'step out of' what can become a negative loop elaborated on and complicated by our imaginative thinking. Our minds are extraordinarily clever, and of course, we could not do without them, but equally, the mind and its thinking can lead us into all sorts of difficulties and it is useful to know this. Instead, it is possible to choose to focus on the present and the good in our lives. So the process here is repeatedly bringing the mind back to what is nourishing and helpful for us.

For example, it is possible to learn to use the five senses more fully in an intentional way in any pleasurable situation to help resource and increase our sense of wellbeing. This might take the form of feeling the weight and warmth and smell of beloved pet or a child or grandchild as they sleep in our lap. It might be feeling the sensation of the sun or breeze on our face when we are out walking, noticing the movement and sound of the trees, the colours and patterns of shade of light. Our minds tend to jump around anyway, and the more anxious or low or stressed we are, the 'jumpier' our minds become. This process of repeatedly bringing awareness to what is supportive of our wellbeing can be thought of as training the 'attentional muscle' in the brain to help shift focus whenever we feel it would be helpful to do so. And just like a muscle, it takes a while to build up!

41.4 Connect with Other People

Healthy relationships are key to our wellbeing. None of us exists in isolation and our lives are inextricably linked to the lives of others. The quality of the relationships that we have throughout our lives impacts us in vital ways, including the capacity to flourish and our longevity. One of the most important ways to care for oneself is to take care of the important relationships we have. In practical terms, this means prioritising relationships with our loved ones and trusted friends, the people who we can rely upon and who make us feel good. It can feel as though in the short term, in order to catch up on work, it might be better to delay or cancel social arrangements, but in the longer term, this can lead to the gradual erosion of friendships and the relationships that support wellbeing. It is a rare occasion that any of us reach the end of the to-do list; there is always more to be done. And of course, there comes a time for all of us, when we no longer get to choose which tasks we leave unfinished.

If work seems to be taking over your life, set the alarm on your phone for a time when you (and your practice team) will begin 'wrapping up' the work day and another for when everyone should have left the building. Commit to the time that you will be home by and let your flatmates/partner/children know. Whilst this may be a challenge in a busy dental practice, the benefits to team morale will be worth it, and if you are leading the team, this will foster a feeling of value for team members. If you cannot make this commitment for 5 days a week, try it for three. See if you can make something like this work for you and your team and seek out allies in this process. Shine a spotlight on, and celebrate small acts of kindness towards each other and towards patients. These acts of kindness contribute to the concept of the practice as a small community, making all team members feel valued. Be prepared to be creative and playful in the service of your own wellbeing and the people that you share your life with, whether those happen to be your colleagues, your patients or family members.

41.5 Exercise and Activity

This is an important part of a wellbeing strategy for all of us, and the endorphins released during exercise are crucial to feelings of wellbeing. There is an amazing array of activities that can be classed as exercise, for example, running, cycling, swimming, walking, yoga, pilates, Tai Chi, Qi Gong, meditation, golf, the list goes on and on! Importantly, a lot of these activities can be done outside or with other people, both factors that we know can enhance the positive effect of the activity itself. In the context of a busy work life, walking in particular confers many psychological and physical health benefits because of the flexibility it offers. A brief period of walking could be fitted in as an individual or team activity where it may offer, in combination with 'focusing in the now', an opportunity to 're-calibrate' and restore oneself at some convenient point in the working day.

Many people use activity as a way of contributing to their mental wellbeing. More physically exerting activities (and these could range from walking to running or cycling depending upon your level of fitness or simply what is required at the time) can be used to work off any anxious energy that may accrue, or indeed to energise oneself. Something more restful and mindful, for example, yoga or Qi Gong, may be used to soothe and restore and settle.

41.6 Sleep

Exercise can also help with sleep provided it is not immediately before you go to bed, when it has a stimulating effect. Likewise, keep an eye on your caffeine intake and eating very late, both of which can interfere with sleep. Alcohol may help you to get off to sleep but sometimes results in wakefulness and dehydration later on. Keep your bedroom dark and not too hot and do not be tempted to check your phone when trying to sleep or on first waking. Try using earplugs if there is a lot of noise pollution where you live. It's also helpful not to vary your wake time too much at the weekend. Lie-ins are helpful, but they can disrupt sleep cycles if you usually get up early on work days. Find the balance of what feels right for you in your life.

41.7 'In the Moment' and 'on the Spot': Quick Strategies to Recover 'Balance' in Clinic

It is not uncommon to have moments when temporarily and fairly briefly we feel 'thrown off balance', somehow, and the sense of being a competent professional deserts us. This experience may take various forms: shaking hands, feeling suddenly quite anxious about something in the clinical encounter, a sense of uncertainty about how to proceed or if patients or colleagues are being challenging and we do not quite know what to say.

41.7.1 Reminding Yourself that You Are Human!

These things happen to everyone and are unpleasant for all of us when they do, but it's important to understand that this is all part of being human. They do not tell us any fundamental truths about us as a person or our capacity as a professional (no matter what our thinking might be leading us to believe). Equally, it's not our fault; we do not need to blame ourselves or to feel ashamed as though these moments of vulnerability are a personal failing.

41.7.2 Taking a 'Mindful Moment' and Slowing Your Breathing

Building on the ideas of the 'focusing on the now' section above (aka extricating yourself from a vortex of unhelpful thinking) is learning to bring your attention down, out of your thinking mind, and to focus on the pattern of fluctuating physical sensations in the body. The examples below need only be brief, and if you are having a tough day, do not wait until things feel unbearable; punctuate your day with these brief acts of self-care to resource and restore you.

If you have the chance to have a cup of coffee in between patients, you could try focusing on the sensory qualities involved in holding the cup, the warmth and appearance of the coffee in your cup and the sensations and the flavour of the coffee as you drink. Being present (using all of your senses) for handwashing is very useful. Focus on feeling the temperature and touch of the water on your hands, the smell of the soap and the appearance and the sound of the water as it splashes in the sink.

Alternatively, you could feel into the sensory quality of your feet connecting with the solidity of the ground beneath you and the physicality of your body extending upward, all the way from your feet, through your legs, buttocks and the gentle curve and uplift of the spine to the crown of your head. Then, as best you can, try feeling into the sense of heaviness and solidity that the body is offering in that moment. Then, when it feels right, see if it's possible for you to slow and slightly deepen your breathing for a few breaths. Slow, regular breathing is part of a physiological 'calming down' process that can be actively used to help steady oneself and calm the mind.

Try not to get into a struggle with the breath, though! If it feels like this is beginning to happen or if focusing on the breath is too difficult for you, then try the Mindful Self-Compassion break below. You can explore and experiment and see what techniques or combinations of technique work best for you. There are no hard and fast rules. And do not worry if your mind wanders off in many and multiple directions during the practice of these exercises – that's to be expected. The important thing is to notice this and bring your attention back to the present exercise, time and time again – strengthening that attentional muscle.

41.7.3 Taking a Mindful Self-Compassion Break

This brief practice has three stages and is intended to be used when you are feeling bothered, upset or otherwise troubled (suffering). The idea is that this practice does not necessarily remove what has upset you, but that it is possible to offer yourself some care and comfort because you are upset, as a good friend might do for you if they were present. This is the outline of the practice but it is best to listen to the guidance (link provided below) before doing it on your own so that you know how it unfolds. The first stage is to acknowledge that there is something unpleasant going on for you. The second stage is to call to mind the notion of common humanity and the fact that it is simply part of the human condition to suffer. This is to reduce the sense of isolation, self-blame and disconnection that is sometimes experienced when difficult things happen. The third stage is to use some comforting form of words that enlists us as our own best friend in that moment. In the guidance, there is also an option of using some kind of soothing self-touch for comfort. These actions can be brief and discreet but surprisingly effective, for example, rubbing the back of the hand.

41.8 Conclusions

We really hope this chapter gives some food for thought and complements the other articles in this issue, with practical and useable ideas on these key areas of wellbeing for you and your teams. There are many wonderful resources that expand on these ideas, some of which are included in the resources section at the end.

As you sit here now, having read this chapter from start to finish, perhaps think about one thing you can first commit to trying, or doing more of, as a starting point. You could even think about inviting other team members to do the same. Write it down and come back to this in a few days. Reflect on how it went, what helped, what got in the way and what else might be needed to support you taking this intended action. And remember, we are all human!

Useful Resources

LGBTQ+ dentists: https://gladd.co.uk/

BAPIO: https://www.bapio.co.uk/

African and Caribbean Dental Association UK: https://acda-uk.org/

Christian Dental Fellowship: https://www.cdf-uk.org/

UK Sikh Doctors Association: https://sdda.org.uk/

Muslim Doctors and Dentists Association UK: https://en-gb.facebook.com/MuslimDoctorsAndDentistsAssociationUK/

Jewish Medical Association UK: https://jewishmedicalassociationuk.org/

Russ Harris' book: *The happiness trap: How to stop struggling and start living*. A good self-help book that everyone should read!

Mindful Self-Compassion break, Dr Kristin Neff: https://self-compassion.org/exercise-2-self-compassion-break/

Wellbeing support for the dental team: https://www.supportfordentalteams.org/. This is an amazing UK-wide resource developed by colleagues and containing links for help with:

- Addictions
- Financial concerns
- Personal life
- Domestic abuse
- Caring responsibilities
- Bereavement

NHS 5 steps to mental wellbeing: https://www.nhs.uk/mental-health/self-help/guides-tools-and-activities/five-steps-to-mental-wellbeing/

NHS: menopause: https://www.nhs.uk/conditions/menopause/

For urgent concerns related to your wellbeing or safety, your GP or local A&E can help, as well as the following organisations:

Samaritans: call 116123, or visit https://www.samaritans.org/.

This article was originally published in BDJ Team *in November 2022.*

Pull-quote:

Shine a spotlight on, and celebrate small acts of kindness towards each other and towards patients. These acts of kindness contribute to the concept of the practice as a small community, making all team members feel valued.

Effective Clinical Communication 42

Aengus Kelly, Jim Carey, Morag Powell, and Ewen McColl

Learning Points
- Understand the importance of good communication with patients and colleagues in optimising clinical treatment.
- Recognise techniques in improving communication and ways in which communication varies depending on the clinical situation or the audience.
- Appreciate how to support patients in their discussions and interactions to ensure clear understanding prior, during or after treatment.

42.1 Introduction

Effective communication is central to every element of clinical practice from first contact with reception to the point the patient leaves the building. Whilst all team members are aware of the importance of good communication, it is an area that we often overlook in our personal development as clinicians.

For the patient, it is routine to develop trust in the dental team on the basis of their communication skills, where effectiveness in interactions is 'a proxy for clinical expertise' [1]. Healthcare educators have known for some time that enhancing clinical communication skills can result in consultations that are more effective, efficient, accurate and supportive [2, 3]. The GDC's Development Outcome A specifically encourages registrants to update these skills as part of their CPD requirements [4]. Clinical communication differs from usual interactions in many ways, including the language we use, the control and dynamics of when the participants

A. Kelly
Devonport Dental Education Facility, Peninsula Dental Social Enterprise, Plymouth, UK

J. Carey · M. Powell · E. McColl (✉)
Peninsula Dental School (University of Plymouth), Derriford Dental Education Facility, Plymouth Science Park, Plymouth, UK
e-mail: ewen.mccoll@plymouth.ac.uk

E. McColl, A. Alani (eds.), *Practical Tips in Clinical Dentistry*, BDJ Clinician's Guides, https://doi.org/10.1007/978-3-031-90355-7_42

take turns to speak and the different sorts of expertise held by each participant [5–7]. It also differs in the cultural conventions. For example, in the dental surgery, it is expected that one might be asked, and expected to answer, intimate and personal questions by a relative stranger. Clinical communication has been described as similar to intercultural communication: It is inherently like speaking in another language or to someone from another country [8].

In dentistry, we routinely need to explain complex procedures and disease processes to patients who are often distracted by anxiety, pain or a concern about the costs of treatment. The challenge for clinicians to communicate effectively becomes greater in these circumstances. Even prior to the COVID-19 pandemic, many patients were having to wait to access routine dental care, and this situation has become more acute, with large numbers seeking appointments for acute problems [9]. Since the Montgomery Supreme Court ruling in 2015, the expectation that indemnifiers and the GDC have is that dental clinicians ensure patients demonstrably 'understand' their treatment options and plan [10, 11]. These challenges highlight the importance of expert communication in everyday practice that is often characterised by busy working days and relatively brief appointments.

In this chapter, we provide some tips and techniques that we have found useful in developing our clinical communication skills, which as with other areas of skill development are a work in progress.

42.2 Audit Your Communication

Many clinicians will be already aware of the core clinical communications skills, such as managing expectations, providing jargon-free advice, employing non-verbal communication and active listening, but when seeing multiple patients day in and day out, unwanted habits can form. Ask a colleague or team member to help you audit your communication or seek specific feedback from patients about your empathy, clarity and effectiveness.

42.3 Golden Minutes

The first 2 or 3 minutes of a consultation are 'golden' for communication, as the patient will often have one or more pressing concerns or anxieties. Prioritise giving focused attention and actively listening to the patient from the first contact – it is a key shortcut to fostering trust [6, 12], even in a 10-minute consultation. A good start in the golden opening minutes of interaction can set the tone for the whole patient journey. In 'The Chimp Paradox' [13], Steve Peters describes how a bad or incorrect first impression might take seven further encounters to rectify. According to the 'Four Habits Model for Medical Visits' (4H) [5], it is important to 'Invest in the beginning', whether it is a new or returning patient or a short or an extended appointment. The better we know our patient, the easier it will be to adapt our communication to their needs – jargon for one may not be jargon for another. Patients often do not reveal all their concerns without prompting [14] and eliciting these effectively may result in a shorter appointment [15] – a return on your investment. To be prepared to greet each patient with the same level of performance and enthusiasm, consider how you transition emotionally, or 'decompress', between appointments. For some, a short breathing exercise can function like a 'reset' button [16] – consider what might be most effective for you. If you are consciously prepared for each patient interaction, you are more likely to respond professionally than to react emotionally [13].

42.4 Be Curious and Pause

One consequence of the Montgomery ruling is that dental professionals are required to appreciate the specific preferences and values of their patients and to ensure that patients understand the options and implications of treatment decisions [10, 11]. This is potentially challenging when under time pressure and may be most efficiently achieved by being genuinely curious about the patient's life and leaving space for them to tell you. An open question to a patient is most valuable when the clinician then pauses for a response, even if only for a couple of seconds. Research across health disciplines reveals that patients are routinely interrupted when presenting their story, often early in the process [17]. This can damage rapport and trust [12] and potentially lengthen the time taken to elicit the patient's concerns and needs. Pausing creates the space for a response but also indicates the expectation of a response. The more engaged the patient is in the interaction, the more likely it will be that they will perceive they have a stake, or control, in the clinical interaction [6, 18]. Ultimately, giving the patient more space to talk to you without unnecessary interruption will facilitate shared decision-making. The empowered patient is also a patient who has taken on more responsibility for decisions made.

42.5 Is There Something Else?

Patients will often attend with a shopping list of queries and concerns. Although there may not be time to address all of them in a single consultation, it is useful to know the full agenda so that appropriate time can be scheduled. Ideally, a well-structured history [2] will elicit the full list of concerns, but how we ask questions can directly impact how fully patients express their unmet concerns in primary care [14]. In a primary care study by Heritage, it was significantly more effective to ask the patient if there was 'something else' they were concerned about rather than 'anything else'. 'Anything' appears to cue a 'no' response, 'something' encourages the patient to give you the full shopping list. Some patients will feel reluctant to ask questions or discuss concerns and so perceiving the clinician as receptive to questions may help. Patients with unmet concerns will tend to feel less satisfied with the encounter.

42.6 Express Yourself Positively

Even as enhanced PPE requirements begin to ease and the COVID-19 pandemic becomes less acute, most of our clinical interactions with patients continue to take place from behind a mask. This restricts the opportunity patients have to receive our intended message, as some of our meaning will be lost with a muffled voice and less visible non-verbal communication. This is exacerbated when we try to explain things whilst seated behind a supine patient. The net result is that, although we may *intend* to be empathetic and attentive, the patient may perceive a more blank and emotionless interaction. The solution may be to turn up the volume on how we express ourselves. Vocalise your empathy ('Oh dear!'), be more demonstrative with the encouraging nods and take care with your tone of voice. The usual regulators of conversation are dampened, so our eyes need to work harder to convey empathy. If you are actively listening to a patient, make sure the patient knows: Acknowledge both the emotion and the content of their concern [19]. When our non-verbal communication is limited, the words we use become correspondingly more important. Framing oral health messages positively may help foster rapport and patient engagement. For example, informing a patient that their gums are '60% plaque-free' might be more encouraging than describing a 'plaque score of 40%', even if the treatment goal is the same.

42.7 Let Me Say It Again

One of the distinguishing features of clinical communication is the need for repetition. Early research into patients' retention of information suggested that approximately 50% of information provided in a clinical appointment was not retained [20]. Of perhaps greater importance now is that patients understand the key information they are given [11]. In his book 'Thinking Fast and Slow', Kahneman [21] proposes that there are two modes of thinking and that when under stress, we tend to revert to 'fast', intuitive thinking. Thinking in 'fast' mode makes it more challenging to absorb information and to make well-reasoned decisions. Many dental patients are sufficiently stressed (by anxiety, pain or by undergoing an invasive/operative procedure) to be inclined to fast thinking. Things that help include using clear, simple language; describing the structure of the appointment in advance ('signposting'); and repeating the core information or message [2].

42.8 Did They Understand?

The fourth habit in the 4H model is to 'Invest in the End' of the appointment [5]. Where you have given important instructions or advice, or have agreed a treatment plan, it is essential to avoid the risk of misunderstandings and miscommunication [22] by engaging the patient in dialogue. When information-sharing is an interaction, like a two-way game of frisbee [2], it is easier to encourage the patient to repeat the key information back in their own words to demonstrate understanding. It may be necessary to repeat the information-sharing in a different format (e.g., an online video, a printed leaflet, a physical model), or with a different emphasis (visual, auditory, etc.), but this additional time will be an excellent investment for an effective course of treatment. Take care that any recommended sources of information are accurate and trustworthy. Ask the patient how they would prefer to have things explained, but also try to adapt your explanation to their worldview. For example, one might describe the incidence of anaphylaxis with penicillin (1 in 10,000) roughly in terms of one football supporter in the crowd at a busy Plymouth Argyle football match.

42.9 The Team and Triadic Communication

The task of effective clinical communication begins at the first point of contact. The entire dental team needs coordinated and consistent messaging when interacting with patients. The dental team can also be used more strategically to enhance the engagement of patients in their own treatment conversations (Fig. 42.1) [23]. The dental nurse can be an excellent partner when it comes to chairside communication and should be encouraged in this role. A 'triadic' interaction with the patient can see the dental nurse act in a range of communication roles. These can include reinforcing the main message, filling in gaps in information-sharing or helping engage the anxious or embarrassed patient in interaction [23]. Paramedics and emergency care specialists talk 'through' the patient, keeping them involved in the interaction even

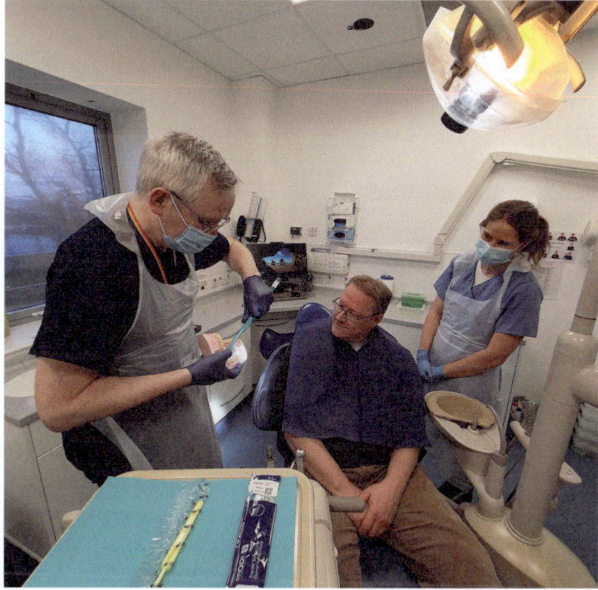

Fig. 42.1 Effective clinical communication requires the dental team to engage with the patient (Source: authors)

when they cannot actively reply. Calling out notes or a charting to your dental nurse is a great opportunity to indirectly speak to the patient too.

42.10 Relationship-Based Health-Centred Dentistry

Theodore Roosevelt is famously quoted as saying 'people don't care how much you know until they know how much you care'. [24] When we look at this in the context of dentistry, patients need to have trust and understanding from the professionals that they are encountering, to allow them to get a feeling that we genuinely do care about them. Relationship-based health-centred dentistry focuses on developing this trust and understanding with patients through our communication with them. One means of creating this trust and understanding is using the tool of co-diagnosis or co-discovery with our patients. This concept can be attributed to the late Dr Bob Barkley and the work he did around developing the dentist-patient relationship [25]. Co-diagnosis is the communication skill of explaining to a patient what you are screening them for and then comparing their diagnosis to health. A good example of this use is when screening the patient for periodontal disease and taking time to explain to the patient what the different codes that you are calling out to your nurse mean – prior to you completing the screening. You do this in layman's terms so the patient can easily understand the different scores, which then helps with the patient 'owning' their diagnosis. Consequences and benefits of treatment are then explained to the patient, which is all tied together with the production of the written treatment plan. This is framed by the patient as the clinician caring about their diagnosis and seen as the clinician wanting to take the patient back to health. With this communication approach, the patient feels that the clinician has taken the time to fully explain the health screening that they have undergone and are more inclined to accept treatment and adopt any behaviour change that is suggested. The patient is more inclined to build a relationship with the dental professional as they feel their individual needs have been catered for.

42.11 Conclusions

The classic school-day adage of *Festina lente*, or 'Make haste slowly', serves as a summary top tip to improve our clinical communication. Create the space for our patients to tell their story. Expect them to be involved in a two-way conversation, and in any decision conversations. Think strategically about how we plan our consultations, deliberately investing time in the beginning and the end. Young or old, experienced or a recent graduate, a periodic audit of performance in communication can benefit every clinician. Those who work in pro-social professions tend to have an aptitude for communicating. The clinical context provides different, specific challenges and consequently, these skills need continuous work. As we improve these skills, the evidence suggests that we will gain benefits in time management, engaging our patients in shared decision-making and smooth, effective practice.

References

1. General Dental Council (GDC). Research into a shared understanding of professionalism Bringing together patients and dental professionals. 20 December 2021. https://www.gdc-uk.org/about-us/what-we-do/research/our-research-library/detail/report/research-into-a-shared-understanding-of-professionalism. Accessed January 2023.
2. Silverman J, Kurtz S, Draper J. Skills for communicating with patients. 3rd ed. CRC Press; 2013.
3. Rao JK, Anderson LA, Inui TS, Frankel RM. Communication interventions make a difference in conversations between physicians and patients: a systematic review of the evidence. Med Care. 2007;45:340–9.
4. General Dental Council. Enhanced CPD scheme 2018. https://www.gdc-uk.org/education-cpd/cpd/enhanced-cpd-scheme-2018. Accessed January 2023.
5. Frankel RM, Stein T. Getting the most out of the clinical encounter: the four habits model. J Med Pract Manage. 2001;16:184–91.
6. Coleman H, Burton J. Aspects of control in the dentist-patient relationship. Int J Soc Lang. 1985;51:75–104.
7. Tuckett D. Meetings between experts: an approach to sharing ideas in medical consultations. New York: Tavistock; 1985.
8. Kleinman A. The illness narratives: suffering, healing, and the human condition (new edition). New York: Basic Books; 2020.
9. BBC News. Patients in pain as many struggle to find dental care. 9 May 2022. https://www.bbc.co.uk/news/health-61340244. Accessed January 2023.
10. DDU. Guide to consent to dental treatment. 14 September 2022. Available at: https://www.theddu.com/guidance-and-advice/guides/quick-guide-to-consent. Accessed January 2023.
11. General Dental Council. Standards for the dental team. Principle Three: Obtain valid consent. 2013. https://standards.gdc-uk.org/pages/principle3/principle3.aspx. accessed January 2023.
12. Yuan S, Freeman R, Hill K, Newton T, Humphris G. Communication, trust and dental anxiety: a person-centred approach for dental attendance behaviours. Dent J (Basel). 2020; https://doi.org/10.3390/dj8040118.
13. Peters S. The chimp paradox: the mind management programme to help you achieve success, confidence and happiness: the acclaimed mind management programme to help you achieve success, confidence and happiness. London: Vermillion; 2012.
14. Heritage J, Robinson JD, Elliott MN, Beckett M, Wilkes M. Reducing patients' unmet concerns in primary care: the difference one word can make. J Gen Intern Med. 2007;22:1429–33.
15. Levinson W, Gorawara-Bhat R, Lamb J. A study of patient clues and physician responses in primary care and surgical settings. JAMA. 2000;284:1021–7.
16. NHS. Breathing exercises for stress. 2022. https://www.nhs.uk/mental-health/self-help/guides-tools-and-activities/breathing-exercises-for-stress/. Accessed January 2023.
17. Beckman HB, Frankel RM. The effect of physician behaviour on the collection of data. Ann Intern Med. 1984;101:692–6.
18. Torper J, Ansteinsson V, Lundeby T. Moving the four habits model into dentistry. Development of a dental consultation model: do dentists need an additional habit? Eur J Dent Educ. 2019;23:220–9.
19. Neumann M, Bensing J, Mercer S, Ernstmann N, Ommen O, Pfaff H. Analyzing the 'nature' and 'specific effectiveness' of clinical empathy: a theoretical overview and contribution towards a theory-based research agenda. Patient Educ Couns. 2009;74:339–46.
20. Ley P. Communication with patients: improving satisfaction and compliance. London: Croom Helm; 1988.
21. Kahneman D. Thinking fast and slow. London: Penguin; 2012.
22. Morgan S. Miscommunication between patients and general practitioners: implications for clinical practice. J Prim Health Care. 2013;5:123–8.

23. Kelly A. The ceremonial (dis)order of the clinic: mapping engagement in dental interactions. 2015. PhD Thesis. Available at: http://www.tara.tcd.ie/handle/2262/81824. Accessed January 2023.
24. GoodReads. Theodore Roosevelt Quotes. https://www.goodreads.com/quotes/34690-people-don-t-care-how-much-you-know-until-they-know. Accessed February 2023.
25. Barkley R. Successful preventive dental practices. Createspace Independent Publisher; 2010.

Managing Medical Emergencies in Primary Care

43

Christian Wiggin and Ewen McColl

Learning Points

- The GDC advises annual medical emergencies and basic life support training.
- Dental professionals will encounter medical emergencies in primary dental care every 1–2 years.
- 'Hands-on', practical simulation training is the preferred method of training.
- Hypoglycaemia, vaso-vagal syncope, angina and non-specific collapse are the most common medical emergencies in dental practice.

Practical Tips in this Chapter

1. **Planning and preparation:**
    (a) 'Failing to plan is planning to fail'.
    (b) Know your patients and anticipate their potential medical needs.
    (c) Equipment and drugs.
2. **Training:**
    (a) Training and simulation are essential.
    (b) Prepare for the worst and help increase mental resilience and confidence in your staff.
    (c) Know your equipment and where it is.
    (d) Involve *all* members of the team.
3. **Use checklists.**
4. **Logistics:**
    (a) Create space.
    (b) Create a plan for ambulance service: access and egress.

C. Wiggin
Critical Care Paramedic, Faculty of Intensive Care, Exeter, UK

E. McColl (✉)
Peninsula Dental School, Plymouth, UK
e-mail: ewen.mccoll@plymouth.ac.uk

E. McColl, A. Alani (eds.), *Practical Tips in Clinical Dentistry*, BDJ Clinician's Guides, https://doi.org/10.1007/978-3-031-90355-7_43

5. **Leadership:**
   (a) Create a team leader.
   (b) Be assertive.
   (c) Share the mental model: Include the team in decision-making.
6. **Take notes.**
7. **Post incident: debrief and create honest feedback.**
8. **Sedation: Specialist emergency medical training is essential.**

43.1 Introduction

Recent evidence indicates dental professionals will encounter medical emergencies in primary dental care approximately every 1–2 years [1]. The General Dental Council (GDC) recognises this and mandates that it is essential that *ALL* registrants are trained in dealing with medical emergencies, including resuscitation, and possess up-to-date evidence of capability clarifying that all registrants must follow the guidance set out by the Resuscitation Council UK (RCUK) [2]. Considering that conditions contributing to medical emergencies encountered by the dental practitioner are increasing in prevalence in the United Kingdom [1] and, for example, those living with diabetes are expected to rise in number to 10% of the population by 2040 [3], it is becoming increasingly important for dental teams to have effective plans in place to manage dental emergencies in a systematic, structured and, most importantly, effective manner.

Dental surgeries are not primarily designed to manage medical emergencies so expert input can help in management when such situations arise, often when least expected. These top tips, written by a pre-hospital air ambulance professional with over 20 years' experience managing life-threatening emergencies and a dental professional with 30 years' dental experience and significant experience of managing medical emergencies, aim to equip dental practitioners with some useful tools intended to make the planning, identification and management of medical emergencies and resuscitation easier.

43.2 Planning and Preparation

43.2.1 'Failing to Plan is Planning to Fail'

Considering the GDC requirements and likelihood of encountering a medical emergency, it is advisable to plan and prepare for the eventuality to ensure patients receive effective and timely management. It is also important to ensure staff have the confidence and appropriate tools and skills to intervene.

The development of a local guideline that is regularly updated, readily available and understood by the whole team is an essential recommendation. This plan should identify the equipment, locations, logistics and management for anticipated medical emergencies and give guidance for staff managing medical events that are outside of their regular expertise. They should be updated regularly to reflect RCUK guidelines and may include the development of checklists and treatment plans for likely medical emergencies.

43.2.2 Know Your Patients and Anticipate their Potential Medical Needs

By knowing your patients' health needs and their previous medical history before commencing treatment, dental staff will hopefully be able to identify developing medical events before they become emergencies. Prevention is always better than cure and communication and recognition of a patient behaving differently to normal can be key.

43.2.3 Equipment and Drugs

The RCUK have recommended a minimal dental care equipment list for medical emergencies [4] that includes self-inflating bag (or bag-valve-mask) and defibrillator. This equipment must be easily accessible and all staff should be familiar with its location, function and how to use it [5]. Emergency drugs should be kept with this equipment. Guidance on what drugs should be contained in emergency drug kits can be obtained from the Department of Health and via the British National Formulary [6].

43.3 Training

The Resuscitation Council UK state there should be regular practice and teaching using simulation-based cardiorespiratory arrest scenarios [5]. This can only really be achieved by face-to-face teaching and 'hands-on' practice. However, in a cross-sectional survey of dentists, dental hygienists, dental therapists and dental specialists in 2019, whilst 89.2% reported undertraining annual medical emergency training, only 62% of these received face-to-face basic life support training. Only 50.5% of respondents received face-to-face medical emergencies training, 48% received face-to-face training involving medical emergencies roleplay and 32% received training involving a simulation manikin [7]. Worryingly, against GDC recommendations, 2.3% of participants in a 2019 study only undertook training every 2 years, putting them at risk from a medico-legal perspective should an adverse incident occur [7].

43.3.1 Training and Simulation Are Essential

Whilst theoretical teaching is undoubtably important, simulation is certainly the preferred method of learning with 93% of participants in a cross-sectional survey in 2019 preferring practical-based with interaction, roleplay and/or simulation [7]. Practical simulation, as the recommended method of teaching basic life support and medical emergencies [5], is not possible 'online' and goes beyond practising chest compressions on a mannikin.

It is known that the most common medical emergencies managed by dental professionals include vaso-vagal syncope, hypoglycaemia, angina and non-specific collapse [7, 8]. These conditions come on relatively quickly. Often, a patient feels ill beforehand and often, these patients go somewhere quiet, such as the toilet, to recover without causing further embarrassment. Simulation should include practising with full-size mannikins in difficult access locations in order to prepare staff for a real event. The authors' experience is that real-time simulation in the dental practice, with all team members present, is absolutely essential.

It is rare for a patient to go into cardiac arrest without some symptoms preceding the event. Cardiac arrest may well be avoided if the patient is located, identified and managed before the medical emergency develops into a full cardiopulmonary arrest. Simulation should be structured to consider this.

43.3.2 Prepare for the Worst and Help Increase Mental Resilience and Confidence in Your Staff

By simulating medical emergencies and resuscitation in challenging locations, with full-size, heavy mannequins and led by experienced trainers in resuscitation, dental staff will develop confidence at overcoming the unexpected and increase their mental resilience to managing an event and processing it after the event. 'Train hard – fight easy' is a well-known military term and relates directly to the management of medical emergencies that often require an assertive and dynamic, medical response to prevent deterioration.

Medical emergencies are extremely stressful for those managing them, particularly when they happen suddenly and the medical team is not accustomed, or practised, at managing them. In these events, the 'bandwidth' of clinicians will be significantly reduced. This should be anticipated and is a normal event. The physiological response is well described by Professor Grossman who describes an escalating loss of fine motor skills, followed by loss of gross motor skills, tunnel vision, dissociation and breakdown of mental performance as physiological stress increases [9].

Professor Grossman advises on being very aware of this and recommends a technique of square breathing (breathing in for 4 s, holding for 4, breathing out for 4 and holding for 4) that actively stimulates the parasympathetic nervous system and reduces this physiological response. By improving the ability to perform fine motor tasks (such as taking a blood glucose reading or opening the zip on a bag), the function of the responding team will be improved. By training for the worst, being aware of your physiological response and anticipating the fact that the very simplest of tasks will become very difficult, management of these emergencies will become easier.

43.3.3 Know Your Equipment and Where It Is

Considering the reduction in bandwidth of the medical team when faced with a true emergency, it is essential that planning for such events includes knowing exactly where the emergency medical equipment is and how to use it. It sounds obvious when preparing but an easily accessible and well-laid out set of equipment will be invaluable when managing an emergency (Fig. 43.1).

43.3.4 Involve All Members of the Team

Dental surgeries are comprised of teams. In a medical emergency, all members of the team are likely to be needed. Medical emergency and basic life support training should include all members of the team, from reception staff to senior dentists. A 'team' response to medical emergencies and resuscitation should be practised so all are aware of their roles, many of which are interchangeable. Including all team members in medical emergency training not only enhances team cohesion but will improve outcomes for patients should an emergency arise.

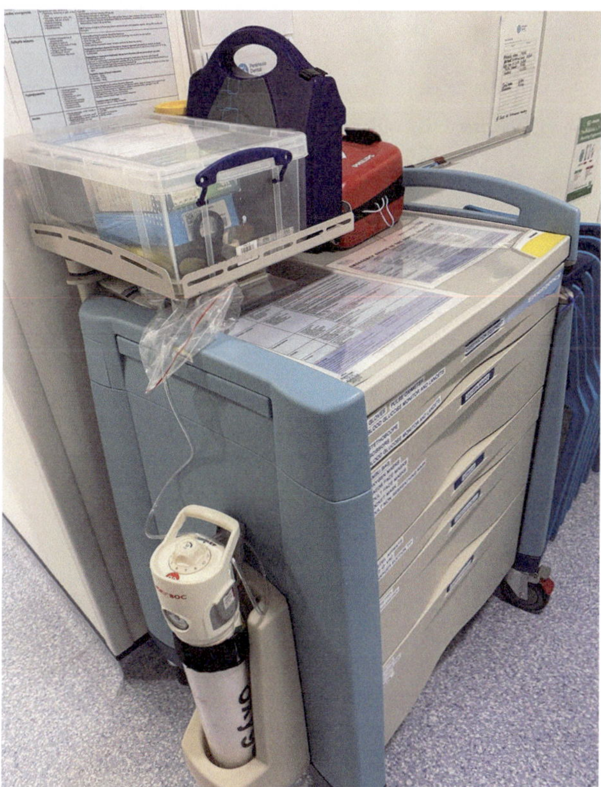

Fig. 43.1 The medical emergency trolley

43.4 Use Checklists

Checklists are a common tool used by professionals and laypeople around the world to manage serious medical events. Even high-performing critical care helicopter teams use checklists to manage anticipated medical emergencies. Checklists are used to share mental models, prevent omissions of care and provide structure to the management of a medical emergency.

The Resuscitation Council UK has a clear list on likely medical emergencies that may be encountered by a dental team. By proactively designing checklists for each of these emergencies and training with these checklists, teams can create order and structure when mental bandwidth is tested. Figure 43.2 shows an example of a medical emergency trolley with pouches created for each medical emergency, which include checklists (which include identification, assessment, management and appropriate drugs, with dosages) associated with that condition.

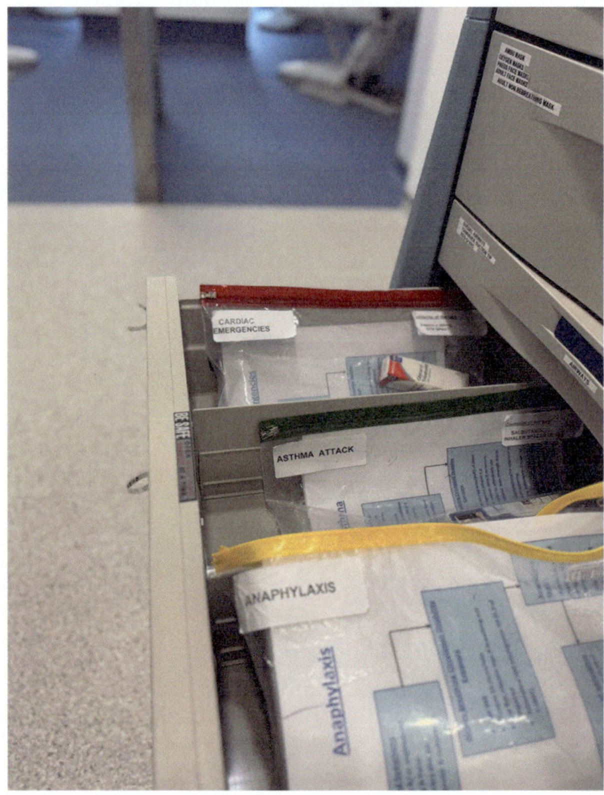

Fig. 43.2 Checklist and pouches for efficient management of medical emergencies

43.5 Logistics

43.5.1 Create Space

Considering that not all patients collapse on the floor in the centre of a room, it is important to plan for the eventuality that a patient may need to be moved in order to optimise care. This may require a certain amount of assertive movement of both the patient and furniture to create 360-degree access to the patient. It is important for the dental team to 'own and control the environment' in an emergency. Training and simulation are useful for this and can often be a fun, but effective way for the team to plan for medical events that occur in unusual locations within their surgery.

43.5.2 Create a Plan for Ambulance Service: Access and Egress

An appropriate and early call to the ambulance service is important. An ambulance may take a long time to arrive and planning ahead is essential. When they arrive, in order to expedite care, it is important to consider where they can park, how they will get in (with a trolley) and quickly gain access to the patient. Much of this can be planned ahead of the incident, and the extent of consideration to the logistics of this will vary depending on the individual challenges of each dental surgery. The importance of the consideration to logistics cannot be overemphasised; given the relief you will feel when the paramedics arrive, expediting this in planning is key.

43.6 Leadership

43.6.1 Create a Team Leader

The first moments of any emergency will be chaotic as the patient is identified, accessed and assessed. But as the situation evolves, it is recommended that someone takes responsibility for acting as the team leader for the event. It is likely to be the most senior person on site but can be any team member. If it is a complex case, the medical lead may well be focused on the patient so might not be the most appropriate person. The team leader who emerges should be recognised as such by the team and act as conduit between the team treating the patient and the team organising logistics and patient notes and liaising with emergency services. The team leader should have the role of oversite of the whole medical scenario and ensure an effective plan is made, communicated and understood by the whole team.

43.6.2 Be Assertive

True medical emergencies are challenging in every respect and will require all team members to step outside their comfort zone. This may require the team to remove patients' garments as appropriate, confirm a cardiac arrest (which is quite a considerable decision), bodily handling of a patient and potentially managing distressed relatives. Dental teams should consider this when training and mentally prepare themselves to perform tasks and procedures that are far outside their normal scope of practice. Leadership of these teams will often require someone to be assertive and motivate their teams to perform these tasks with reassurance they are doing the right thing. First responders are rarely criticised for being over-assertive but often fail to do tasks (such as removing a bra in cardiac arrest) due to lack of confidence and mental preparedness. Planning and training can help avoid this lack of assertion.

43.6.3 Share the Mental Model: Include the Team in Decision-Making

Communication with the whole team is key. Checklists are really useful to optimise this and practical training should include them. The team leader should ensure that their thoughts and decisions are communicated with the team and encourage the team members to share their thoughts before making the final decision. Often, the quiet team members will have a great idea but the team dynamics make it difficult for them to share this with the team leader.

43.7 Take Notes

Whilst this may not be required, or may not be possible in the first few minutes, try and start taking notes that can be handed over as early as possible. These include timings and patients' previous medical history and medications. It is invaluable to ambulance teams to know what happened before and during the event as it will help guide their treatment and help decide on the appropriate patient pathway of care. The paramedics are part of the team, and facilitating their care of the patient is a sure way of improving outcomes.

43.8 Debriefing

43.8.1 Debrief and Create Honest Feedback

When training medical professionals for medical emergencies and cardiopulmonary resuscitation, it is advisable to use an experienced and credible instructor to deliver the training. It is known that significant cardiopulmonary resuscitation quality deficits exist among healthcare providers [10]. Credible trainers can offer realistic simulations with useful feedback and debriefing, improving team performance. Effective debriefing of simulation has been shown to serve as a powerful tool to improve rescuer training and care for cardiac arrest patients [10].

A true medical emergency is stressful for all concerned. A good plan should consider the mental health of the medical team at all times. The Resuscitation Council UK advise that serious events, including cardiac arrests, should always include a full 'debriefing' of staff. This allows them to reflect on the treatment given and permits discussion of whether anything might have been done differently [5]. There are many guidelines on how best to do this, but it is generally advisable that immediately post incident, all staff are gathered together and given the opportunity to discuss the events and vocalise any issues or concerns they have as soon as possible. A more formal, structured debrief later may be required and learning points identified. Dealing with a medical emergency will affect all staff members differently, and as with any such stressful situation, it is always good to discuss our feelings in a non-judgemental manner.

43.9 Sedation

43.9.1 Specialist Emergency Medical Training Is Essential

When a dental surgery offers more advanced care options, such as sedation, the RCUK recommends that a more advanced trainer or attendance at a designated course may be appropriate [5]. Intravenous sedation specifically includes the administration of anxiolytic drugs that may have complex, potentially serious, side effects. A specialist trainer, experienced in sedation (inhalation and IV), can offer training to manage these side effects and improve the confidence and ability of staff to help manage these events. The planning for dental emergencies will have to be modified to acknowledge these risks.

43.10 Conclusion

Medical emergencies may arise when least expected. By utilising these tips, the dental team will be in the best position to deal with such events effectively and efficiently, optimising outcomes for patients.

References

1. Müller MP, Hänsel M, Stehr SN, Weber S, Koch T. A state-wide survey of medical emergency management in dental practices: incidence of emergencies and training experience. Emerg Med J. 2008;25:296–300.
2. General Dental Council. Medical emergencies. https://www.gdc-uk.org/standards-guidance/standards-and-guidance/gdc-guidance-for-dental-professionals/medical-emergencies. Accessed November 2023.
3. Diabetes UK. Global prevalence of diabetes set to affect one tenth of humanity by 2040. 2016. https://www.diabetes.co.uk/news/2016/nov/global-prevalence-of-diabetes-set-to-affect-one-tenth-of-humanity-by-2040-94931987.html. Accessed November 2023.

4. Resuscitation Council UK. Quality standards: primary dental care equipment. 2020. https://www.resus.org.uk/library/quality-standards-cpr/primary-dental-care-equipment-list. Accessed November 2023.
5. Resuscitation Council UK. Quality standards: primary dental care. 2020. https://www.resus.org.uk/library/quality-standards-cpr/primary-dental-care. Accessed November 2023.
6. National Institute for Health and Care Excellence. Prescribing in dental practice. https://bnf.nice.org.uk/medicines-guidance/prescribing-in-dental-practice/. Accessed November 2023.
7. Edwards D, Sin M. Prevalence of medical emergencies in primary within the UK. Br Dent J. 2023;235:721–6.
8. Girdler NM, Smith DG. Prevalence of emergency events in British dental practice and emergency management skills of British dentists. Resuscitation. 1999;41:159–67.
9. Grossman D. On combat: the physiology of deadly combat in war and peace. Human Factors Group Inc.; 2004.
10. Dine CJ, Gersh RE, Leary M, Riegel BJ, Bellini LM, Abella BS. Improving cardiopulmonary resuscitation quality and resuscitation training by combining audio-visual feedback and debriefing. Crit Care Med. 2008;36:2817–22.

Incorporating Research into Primary Care

44

Zoë Brookes, Ian Mills, Robert Witton, and Ewen McColl

Learning Points

- Understand how research in primary care can be beneficial for fulfilment and career advancement.
- Recognise the various avenues for research involvement in primary care.
- Identify avenues for further training and education to become proficient in conducting and delivering research.

44.1 Introduction

The COVID-19 pandemic has had a significant impact on all aspects of society, with dentistry facing specific challenges in maintaining access to dental services within a safe environment. One of the key challenges in early 2020 was the lack of knowledge and understanding around the risks of transmission of a novel coronavirus in the dental setting. The lack of credible research, particularly within the primary care setting, led to challenges in developing reasonable and informed guidance to support the profession. As a consequence, research from other settings was translated to dentistry that was viewed by some as inappropriate. Dental academics were keen to contribute, but with limited research capacity, particularly within primary care, the lack of empirical evidence undoubtedly hampered progress in dealing with the threat of coronavirus.

In the United Kingdom, over 90% of dental care is provided within general dental practice, yet only 2% of current published research relates to primary care [1]. Evidence-based dentistry (EBD) is a vital aspect of delivering high standards of

Z. Brookes · I. Mills · R. Witton
Peninsula Dental School, University of Plymouth, Plymouth, UK

E. McColl (✉)
Peninsula Dental School, Plymouth, UK
e-mail: ewen.mccoll@plymouth.ac.uk

E. McColl, A. Alani (eds.), *Practical Tips in Clinical Dentistry*, BDJ Clinician's Guides, https://doi.org/10.1007/978-3-031-90355-7_44

care for our patients, and this should be informed, wherever possible, by high-quality empirical research. The majority of research is conducted in academic settings or secondary care, and this may not necessarily translate to primary care [2].

Primary care dental services provide the ideal environment for clinical research given the wide range of patients and applicability of research findings to real-world circumstances. In our experience, busy practitioners often find it difficult to get going with research in practice whilst recognising the value of being involved in research. In this short paper, we hope to give some tips on how to get involved in research in primary dental care.

44.2 Why Bother?

Working in general practice can be extremely challenging, particularly at the present time. The thought of taking on additional responsibilities, such as research, may seem like an unnecessary burden. However, there are many positives in getting involved with research in primary care and some of the benefits include:

- Developing new skills and knowledge.
- Working as part of a wider team.
- Involvement of staff and patients.
- Variety within your working week.
- Professional fulfilment through advancing knowledge of the profession.
- Potential for future career advancement including publication.
- Point of difference in terms of practice promotion or staff recruitment.

44.3 What Level of Involvement?

You can become 'research active' at many different levels, and for many, this may be a convenient way to get started and make contact with more established researchers.

- **Research participant**—Get involved as a participant in an existing study or trial. Many researchers are keen to recruit participants in a variety of projects.
- **Data collector**—Participate in a study by collecting data for a colleague, perhaps through a questionnaire at the practice or collection of clinical data.
- **Collaborator**—More active involvement as a member of the research team, perhaps providing clinical expertise and advice or interpretation of results and their relevance to the clinical setting.
- **Clinical lead (CL)**—Direct involvement in the design of the study including funding application and research and ethics, as well as clinical input, analysis, interpretation of findings.
- **Principal investigator (PI)**—Responsible for all aspects of the study and likely to be undertaken by experienced researcher or someone in academic post.

44.4 Getting Started

It can be difficult to know where and how to start, and the importance of professional networks cannot be understated. 'Local knowledge' is always a good place to start and colleagues will often be able and willing to signpost you accordingly. Groups, such as the LDC, BDA Section, FGDP/CGDent and IPG, will often be able to help.

- **Find a supportive practice**—It can be difficult to conduct research in isolation, particularly if your practice is not engaged or supportive. There are others who are, and colleagues will often be delighted to act as a mentor. Dental body corporates will potentially have research opportunities due to their size and management structure, and it is always worth enquiring.
- **Dental school—**The majority of dental research is linked to universities or dental schools, and many academics are keen to collaborate with colleagues in primary care. It is worth contacting the research lead or a named academic at the school, and you may be pleasantly surprised at just how keen they are.
- **University—**Contact your nearest university as they may be grateful of your input with ongoing research projects by providing clinical expertise, also in non-dental disciplines.
- **College of General Dentistry** (formerly FGDP UK)—CGDent provides support, advice and information on research in general dental practice (https://cgdent.uk/research/). An introduction to research for primary dental care clinicians was previously published in 2010 and can be accessed online: https://cgdent.uk/standards-guidance/.
- **Society for Academic Primary Care (SAPC)**—The SAPC has a special interest group—'Academic Primary Dental Care Group'—that provides an academic platform to nurture academic careers in primary dental care: https://sapc.ac.uk/special-interest-group/dental-care.
- **Centre for Evidence-Based Dentistry (CEBD)**—Excellent resource and often runs introductory short courses on research: https://www.cebd.org/.
- **National Institute for Health Research (NIHR)—**The NIHR provides extensive information, advice and support on research in addition to providing funding for training opportunities: https://www.nihr.ac.uk/explore-nihr/specialties/primary-care.htm.
- **Local Clinical Research Network** (**CRN**)—Approach your local CRN for advice and support. The NIHR Clinical Research Network provides researchers with the practical support they need to make research happen. It supports the set-up and delivery of clinical research in the NHS and in other health and care settings through the Study Support Service, including staff once funding has been secured: https://www.nihr.ac.uk/explore-nihr/specialties/oral-and-dental-health.htm. There may be other local groups such as Northern Dental Practice-Based Research Network that can offer advice and support in getting research going in your practice: https://blogs.ncl.ac.uk/northerndentres/.

- **Research groups/societies—**Join research societies, present your work, get feedback and meet like-minded research enthusiasts who will help you make things happen, for example, the IADR/BSODR (https://bsodr.org.uk/) and British Society of Periodontology and Implant Dentistry (https://www.bsperio.org.uk/, ADEE https://www.adee.org/).
- **Existing trials—**There are several national multi-centre randomised controlled trials currently taking place in primary dental care, for example, *Pulpotomy for the management of irreversible pulpitis in mature teeth (Pulpotomy for Irreversible Pulpitis, PIP Trial)* and *ENHANCE-D, Enhancing Dental Health Advice*. Search the NIHR site for 'dental' within https://fundingawards.nihr.ac.uk/. Such studies can only take place if primary care dentists are willing to take part in research and they need you.

44.5 Training

Dental graduates and foundation trainees are likely to have knowledge and experience of searching the literature, critical reading and clinical audit but may not have been exposed to research. There are an increasing number of academic opportunities for the dental team, but they are often poorly understood and the opportunities underappreciated. Your own knowledge and experience should not be undervalued, and you can make a significant contribution in helping translate research into clinical practice.

- **Intercalated degree**—An intercalated degree during your undergraduate training (BSc or MSc) will give you basic research skills training, a more competitive CV and a taste of whether research is for you.
- **NHS Good Clinical Practice (GCP) training**—If you are interested in research, it is well worth undertaking this training at an early stage: https://www.nihr.ac.uk/health-and-care-professionals/learning-and-support/good-clinical-practice.htm.
- **Academic Dental Foundation (DFT)** posts are available to combine DFT with basic research training and information is available at https://www.copdend.org/postgraduate-training/dental-foundation-training/872-2/. Research opportunities have also been created within Dental Core Training (DCT). See https://www.copdend.org/postgraduate-training/header-dental-core-training/.
- **NIHR** offer part-time integrated training pathway within an academic institution, whilst continuing clinical practice, as an Academic Clinical Fellow (ACF) with 25% protected educational/research time for masters level training (https://www.nihr.ac.uk/funding/nihr-academic-clinical-fellowships-in-dentistry-2022/28684) or as an Academic Clinical Lecturer (ACL). The latter requires a PhD but involves further academic and clinical training, with 50% protected educational research time to become established as an independent research leader: https://www.nihr.ac.uk/funding/nihr-clinical-lectureships-in-dentistry-2022/28686.

- **University**—There are opportunities to undertake part-time masters training in clinical specialist areas, involving an element of research, or doctoral training to gain a PhD whilst continuing to work in primary care. If a PhD is something you could consider whilst working in primary care, send your CV; funding may be available. Experts in your field of interest will also become apparent through your engagement with the literature and looking through university research pages.
- **Chief Dental Officer's Clinical Fellow Scheme in England**—The Clinical Fellow Scheme was established in 2017 by the Chief Dental Officer for England. It provides dentists with dental leadership opportunities, who have not held a senior leadership role in dentistry, a unique opportunity to spend 12 months in a national healthcare-affiliated organisation outside of dentistry practice to develop skills in leadership, management, strategy, project management and health policy (https://www.fmlm.ac.uk/programmes-services/individual-support/clinical-fellow-schemes/chief-dental-officers-clinical-fellow-scheme).

44.6 Read the Literature

- Read dental journals regularly. This will keep you up to date, help develop your critical reading skills, expand your knowledge of research methods and provide good examples of academic writing.
- It can be difficult to keep on top of the literature and you may need to be selective in what you read: *Evidence-Based Dentistry* (https://www.nature.com/ebd/) and Dental Elf (https://www.nationalelfservice.net/dentistry/ are excellent resources).
- Search Medline, PubMed, EMBASE and other databases regularly on your topics of interest. Topic alerts can be created automatically to keep you up to date on published articles within a particular subject.

44.7 Define Your Research Interest

Oral health research is rich and varied with many topics to explore and methods to utilise: from dental materials to behavioural science, from therapeutics to epidemiology and from clinical techniques to patient-reported outcomes. The possibilities are limitless, but it will help considerably if you consider the following:

- Choose a topic that you have some knowledge, interest or feel passionate about.
- Develop a research question that is focussed and SMART; use 'PICO' (https://www.cebd.org/practising-ebd/question/).
- Base your research interests on real-life clinical problems that you have experienced or have relevance to everyday practice.
- Remember, despite your passion, only certain areas will get funded. Learn what the research priorities are in dentistry (https://www.jla.nihr.ac.uk/priority-setting-partnerships/oral-and-dental-health/top-10-priorities.htm) and read the

NHS long-term plan (https://www.longtermplan.nhs.uk/publication/nhs-long-term-plan/). How does your research fit with these?
- Aims and objectives are the most important part of project planning—Define these first and conduct clear, focussed hypothesis-driven research rather than a fishing expedition to see what you might find.

44.8 Funding

Leading your own research in primary care can be expensive in terms of time and resources, and the majority of research projects require funding. Research conducted within training posts may be funded, such as NIHR, but most projects need to be supported by grants.

- Start small and work your way up; you need publications, preliminary data and national/international collaborations to be competitive with large grants. There are lots of small grants available in dentistry, especially for early career researchers (ECRs), and some focussed on primary care, for example, Oral and Dental research Trust (ORDT; https://www.odrt.org.uk/) and Royal College Surgeons of England (https://www.rcseng.ac.uk/standards-and-research/research/fellowships-awards-grants/).
- Large grants are few and far between for oral and dental research, but it may be worth monitoring funding calls for larger charities such as the NIHR, Medical Research Council (MRC; https://mrc.ukri.org/), Biotechnology and Biological Sciences Research Council (BBSRC; https://bbsrc.ukri.org/), British Heart Foundation (BHF; https://www.bhf.org.uk/) and Cancer Research UK (CRUK; https://www.cancerresearchuk.org/) and consider how your research interests might fit within the research criteria.

44.9 Have a 5- and 10-Year Career Strategy

- Write down what you want to be doing in 5 or 10 years; if it looks like you want a mixed portfolio career involving research, then make a map of how to get there.
- Be patient; research does not give immediate rewards with results or immediate financial rewards; most of the benefits to you and patients are long term.
- Be proactive, knock on doors and do not expect people to do it for you.

44.10 Conclusion

There are numerous avenues for primary care oral health professionals to get involved in research. On the individual level, this can contribute to career development and achievement providing further impetus to explore the scientific basis for treatment provision and how these can be improved. The wider impact of primary care-based research includes greater applicability of evidence to include greater relevance of research to the general population.

References

1. Clarkson J. Experience of clinical trials in general dental practice. Adv Dent Res. 2005;18:39–41.
2. Committee of Vice Chancellors and Principals. Clinical Academic careers: report of an independent task force, 1997. London: CVCP; 1997.

Clinical Governance in Primary Care

45

Rebecca Anderson, Robert Witton, and Ewen McColl

Learning Points

- Understand how a clinical governance framework improves patient treatment and outcomes.
- Recognise how the various clinical governance tools available (such as audit) and how they apply to the daily improvement of patient care.
- Appreciate the importance of complaints handling in developing and improving care delivery.

45.1 Introduction

Clinical governance can in simple terms be described as everything and anything related to quality of outcomes in the clinical environment. More technically, clinical governance can be defined as a framework through which UK National Health Service (NHS) organisations and their staff are accountable for continuously improving the quality of patient care [1]. Whilst the pillars of clinical governance are often quoted as clinical effectiveness, risk management, patient experience and involvement, communication, resource effectiveness, strategic effectiveness and learning effectiveness, in this chapter, we will describe in our opinion key areas related to primary dental care and its delivery [1].

R. Anderson
Peninsula Dental Social Enterprise CIC, Plymouth, UK

R. Witton
Peninsula Dental School (University of Plymouth), Plymouth, UK

E. McColl (✉)
Peninsula Dental School, Plymouth, UK
e-mail: ewen.mccoll@plymouth.ac.uk

E. McColl, A. Alani (eds.), *Practical Tips in Clinical Dentistry*, BDJ Clinician's Guides, https://doi.org/10.1007/978-3-031-90355-7_45

45.2 Use of Guidelines and Standards

Guidelines and standards exist to support and assist all dental team members in delivering safe, high-quality and effective care to patients, but the different terms can sometimes lead to confusion [2]. *Standards in dentistry* define each as [3]:

Clinical guidelines are systematically developed statements to assist practitioner and patient decisions about appropriate healthcare for specific clinical circumstances.

A **standard** is a definable measure against which existing structures, processes or outcomes can be compared.

Guidelines and standards have subtly different purposes. Guidelines provide recommendations in the management of oral conditions that take into account the context in which the care is being provided, the best available evidence and what good practice looks like and recognise that it is not practical or reasonable to expect every patient to receive identical healthcare [3]. Every patient is unique and care should be delivered that meets their individual oral healthcare needs, taking into account a range of factors.

Clinical standards are specific and measurable [3]. They define specific elements of clinical care that need to be correct to optimise outcomes for patients. Standards often represent a minimum essential level of patient care, and they may additionally be enforced through systems of governance to promote accountability and patient confidence.

The differences highlighted are described in detail in CGDent's *Standards in dentistry*, which can be accessed online for free at https://cgdent.uk/wp-content/uploads/2021/08/Standards-in-Dentistry-2018-text.pdf.

There are a plethora of guidelines and standards continually being developed and/or updated, and it can be challenging keeping up to date with the latest versions. Membership of professional organisations, attendance at CPD events and reading key dental journals can be an effective way of keeping up to date, and many organisations now have social media accounts that regularly share updates for the dental profession such as the British Dental Journal and the British Dental Association.

45.3 Audit: A Tool for Improvement

Clinical audit is a key requirement for all healthcare settings and an expectation of dental regulators across the four UK nations. Performing clinical audit can sometimes feel like a burden but it is essential for establishing and maintaining standards in clinical care. Clinical audit can be defined as 'the systematic review of activity in practice against standards, in order to improve patient care'. [4] Whilst traditionally audit has been regarded as a quality assurance process, it is increasingly being recognised as one of the fundamental tools in quality improvement, the difference being improvement deliberately intends to bring about immediate, positive change in the system rather than merely observing a defined standard.

Using audit for quality improvement can be a force for good in practice, and involving all members of the dental team can foster a spirit of common purpose and ownership in roles and responsibilities, ultimately improving patient care but also benefitting the working culture of a practice and improving its effectiveness and efficiency. A recent guide has been published providing tips on carrying out audit and the various elements that comprise audit activity [4].

A good way to embed audit into the fabric of practice is to include it as part of the practice's annual quality improvement plan, which sets out the framework for how the practice meets regulatory compliance and demonstrates quality is at the heart of the service. Having a clear plan for service improvement can also help to reassure patients and members of the public that service standards are continually reviewed and that the practice is a progressive and forward-thinking provider. For those interested in the various quality improvement tools, the West of England Academic Health Science Network has produced an excellent guide [5].

45.4 Risk Management

Identifying and managing risks in dental practice is an increasingly complex area covering a diverse range of topics. Risk assessment is a systematic examination of work activities to identify what could go wrong and cause harm and whether adequate controls are in place [3]. The BDA provides comprehensive information to assist practices in meeting these requirements through advice, model polices and protocols and changes in policy made by regulators (www.bda.org).

One particular area of risk management that warrants further attention is learning from clinical incidents to help develop a culture of patient safety. Whilst this is routine in large healthcare organisations, it is still underdeveloped and implemented in primary dental care [3, 6]. Identification of clinical incidents, their reporting and monitoring is fundamental to clinical risk management and preserving patient safety. Being open, transparent and honest when things go wrong is a professional responsibility and the cornerstone of ethical practice. It is important to learn from incidents to prevent their reoccurrence and to instigate changes to systems, processes or staff training through a process of root cause analysis to improve clinical outcomes and prevent harm. In addition, all staff should understand their professional responsibilities to raise concerns about the quality of care if they feel they are below acceptable standards without fear of personal reprisal or blame.

There is increasing research and policy interest in this area, and it is likely patient safety reporting in primary dental care will become easier, better defined and routine in years to come [3].

45.5 Complaints Handling

All members of the dental team strive to achieve optimal outcomes for their patients, often under the most challenging of circumstances that may be clinical, operational or where patient expectations exceed the outcome that can be reliably predicted.

Understandably therefore, our first instinct upon receipt of a verbal or written complaint may be to take the matter personally and respond defensively.

Successful complaint handling involves the whole team, from 'front of house' right through to the responsible person who signs off the final response; amongst the key elements are prompt acknowledgement, the provision of a copy of the practice complaints protocol and keeping lines of communication open. It's counter-intuitive but making it easy for patients to complain at practice level gives an early opportunity to achieve local resolution and reduce the risk of escalation to third parties.

Get early-stage guidance and support from your defence organisation, particularly if the patient is seeking compensation. On a practical level, it is important to aim to understand the concerns from the patient's perspective and what they are looking for by way of satisfactory resolution. This may not always be reasonable or feasible, but at least you have a good starting point to resolve the complaint.

In many cases, a simple clarification of a misunderstanding or the offer of a second opinion to explain any biological complication and to discuss further options may be sufficient. If things haven't gone so well, the duty of candour requires that the patient receives an honest explanation, and you should set out what you are able to do to remedy the situation.

Receipt of a complaint does not necessarily mean that the relationship between the patient and dental professional is irretrievably broken—although this may sometimes be the case. As in other public-facing areas of life such as the retail and service sectors, where complaints are well handled and equitable solutions found, patients can often become great advocates for the practice.

Whilst complaints offer an opportunity for reflective learning and improvement, they can, at the time, be stressful for hard-working dental professionals to deal with. These stresses can be mitigated by a well-trained team approach and accessing support networks including those provided by your defence organisation. Above all else, keep things in perspective and don't try to deal with them in isolation.

45.6 Patient Involvement

Engaging with patients effectively is key to achieving the best possible outcomes in patient care. It is, therefore, important to ensure that patient involvement remains at the forefront throughout the whole of the patient journey. It is human nature for us to be more receptive and feel more positive towards an experience, when we believe that our views are being listened to and our opinions are valued.

The concept of shared decision-making is widely recognised across the profession as being fundamental to providing high-quality patient care. Evidently, it plays a significant part in the regulatory assessment framework adopted by the Care Quality Commission (and similar bodies in the other UK nations) forming several parts of the Key Lines of Enquiries (KLOEs) that demonstrate a service is both responsive and well led. So how do we ensure that we portray a positive and open approach that will empower patients to play an active role?

It is important to remember that one size does not fit all and that patients engage in different ways. With that in mind, try to devise and encourage as many different mechanisms and forums for patients to provide their views, opinions and feedback as possible. Encourage open channels of communication for receiving both positive and negative feedback.

Make patient surveys easily accessible by providing them in both electronic and paper formats available in reception areas, including Web links on patient letters and emails and promoting through social media to gather volumes of anonymous feedback that when collated can help to identify reoccurring themes and trends. Promote patient participation at regular patient focus groups, which can be held either in person or remotely. This provides a forum for patients to give their personal experiences but also allows an opportunity for channelling questions directly.

Not only is it important to engage and listen to patients' feedback but it is even more important to learn from patient experiences and use them to elicit positive change. Utilise the feedback gathered from patient surveys, focus groups and the learning outcomes from complaint investigations and disseminate them to all members of the team. Create a culture of celebrating successful outcomes and acknowledging and learning from when things have gone wrong.

45.7 Data Protection

The General Dental Protection Regulation (GDPR) came into force in 2018 and changed the landscape of data protection. What are the key aspects?

Appoint a Data Protection Officer (DPO): Practices that provide NHS services must appoint a DPO 'to monitor internal compliance, inform and advise on your data protection obligations, provide advice regarding Data Protection Impact Assessments (DPIAs) and act as a contact point for data subjects and the Information Commissioner's Office (ICO)'.

The ICO state that the DPO must have expert knowledge in the area of data protection and may be an existing member of staff, an external employment or shared with another organisation.

Review Privacy Notices: Ensure that you are providing the required information to patients regarding how you will manage their personal data. This should include:

- The legal purpose for processing.
- Retention periods.
- Who the information is shared with.

Subject Access Request: Review the process for subject access requests and ensure that it meets the requirements under GDPR, which can be found on the ICO website [7]. Make sure the process is clearly communicated to patients.

In these top tips, we build on the clinical tips discussed previously, expanding on routes to quality improvement in day-to-day practice. As with clinical tips, the aspiration is to improve outcomes for patients and improve satisfaction in day-to-day clinical work for all team members.

45.8 Conclusions

Clinical governance reduces negative outcomes and adverse incidents that makes the clinical environment safe for care providers and their patients. Ultimately ensuring a robust and responsive clinical governance framework has a positive impact on the well-being and quality of life of individuals associated with dental treatment provision.

References

1. Rosen R. Clinical governance in primary care: improving quality in the changing world of primary care. BMJ. 2000;321:551–4.
2. Roberts-Harry E. Guidelines are not standards. Br Dent J. 2021;230:688.
3. Moles D, Tredwin C, McColl E, Witton R, Burns L. Standards in dentistry. London: Faculty of General Dental Practice (UK); 2018.
4. Hook H. A guide to clinical audit for the dental team. BDJ Team. 2020;7:34–7.
5. West of England Academic Health Science Network. Quality Improvement (QI) Tools. https://www.weahsn.net/toolkits-and-resources/quality-improvement-tools-2/. Accessed March 2022.
6. Bailey E, Dungarwalla M. Developing a patient safety culture in primary dental care. Prim Dent J. 2021;10:89–95.
7. Information Commissioners Office. https://ico.org.uk/. Accessed March 2022.

Leading a Team in Primary Care Dentistry

46

Janine Brooks and Ewen McColl

Learning Points

- Understand the relevance of leadership and the many different ways in which leadership can be applied to everyday dentistry.
- Recognise good leadership as a core aspect of professionalism that promotes and supports our work as healthcare providers.
- Appreciate the different ways in which leadership can be developed and that developing leadership skills and techniques provides self-fulfilment.

46.1 Introduction

The General Dental Council (GDC) in *Preparing for practice* [1] group the key learning outcomes into four domains. These categories fit with those that will be required by the GDC throughout registrants' practice, and mastering these skills is a lifelong commitment:

- Clinical.
- Communication.
- Professionalism.
- Management and leadership.

The GDC highlights the challenges of developing good leadership skills:

Good management and leadership skills are vital to effective delivery of high-quality patient care. This includes management of time, resources and effective

J. Brooks
Bedford Heights, Brickhill Drive, Bedford, England, UK

E. McColl (✉)
Peninsula Dental School, Plymouth, UK
e-mail: ewen.mccoll@plymouth.ac.uk

E. McColl, A. Alani (eds.), *Practical Tips in Clinical Dentistry*, BDJ Clinician's Guides, https://doi.org/10.1007/978-3-031-90355-7_46

team working. Upon registration, a professional would not be expected to be fully competent in a management and leadership role—this will take time and experience [1].

Whilst all domains above are intrinsically linked, there are many courses and professional journals on the first three domains but less so the domain of management and leadership. However, if you look outside the immediate dental field, there is a vast quantity of academic and practical expertise that can be accessed. Indeed, it is challenging to 'learn' leadership as much of this development depends on experiential learning, though an understanding of leadership concepts helps frame those experiences in terms of leadership development. You may be a natural leader but you can always learn to be an excellent leader. Leadership is probably one of the most complex and complicated skills a dental professional will ever master, and yet it is rarely touched upon during training, with limited opportunity to develop these skills practically. Effective leadership is key to the success of any organisation, none more so than a dental practice.

Bennis [2] notes that 'leadership is the most studied and least understood topic of any in the social sciences' and 'never have so many laboured so long to say so little'.

With that in mind, in this short paper, we offer our perspective of key elements of leadership in dentistry relevant to all members of the dental team. This is borne of experience in a wide range of leadership roles spanning almost all areas of dentistry—from primary care to running large clinical teaching facilities, and specialist practice.

Whilst leadership and management are closely linked, it is worth differentiating without getting fixated with definitions. Leadership is often described as having a vision and encouraging others to share and work towards this vision; leaders see the path. Management is enabling the processes to achieve this vision; managers navigate the path. In military terms, it is often stated you can lead soldiers into battle but you cannot manage them into battle. It is interesting that the Royal Military Academy Sandhurst—the UK's officer-training academy—have as their motto 'Serve to Lead', highlighting service to others allows us to lead. Indeed, when we think of great leaders, their leadership skills are often forged in war or conflict. Of course, there are also visionaries outside the theatre of war—think of Anita Roddick, Steve Jobs, Elon Musk and Richard Branson. Fortunately, dentistry is not war but the concepts of leadership and service to our patients have important parallels in getting the most out of any team.

Leadership is one of the 16 'crucial proficiencies in the twenty-first century' identified by the World Economic Forum, 10 of which are non-technical [3]. If you really want to be a successful dental professional, you really need to hone your leadership skills. Times have changed in the world of leadership; it's no longer about telling; it's about creating an environment where the leader gets the best out of the whole team. See Table 46.1 [4].

Below, we give examples of essential leadership skills in dentistry, which help ensure a more fulfilled workplace and improved outcomes for our patients who we serve.

Table 46.1 Information sourced from Myatt M. *Hacking leadership* [4]

Twentieth-century paradigm	Twenty-first-century paradigm
Have a leader	Create a culture of leadership
Invest in tools	Invest in people
Play the game	Change the game
Compete	Collaborate
Driven by profit agenda	Driven to create value
Reward potential	Reward contribution
Manage risk	Manage opportunity

46.2 Lead By Example: That Means Being Authentic, Not Do As I Say but Do As I Do

An example from clinic may be if you are the practice principal and you are late every day, it will be challenging for you to address lateness of other staff members when this impacts on patient care. It is thus of paramount importance to reflect on your own behaviours and lived values if you are in a leadership position. How might others perceive such a leader's behaviour?

Similarly, if you as the leader of a team park in the reserved patient's parking space every day but expect others not to, how might this be perceived? What sort of example are you setting? This type of behaviour would quickly undermine the ability of an individual to lead; others would soon lose respect and begin to turn away from that person, with a breakdown in team cohesion.

46.3 Look After Every Member of Your Team; Everyone Is Important and Has a Role to Play

Every member of the team has different motivations for being in the work environment. Consider what their perspectives may be and discuss this with team members individually and as a group. How does this link in with the vision of the practice and how can you facilitate success for all? Don't forget the non-clinical staff: They are just as important in the smooth running of the practice. Valuing staff isn't always about how much someone is paid; often, it's more about how involved they feel and the degree of control they have over what they do. It will include how much flexibility someone has and the tasks that are delegated to them. A simple thank you for a job well done can go a long way.

46.4 Act as a Professional Role Model: Walk the Talk

A leader sets the vision for a group of individuals. If the practice principal shares with other staff that respect for patients is an important value for the practice and then makes jokes about patients to other staff, that shows they do not respect patients. It also encourages other staff to act in the same way. The dentist who expects their nurse to work late because they regularly run late is being disrespectful and a poor professional role model, plus demonstrating poor time management. Whilst in clinical dentistry everyone expects running over from time to time, consider other team members' circumstances, not just your own. This respect for others and consideration of their life balance beyond the workplace leads to a more motivated and committed team.

46.5 Clinical Leadership: Set the Standards But Give People the Tools to Achieve Them

Developing your team clinically takes time and commitment, but is time very well spent in future proofing the practice, and will encourage team members to stay at the practice. For example, if you have skills as an implantologist, take time to mentor and if practical, supervise some early cases with interested colleagues. This professional fulfilment will encourage staff to remain at the practice and share the clinical load or develop resilience if you are not present in the practice for whatever reason.

If attending conferences, invite wider team members so that they will feel invested in and an important part of the team. Developing every member of staff increases buy in to the shared vision and will pay benefits in the long term. Equality of development opportunities is crucial, not just for clinical facing staff.

46.6 Mentoring, Coaching, Developing Future Leaders: Be the Person Everyone Wants to Follow

Practice meetings—from time to time, allow team members to lead. This shows your trust in the team and your willingness to help others to learn and shine. The team will become more confident and show more willingness to participate. If you do this, always be encouraging and never publicly critical: Support your team and they will support you. Praise in public, constructively criticise in private. Great leaders foster a working environment that includes mentoring and coaching. They learn how to adopt a coaching leadership style that gets the best out of those they lead. Mentoring is about supporting others to grow by signposting and sharing expertise so that the person can find their own ways forward. The best leaders know when to listen and ask the right questions at the right time.

46.7 Trust your People: They Usually Want to Be the Best they Can Be

People rarely go to work intending to do a poor job. We can all stumble but a good leader is there to catch the person who stumbles and set them back on the right road. The more you trust, the greater the reward will be both for the leader and the people they lead. People who are trusted and who feel valued generally go the extra mile and do so willingly.

46.8 Conclusions

Being a leader needs practice and an understanding of how to do it. You may be a natural but understanding concepts and embracing lifelong learning relevant to leadership is essential as your career progresses. Look outside dentistry to get the best information about leadership; read around the topic—there are some great books that help in this journey [5–7] whatever career pathway you choose to follow.

The best leaders are authentic and ethical; they share failures and successes but learn from both in equal measure. Once the leader has set the vision and inspired those around them, they give their managers the tools and the trust to get on with the job. The leader is about motivating and setting the path, supporting their team to stay on the correct path even when the going gets tough. Great leaders have great businesses, and good leadership has a huge impact on the bottom line of the practice whilst ensuring staff remain content and motivated. Great leaders know they can't do it alone; they need others to follow and at times to lead.

Whilst a challenging area in many respects, the rewards are great across the whole dental team and encouraging all to take on leadership roles not only fosters happier staff but optimises outcomes for patients whom we serve to lead.

References

1. General Dental Council. Preparing for practice. Dental team learning outcomes for registration (2015 revised edition). https://www.gdc-uk.org/docs/default-source/quality-assurance/preparing-for-practice-%28revised-2015%29.pdf. Accessed 6 May 2022.
2. Bennis WG. On becoming a leader. New York, NY: Basic Books; 2009.
3. Soffel J. Ten 21st-century skills every student needs. World Economic Forum, 10 March 2016. https://www.weforum.org/agenda/2016/03/21st-century-skills-future-jobs-students/. Accessed 2 Dec 2022.
4. Myatt M. Hacking leadership. Wiley & Sons; 2014.
5. Goleman D. Working with emotional intelligence. Bloomsbury; 1998.
6. Goleman D. What makes a leader? Harv Bus Rev. 1998;76:93–102.
7. Syed M. Black box thinking—marginal gains and the secrets of high performance. John Murray Press; 2016.

Practical Tips on Staying Up to Date in Primary Care

47

Lorna Burns and Ewen McColl

Learning Points

- Be aware of the various avenues to maintain awareness of change within the dental profession
- Understand the interrelationship of accessing information and personal knowledge
- Recognise networking opportunities either face to face or virtually

47.1 Introduction

It is important that dental professionals stay up to date with developments in dentistry such as new guidelines, latest research and technology. However, the myriad of information sources, compounded by a lack of time, can make staying up to date a difficult task. An effective strategy to help you stay well informed and avoid information overload is to streamline electronic communications. Automated systems can be set up to assemble updates from numerous sources into a single digital location, which can be checked at a time convenient to you. This chapter presents some recommendations for streamlining information notifications, which, after the initial set-up, will save time and effort.

L. Burns
Peninsula Dental School (University of Plymouth), Derriford Dental Education Facility, Plymouth Science Park, Plymouth, UK

E. McColl (✉)
Peninsula Dental School, Plymouth, UK
e-mail: ewen.mccoll@plymouth.ac.uk

E. McColl, A. Alani (eds.), *Practical Tips in Clinical Dentistry*, BDJ Clinician's Guides, https://doi.org/10.1007/978-3-031-90355-7_47

47.2 Email Updates

Many information sources can be set up to deliver updates by email. It is best to be selective at first, choosing sources relevant to UK practice, before adding to their number. Below are some suggestions for useful and relevant email updates that you could subscribe to.

- The *British Dental Journal* and sister publications *BDJ in Practice*, *BDJ Open*, *BDJ Team* and *Evidence-Based Dentistry* are all published by Springer Nature on behalf of the British Dental Association (BDA) (Fig. 47.1). Creating an account with the publisher allows you to sign up for email alerts for each of these publications (note these are listed under Medicine). Follow the links to sign up for alerts from the BDJ homepage at https://www.nature.com/bdj/. These alerts will provide readers with news, current affairs, educational and practice updates as well as peer-reviewed research evidence (some content is subject to BDA membership or subscription).
- *Dental Update* and *The Dentist* offer free email alerts, providing news, discussion articles and knowledge and education updates. Much of the content is free or open access. Sign up to alerts from their websites at:
  - *The Dentist* https://www.the-dentist.co.uk/
  - *Dental Update* https://www.dental-update.co.uk/

The British Dental Association (https://bda.org/) as well as the College of General Dentistry (https://cgdent.uk/) both offer email newsletters, even to non-members (note the link to the College of General Dentistry newsletter sign-up is https://cgdent.uk/college-newsletter/). These provide latest news about practice, regulation, compliance and governance. The College of General Dentistry also produces a peer-reviewed journal for the whole dental team, *Primary Dental Journal*

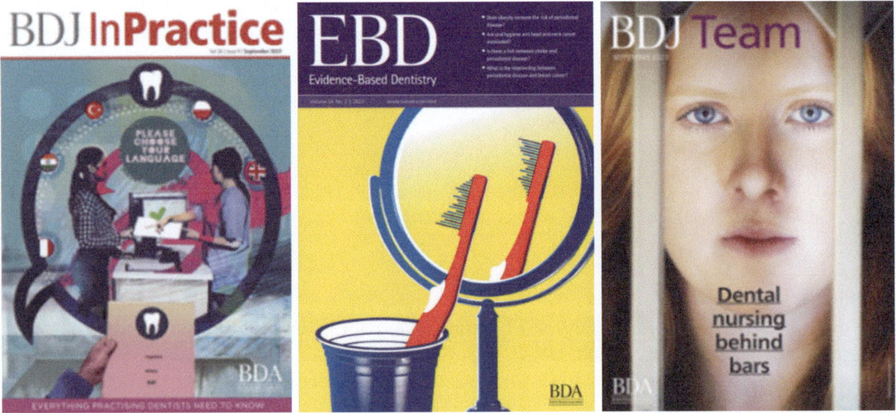

Fig. 47.1 BDJ Portfolio cover montage (to be created by BDJ editorial team, this could include the BDJ too if possible pls)

(https://journals.sagepub.com/home/PRD). This quarterly journal focuses on a particular theme with each issue (e.g., aesthetic dentistry, digital dentistry, oral surgery) and provides knowledge and education articles. Members of the College receive print issues and can access the full online archive of over 1,400 articles. If you are not a member, you can read and download the open access content and purchase individual issues. You can also stay up to date by following the College or the BDA on social media. The College has a new Instagram page https://www.instagram.com/cgdentyoungdental/ specifically curated for dental students and early career professionals, which posts tips and advice and highlights relevant open access articles from the journal.

47.3 Managing Email Updates

Creating numerous email alerts has the potential to overload your inbox, but there are some options for managing the volume of email traffic. First, consider if you prefer to create a designated email inbox for keeping up to date, which is separate from your primary email. This option prevents your own inbox from becoming too busy but requires regular checking. It may be more convenient for email alerts to be filed in a folder inside your primary email account. Most email services allow this function; check the settings for filters, folders or categories.

47.4 Twitter Lists

Twitter (rebranded as X) continues to be widely used by many organisations and is a good source for keeping up to date. If you are an active tweeter, you might consider creating a new profile for your professional interests which will prevent your personal feed from becoming overloaded. There are many key organisations that actively push content on Twitter. These can either be *followed* or you can create a *List* within Twitter, which is a way of organising the content. Key dental publications also tweet their latest papers. These are often at e-publication stage, before the papers appear in an assigned issue. Suggested accounts and their *handles* are given in Table 47.1. You can search for these handles and then either *follow* them or add them to your *List*. To search, include the @ symbol, for example, @TheDentalElf (without spaces).

Table 47.1 Dental organisations' X (Twitter) handles

Keep up to date with practice, news and events	Twitter handle
General Dental Council	@GDC_UK
College of General Dentistry	@CGDent
Dentistry (news website and magazine)	@Dentistry
British Dental Association	@TheBDA
British Association of Dental Therapists	@BADT1963
Keep up to date with research	
British Society for Oral and Dental Research	@BSODR_UK
International Association for Dental Research	@IADR
British Association for the Study of Community Dentistry	@bascd_uk
British Dental Journal	@The_BDJ
Dental Elf (research evidence blog)	@TheDentalElf
JDR Clinical and Translational Research	@JDRClinTransRes
Community Dental Health	@CDHJournal

47.5 Creating Knowledge From Information

The recommendations presented above are strategies for managing information by selecting and combining information streams into a single digital location. These digital items remain explicit forms of information until they have been read and internalised by you, the reader [1]. This is when explicit becomes tacit knowledge. The conversion of knowledge across explicit and tacit forms is illustrated in Fig. 47.2. Whilst information management is concerned with retrieving, assembling and organising information, the discipline of knowledge management is concerned with the creation and exchange of knowledge between individuals and across organisations [2]. Knowledge management practitioners believe that knowledge is created when people interact; therefore, opportunities for professionals to connect and mobilise knowledge are seen as a key strategy [3]. The final recommendation therefore is to seek out networking opportunities with other dental professionals.

Fig. 47.2 Adapted from Nonaka's SECI model of knowledge creation (1994) [1]. This depicts four modes of knowledge creation: Socialisation (when individuals interact), Externalisation (when knowledge is expressed in written form), Combination (when explicit information is organised) and Internalisation (when documented information is learned and understood)

	Tacit knowledge	Explicit knowledge
Tacit Knowledge	**Socialisation** Networking with other professionals for example through attending conferences or afterwards disseminating to the team.	**Externalisation** Creating information artefacts from personal knowledge, for example writing an article for a newsletter.
Explicit knowledge	**Internalisation** Learning from information that is written, for example reading a research paper.	**Combination** Organising explicit information for example creating an folder for email newsletters, or a curated list on Twitter (X).

47.6 Networking

Attending conferences is not only a way of learning about new research, products and technologies. They are also places to connect with other professionals. Whilst conference keynotes and presentations disseminate information, they are often uni-directional. Many conference programmes also include workshop activities, where knowledge exchange can be dynamic, unplanned and multi-way. Some of the key dental conferences in the United Kingdom are:

- British Dental Conference and Dentistry Show. This takes place at the Birmingham NEC in May each year. The sister event takes place in the London ExCeL Centre in October. Both events are inclusive for all members of the dental team.
- Specialist interest societies such as the British Society of Periodontology (https://www.bsperio.org.uk/) often host an annual conference. Other special interest conferences are held by the British Society of Prosthodontics (https://www.bsspd.org/), British Society of Paediatric Dentistry (https://www.bspd.co.uk/), British Society for Oral and Dental Research (https://bsodr.org.uk/) and British Society of Dental Hygiene and Therapy (https://www.bsdht.org.uk/).

Local Dental Committees are a valuable source of networking for dentists with an NHS contract. Dental professionals working in private practice can instead link up with others through regional branches of special interest societies, such as those above. There may also be opportunities to network with other dental professionals through events hosted by one of the UK's dental schools. These may include evening lectures or alumni events.

Networking does not have to be with people outside of the home practice. Knowledge can be mobilised through regular journal club and knowledge exchange activities within the practice. A journal club, for example, would encourage the whole dental team to engage with dental literature. Team members should take it in turns to select and share an article for discussion. Further sharing of knowledge can take place following attendance at a conference or lecture. When keeping yourself up to date, consider what might be useful for other team members, and the best mechanisms for sharing knowledge with colleagues.

47.7 Conclusion

With social media and digital communication, there are various ways in which the individual clinician can keep abreast of developments and network opportunities.

References

1. Nonaka I. A dynamic theory of organizational knowledge creation. Organization Sci. 1994;5:14–37.
2. Payne J, Fryer J. Knowledge management and information management: a tale of two siblings. Bus Inf Rev. 2020;37:69–77.
3. Day A. K is for Knowledge, M is for Mobilisation. Why bother with Knowledge Mobilisation in healthcare? Health Education England, 24 May 2021. Available at: https://library.hee.nhs.uk/about/blogs/k-is-for-knowledge-and-m-is-for-mobilisation.-why-bother-with-knowledge-mobilisation-in-healthcare. Accessed November 2023.

Teamworking: Effective Utilisation of Dental Therapists

48

Morag Powell and Ewen McColl

Learning Points
- Appreciate the benefit of teamworking with dental therapists and supporting them in providing all skills and abilities within their scope of practice.
- Recognise clinical presentations and opportunities that are applicable to a dental therapist and how best to introduce these through collaborative treatment provision.
- Understand the role of a dental therapist may change in the future to aid access to dental care.

48.1 Introduction

The relatively recent publication of Health Education England's (HEE) Advancing Dental Care Review highlighted the underutilisation of dental therapists in general dental practice [1]:

- HEE wants to create opportunities across each of its regions to optimise the skills of dental therapists and facilitate the profession to undertake more simple dental treatments. The London Economics study found that potential net economic benefits and, consequently, service benefits would be associated with a greater flexibility in the use of skill mix by creating an environment where dental therapists could undertake more Band 1 and simple Band 2 treatments, which would free up dentists to undertake more complex treatments.

M. Powell
Dental Therapy and Hygiene, Peninsula Dental School (University of Plymouth), Plymouth, UK

E. McColl (✉)
Peninsula Dental School, Plymouth, UK
e-mail: ewen.mccoll@plymouth.ac.uk

E. McColl, A. Alani (eds.), *Practical Tips in Clinical Dentistry*, BDJ Clinician's Guides, https://doi.org/10.1007/978-3-031-90355-7_48

- They frequently find themselves unable to exploit their full Scope of Practice—often for historic or contractual reasons. The potential for dentists—particularly in primary care—to share workload with DCPs in line with their Scope of Practice and experience is greatly underutilised. This opens opportunities for securing an adaptive workforce, particularly in rural and coastal areas, where dental access is a challenge.
- One of the consistent issues identified by patient engagement events was a lack of understanding among patients of the roles of the whole dental workforce, which has contributed to the situation.

48.2 Aims and Objectives

In this paper, we will discuss six top tips for optimising teamworking with a dental therapist in order to optimise outcomes for patients.

48.3 Understand Your Colleagues' Scope and How to Utilise It

In May 2013, the General Dental Council (GDC) clarified the scope of practice (SoP) [2] for members of the dental team including dental therapists (DTh), which is illustrated in Table 48.1. This guidance is a way of describing what individual team members are trained and competent to do in practising their profession. It describes the knowledge, skills and experience team members can utilise to practise safely and effectively in the best interests of patients. This is currently under review by the GDC with the hope that this will further increase utility of dental therapists, particularly in primary care.

This review is based on recent evidence commissioned by the GDC indicating there was a lack of understanding around the scope of practice document in some registrant groups [3]. This research demonstrated that 9 in 10 dental therapists (91%) and orthodontic therapists (88%) and 8 in 10 hygienists (84%) felt that they knew a great deal or fair amount about the SoP guidance document. In comparison, only around 6 in 10 dentists (61%) and dental nurses (59%) stated that they knew a great deal or fair amount about the SoP guidance document.

The aspiration in Advancing Dental Care is that by optimising the full scope of practice of dental therapists, this would allow dentists to focus on more complex treatments unique to their scope such as endodontics or fixed prosthodontics, facilitating holistic patient care in a well-defined manner, with primary disease control at the centre of patient care. Below, we discuss and clarify some issues that in our experience, there is still some confusion relating to dental therapists' scope.

Table 48.1 Scope of practice

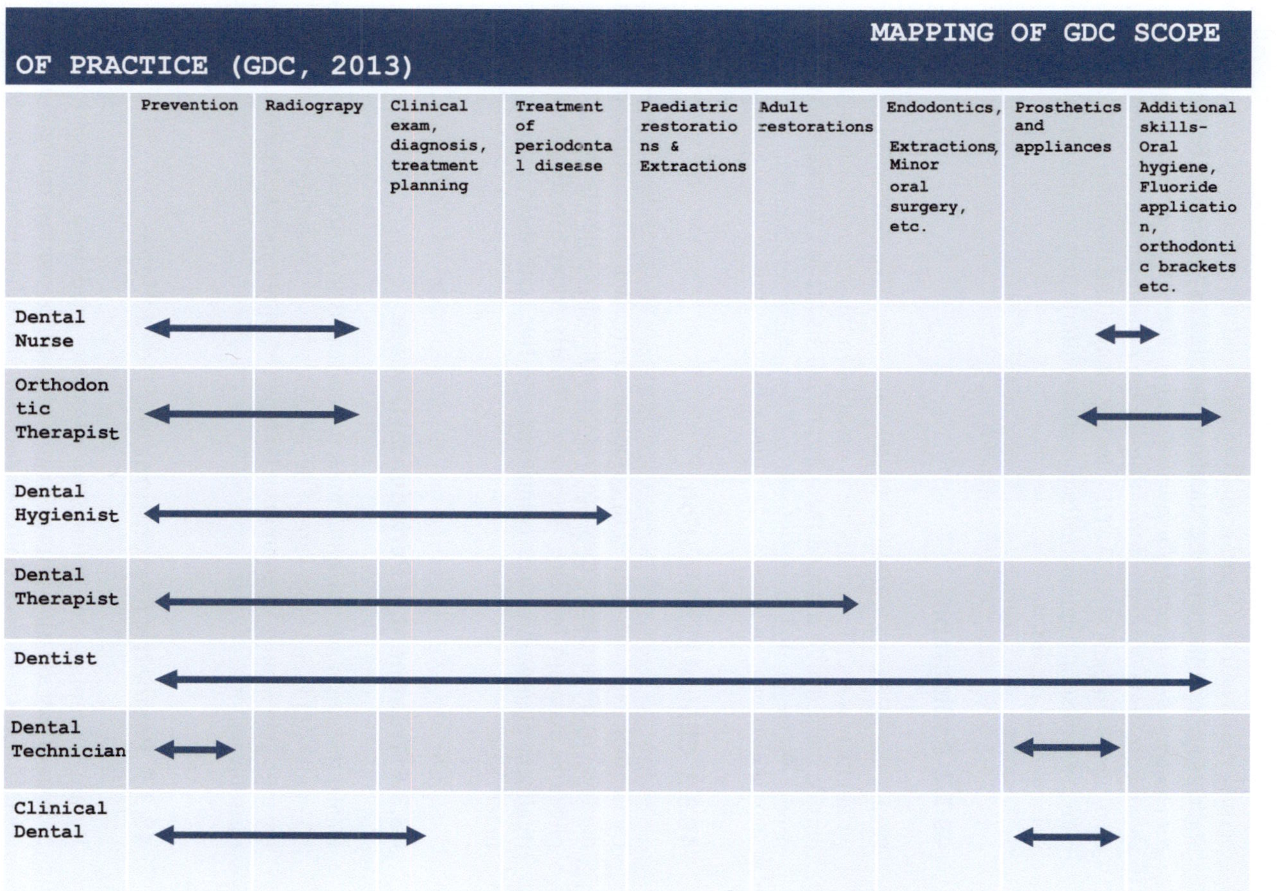

MAPPING OF GDC SCOPE OF PRACTICE (GDC, 2013)									
	Prevention	Radiograpy	Clinical exam, diagnosis, treatment planning	Treatment of periodontal disease	Paediatric restorations & Extractions	Adult restorations	Endodontics, Extractions, Minor oral surgery, etc.	Prosthetics and appliances	Additional skills- Oral hygiene, Fluoride application, orthodontic brackets etc.
Dental Nurse	↔	↔							↔
Orthodontic Therapist	↔	↔						↔	↔
Dental Hygienist	↔	↔	↔	↔					
Dental Therapist	↔	↔	↔	↔	↔	↔			
Dentist	↔	↔	↔	↔	↔	↔	↔	↔	↔
Dental Technician	↔							↔	
Clinical Dental	↔	↔	↔					↔	

48.3.1 Prevention

Prevention is the cornerstone to everything that we do within dentistry. All members of the dental team are trained in this, and all undergraduate dental therapy students are familiar with the standards detailed in *Delivering better oral health: An evidence-based toolkit for prevention* [4]. Preventive advice should be patient specific, include written information for the patient and be followed up at subsequent appointments. Details of disclosing, plaque and bleeding scores, risk assessment, specific oral hygiene instruction and reinforcement of this should be detailed in the patient record.

48.3.2 Radiographs

Dental therapists are trained to justify, prescribe, take and report on radiographs within their scope. Teamworking is essential in this area, and where reporting falls outside the scope of a dental therapist, then consultation will need to occur with a dentist registrant, that is, endodontic radiographic interpretation.

48.3.3 Clinical Examination

Dental therapists are trained to complete a full clinical examination, working to the level of competence they are trained and indemnified to do so. This is completed as standard practice. They are similarly trained to diagnose and prepare treatment plan within their competence, in line with their training and level of indemnity.

48.3.4 Treatment of Periodontal Disease

Dental therapists are trained to meet the current British Society of Periodontology S3 guidance [5] and are aware of the evidence base supporting this guidance. They are trained in a range of equipment both power, ultrasonics and piezon, and manual instrumentation.

48.3.5 Paediatric Restorations and Extractions

Dental therapists are trained to complete paediatric restorations and hall crowns. They are also trained to complete pulpotomies, though in our experience this is of limited utility in modern paediatric practice and they are not trained to complete pulpectomy as it is not in their scope of practice. Dental therapists' scope covers paediatric extractions and many have an interest in paediatric care.

Table 48.2 Preparing for practice. Dental therapy restorative undergraduate learning outcomes [6]

1.14	Restoration of teeth
1.14.1	Assess and manage caries, occlusion and tooth wear, and, where appropriate, restore the dentition using the principle of minimal intervention, maintaining function and aesthetics
1.14.2	Restore teeth using a wide range of treatments and materials appropriate to the patient including permanent and temporary direct restorations, maintaining function and aesthetics
1.14.3	Provide pulp treatment for deciduous teeth
1.14.4	Restore deciduous teeth using preformed crowns
1.14.5	Explain the role of the dental therapist in the restoration of teeth

48.3.6 Adult Restorations

They are trained to provide permanent and temporary direct restorations. This includes extensive caries removal and stepwise techniques and includes all dental materials including Biodentine. In cases where it is suspected clinically and radiographically that the caries removal will affect the pulp, therapists should discuss with a dentist registrant as to the best management of this case. Should endodontic intervention be needed, this is outside the dental therapist's scope; therefore, discussion and case planning with a dentist registrant is essential.

Dental therapists can carry out composite build-ups of teeth but not in cases where vertical dimension is altered in any way.

Dental therapists' scope does not include Nayyar Core-type restorations, that is, that involves placement of a restoration that involves invading the root canal complex and the purpose of which is to act as a core for the construction of a crown.

48.3.7 Occlusal Alteration

Further to the above with regard to composite build-ups and composite restorations, reconfiguring occlusion is out of scope of the dental therapist and any restorations should involve a conformative approach. Dental therapists are trained (Table 48.2) to assess and manage existing occlusion as part of the placement of restorations. In cases where there is any concern around altering occlusion, this needs to be discussed with a dentist registrant who should take over this element of the care. Shared care is essential in such cases.

48.4 Wider Scope Considerations

Dental therapists are trained to take impressions and can take an impression as appropriate to scope and competence. However, dental therapists may only be trained to take alginate impressions as a baseline and further training may be required on appropriately quality-assured postgraduate courses.

They can complete tooth whitening procedures on prescription from a dentist registrant; however, the first cycle of this must be completed with the dentist registrant on the premises. They can take the impressions for the bleaching trays and they can fit the bleaching trays, as this is deemed within scope.

The non-surgical treatment of peri-implantitis is within scope; however, removal of any implant-retained superstructure to gain better access to implants is not within the scope of practice and shared care is essential. For example, if the implant-retained superstructure needs to be removed to facilitate maintenance, this can be done by the dentist registrant. This will then allow the therapist to carry out the Professional Mechanical Plaque Removal (PMPR) including scaling with appropriate implant-specific instruments.

Orthodontics including Invisalign is not within the scope of a dental therapist, and indemnifiers differentiate between the fitting of bleaching trays, which is in scope, from fitting Invisalign trays that is out of scope. In addition, a grey area is the placement of composite 'buttons' for the Invisalign trays, which is currently deemed in scope. However, guidance on this may change when the new scope of practice is published.

Periodontal splinting is another grey area of the scope; however, it is the authors' view that this is within scope when completed as shared care, and the teeth have been assessed by the dentist registrant prior to referring to DTh for composite-type splints in periodontal patients. However, it would be prudent for registrants to confirm the exact position of their indemnifiers in relation to this procedure before completing it on a patient.

48.5 Written Treatment Plans

If patients are being treated under shared care, then written treatment plans are required to be in place for the dental therapist, for all aspects of their scope. The scope of practice is clear that a dental therapist cannot change the direction of a treatment plan; however, they can change the detail. An example of this would be a written prescription for a paediatric restoration can have the details of surfaces and/or materials changed by the dental therapist; however, the direction of this cannot be changed from filling to extraction. It is therefore helpful, if there is question over the restorability of the tooth, to include a statement advising to extract if necessary, if indeed the tooth is unrestorable.

The amount of detail included in the written treatment plan is determined by the dentist registrant and can vary depending on the complexity of treatment proposed. Treatment plans should be patient specific, based on the findings of a clinical examination, and give sufficient detail to allow the dental therapist to know what treatment they are expected to provide.

Taking time to develop a practice treatment protocol with the clinical team can be advantageous for standardisation, particularly if the practice employs a number of dental therapists and associates, as this allows for standardisation of treatments in appointments. This allows both the dentist and the therapist to know what is expected at each appointment, in line with appropriate scope.

Table 48.3 Example of written prescription for local anaesthetic

Patient's name	Xxxxxxxxxx
Anaesthetic	Lignospan special 2% 2.2 mL
Max cartridges	4
Route of administration	IDB and infiltration

48.6 Prescription-Only Medicines

Both injections of local anaesthetic and the provision of high-concentration fluoride products are procedures that are controlled by the Medicines Act 1968 because they involve the use of prescription-only medicines (POMs) [7]. If patients are being treated in a practice setting under shared care and not under direct access, then various prescriptions are required to be put in place for the dental therapist to allow them to complete the required treatment.

For local anaesthetics, either a Patient Group Direction (PGD) is required to be in place or a written prescription needs to be provided by the dental registrant for the anaesthetic. The Human Medicines Regulations 2012 allow independent hospitals, clinics and medical agencies to authorise their own Patient Group Directions. The regulations also allow dental practices and clinics that are registered with the CQC (or the HIW in Wales or the RQIA in NI) for the treatment of disease, disorder or injury and/or diagnostic and screening procedures to authorise PGDs [7]. If providing a patient-specific written prescription, in order to meet legal requirements on prescribing, the dentist registrant must have completed a recent clinical examination of the patient. If a written prescription is required, then this must include the name of the drug, the amount to be administered, the maximum number of cartridges that can be administered and the method of administration, as demonstrated in Table 48.3. In addition to local anaesthetic, high-concentration fluorides also require a similar detailed prescription or PGD in place.

Work is currently being undertaken by British Association of Dental Therapists (BADT) and British Society of Dental Hygienists and Therapists (BSDHT) on Exemptions of the Human Medicines act. The Department of Health has recently consulted on the exemption from the act for DTh specifically for the exemption of local anaesthetics, fluorides and topical antimicrobials. Once these relevant changes are approved and are in place, there will no longer be a need to provide a written prescription or a PGD for these items.

48.7 Chairside Assistance

Much work is currently being undertaken on the subject of chair side assistance by BSDHT, who would like to further promote chairside dental nurse support for all clinicians as part of their ongoing work. A recent survey of BSDHT members identified 30% (145) of dental hygienist respondents were rarely or never provided with chairside support [8].

The CQC have published that they feel there are two aspects to lone working [9], which include:

- Having someone else on the premises so there is support in a medical emergency.
- Whether a clinician needs chairside support from a dental nurse when treating patients.

The CQC currently judge whether lone working is safe by considering:

- The view of the General Dental Council (GDC) professional guidelines: General Dental Council *Standards for the dental team* Principle Six: 'Work with colleagues in a way that is in patients' best interests'.
- The Health and Social Care Act 2008 (Regulated Activities) Regulations 2014, regulation 18 (staffing) and regulation 12 (safe care and treatment).

The guidance provided by the CQC is that DCPs should assess the circumstances and make a clinical judgement about the level of appropriate support required to treat a patient safely.

It is the authors' view that both the employer and the DTh should also consider the safety and wellbeing of the DTh within this clinical judgement. A judgement needs to be taken on whether they regard it as safe practice for the DTh to not have a chaperone and what the potential impact would be on the wellbeing of the DTh if they are lone working. The BSDHT survey found that 49% of respondents agreed that work pressures affected the quality and safety of dental care delivery with 82% attributing time pressures as the main causative factor in errors made. In addition to this, 77% of respondents reported suffering from stress and 66% from anxiety. Recent evidence published in a rapid review [10], commissioned by the GDC, into the mental health and wellbeing of the dental profession acknowledged that there are significant issues with the wellbeing of members of the dental team.

Taking this into account, the question to consider here is, is it feasible for a dental therapist to complete the majority of their scope without chairside assistance? This question is not only limited to DTh and is relevant to DCPs including dental hygienists, therapists, orthodontic therapist and clinical dental technicians. Patient comfort should be considered, along with the need for acceptable levels of cross-infection control with high-volume suction.

In addition to this, from an equality perspective, employers need to consider the fairness of any decision for a DCP to work as a clinician without chairside assistance. Any such decision would exclude the DCP from having a chaperone present in the surgery with them, which is below the accepted standard that a dentist colleague working as an associate would be expected to accept.

Additionally, in order to optimise outcomes for patients, the quality of work provided in Fig. 48.1 would in our opinion not be possible without chairside assistant, so we believe this is essential for the clinician and the patient.

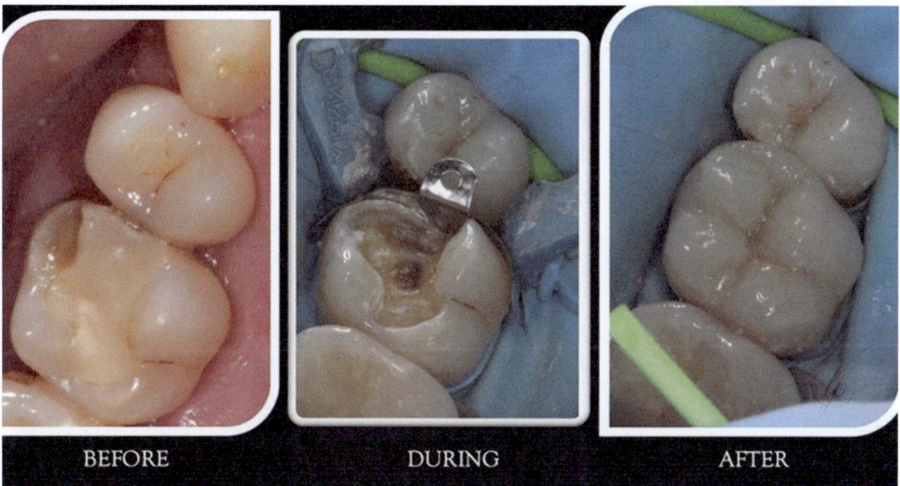

Fig. 48.1 Replacement of a failing composite by a dental therapy student. (Courtesy of Lorena Pivoda, now GDC registered dental therapist)

48.8 Promotion of the Dental Therapist Role to Patients

There is a lack of understanding in the general public of the role of a dental therapist and further work is needed to educate the public in the different roles of the dental team [3].

Recent research, commissioned by the GDC, demonstrated that the public were least likely to be aware of the role of a dental therapist [3]. They were variously thought of as providing advice, exercises or post-surgery recuperation (like a physiotherapist) or assisting those with phobias of visiting a dentist (like a counsellor). People were unsure about their remit and only guessed at the tasks they might undertake. When explained, people were particularly surprised about the extent of tasks a dental therapist could undertake [3].

Therefore, when referring patients to the dental therapist, it is important that you explain to the patient that a dental therapist will be carrying out the treatment as part of shared care. It is also imperative that as part of the introduction to the patient in the surgery that the dental therapist identifies themselves as a dental therapist, so it is clear to the patient what their role is within the team.

An infographic has recently been created by a member of the BSDHT to help promote the role of the dental therapist, specifically aimed at educating patients on the skill set of the dental therapist (Fig. 48.2). This would be an excellent addition to any practice wishing to promote the role of the dental therapist within the team.

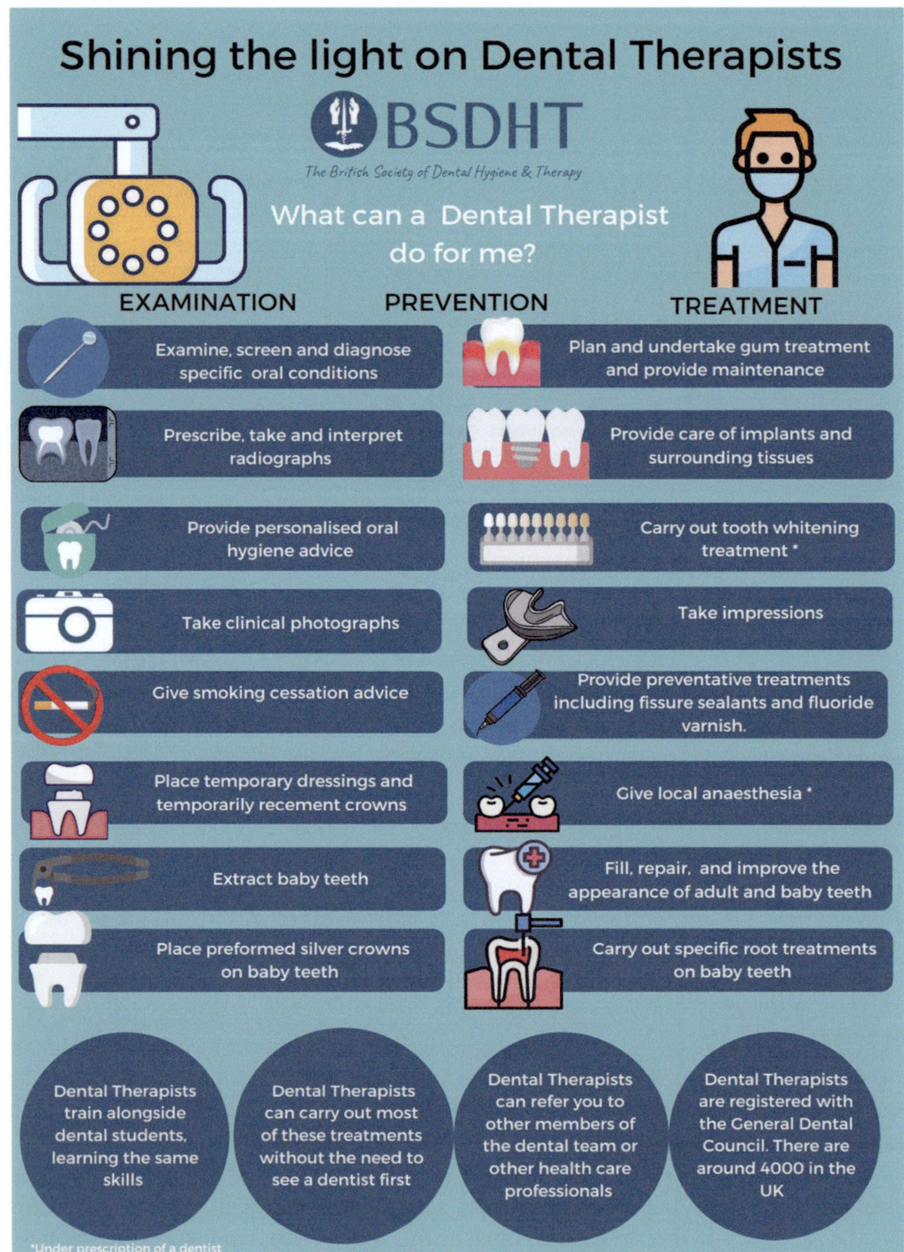

Fig. 48.2 Image courtesy of BSDHT and infographic winner 2022, Kim Chambers

48.9 Conclusion

Dental therapists have a wide skill set often underutilised in practice. Full utilisation of a dental therapist in primary care will inevitably optimise outcomes for patients, and consideration of the above top tips will hopefully go some way to facilitate change or stimulate innovative teamworking to optimise clinical outcomes.

References

1. Health Education England. HEE's advancing dental care review: final report 2021. https://www.hee.nhs.uk/sites/default/files/documents/Advancing%20Dental%20Care%20Report%20Sept%2021.pdf. Accessed 31 May 2022.
2. General Dental Council. Scope of practice. London: General Dental Council; 2013. p. 1–11.
3. IFF Research. Scope of practice review: final report. 2020. https://www.gdc-uk.org/docs/default-source/research/scope-of-practice-guidance.pdf?sfvrsn=7b3d8e58_4. Accessed 31 May 2022.
4. Department of Health. Delivering better oral health: an evidence-based toolkit. 2021. https://www.gov.uk/government/publications/delivering-better-oral-health-an-evidence-based-toolkit-for-prevention. Accessed 31 May 2022.
5. British Society of Periodontology. UK version of S3 treatment guidelines. 2021. https://www.bsperio.org.uk/professionals/bsp-uk-clinical-practice-guidelines-for-the-treatment-of-periodontitis. Accessed 31 May 2022.
6. General Dental Council. Preparing for practice: dental team learning outcomes for registration. 2015. https://www.gdc-uk.org/docs/default-source/registration-for-dcps-qualified-overseas/preparing-for-practice-(revised-2015)-(3)9cfe2565e7814f6b89ff98149f436bc7.pdf?sfvrsn=ab3900f4_7. Accessed 31 May 2022.
7. Dental Protection. Use of anaesthetics and fluorides by dental hygienist. 2015. https://www.dentalprotection.org/uk/articles/use-of-local-anaesthetic-and-fluoride-by-dental-hygienists-and-therapists. Accessed 1 Jun 2022.
8. Stratford D. The perceived impact on performance and patient safety of work-related stress and mental health disorders experienced by dental hygienists and dental therapist members of the British Society of Dental Hygiene and Therapy. Ann Clin J Dent Health. 2022:44–9.
9. Care Quality Commission. Dental mythbuster 13: lone working in a dental practice setting. 2022. https://www.cqc.org.uk/guidance-providers/dentists/dental-mythbuster-13-lone-working-dental-practice-setting. Accessed 31 May 2022.
10. Plessas A, Paisi M, Bryce M, et al. Mental health and wellbeing in dentistry: a rapid evidence assessment. London: General Dental Council; 2021. https://www.gdc-uk.org/docs/default-source/research/mental-health-and-wellbeing-in-dentistry27973e06-eb0f-4ee2-b92f-7fee3d2baf5b.pdf?sfvrsn=511f2ef9_5. Accessed 31 May 2022.

Preventing Musculoskeletal Disorders and Optimising Posture for Dental Professionals

49

Carol Robinson, Dhruti Mysore, Ewen McColl, and Sunitha Bhagavathi Mysore

Learning Points

- Understand posture while standing and operating.
- Recall how to sit correctly when viewing a screen.
- Appreciate the need for appropriate lighting and the maintenance of instruments.
- Recognise the need for seating and magnification.
- Understand the need to stretch and move regularly.

49.1 Introduction

There cannot be many members of the dental team who have not suffered from musculoskeletal aches and pains on a regular basis, but little emphasis is placed on this area of health and its effect on the dental team [1]. Dental professionals are one of the highest risk groups for developing musculoskeletal disorders (MSD) [2]. Neck, back, shoulder and wrist pain are most commonly reported amongst dentists, dental therapists and dental hygienists [3].

To ensure a successful and lengthy career, looking after our health, both physical and mental are vital. Dentistry is a physically demanding profession, with

C. Robinson
Simulated Dental Learning Environment, Peninsula Dental School (University of Plymouth), Plymouth, UK

D. Mysore
Peninsula Dental School (University of Plymouth), Derriford Dental Education Facility, Plymouth Science Park, Plymouth, UK

E. McColl (✉)
Peninsula Dental School, Plymouth, UK
e-mail: ewen.mccoll@plymouth.ac.uk

S. B. Mysore
Physiotherapy, Fatima College of Health Sciences, Abu Dhabi, United Arab Emirates

E. McColl, A. Alani (eds.), *Practical Tips in Clinical Dentistry*, BDJ Clinician's Guides, https://doi.org/10.1007/978-3-031-90355-7_49

clinicians having to adopt static positions for extended periods of time to facilitate for good vision and access. Reduced productivity, frequent absences and early retirement have all been correlated to MSD-related pain [4]. When investigating causes of ill-health retirement within dentistry, MSDs were reported to be the most common cause [5, 6]. Therefore, it is crucial that dental professionals are equipped with tools to prevent and manage MSDs as the long-term consequences can be severe.

In this article, we provide a series of practical tips to minimise MSDs and improve posture for all members of the dental team. The tips are borne from years of experience and observation of serious ill effect when good posture in clinical practice is ignored.

49.2 Understand Posture

Posture is the way you hold your body when moving (dynamic) or at rest (static). There are guidelines for dentists on ergonomics and posture from organisations such as the FDI World Dental Federation and in various papers found in dental journals [7–9]. Mastering the correct posture while standing, operating and sitting at a computer will guarantee long-term health benefits.

49.2.1 Standing Posture

Your spine has three curves, which you need to maintain. You may have to retrain your body to achieve good posture if you have developed unhealthy habits over the years. Standing correctly helps to distribute your weight across your joints, reducing strain and stress (Fig. 49.1). Try this out now:

- Stand with your feet hip width apart, ankle bones under hip bones.
- Do not lock your knees; keep them soft.
- Gently tilt your pelvis backwards and forwards and allow it to settle into a neutral position.
- Shrug your shoulders a few times and bring them down and back so your shoulder joints are over your hip joints, and horizontal.
- Let your arms relax down by your sides.
- Let your neck, jaw and eyes relax, and feel the crown of your head gently lift.

You should already feel taller and more evenly balanced.

49.2.2 Posture for the Seated Clinician

Healthy sitting posture while working is critical for preventing musculoskeletal disorders, as it encompasses a large part of the working day (Fig. 49.2):

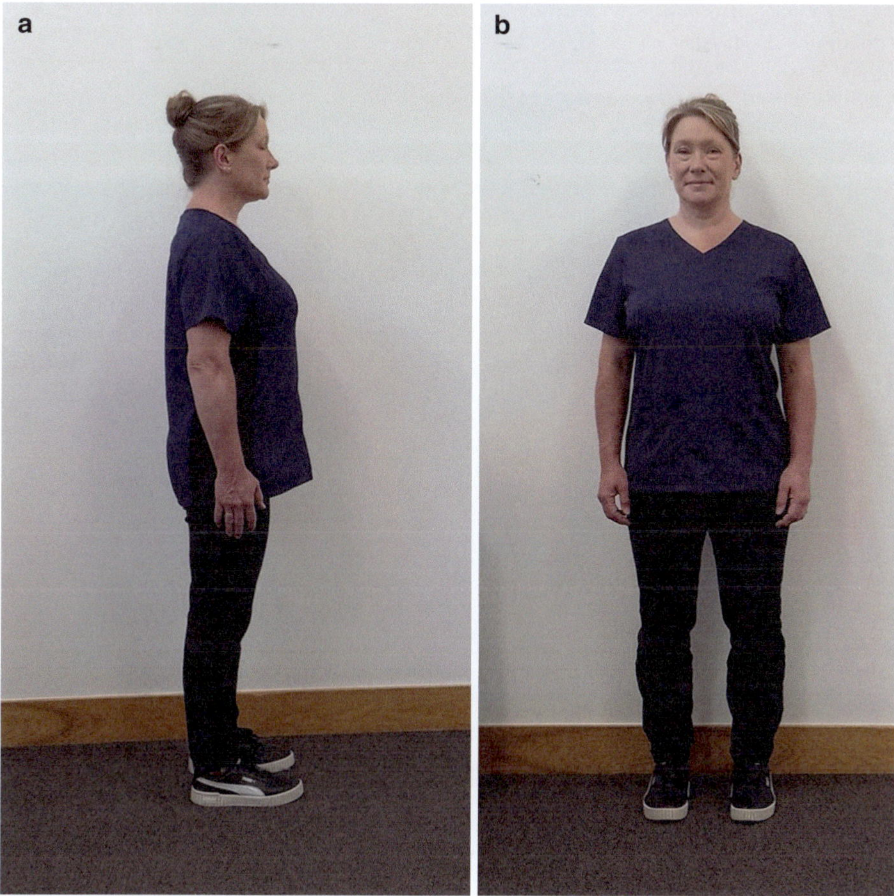

Fig. 49.1 (**a**) Side view of optimal standing posture. (**b**) Frontal view of optimal standing posture. (Courtesy of Peninsula Dental School staff and Carol Robinson)

- Sit in a stable, upright, symmetrical position [8].
- Lower legs vertical.
- Look perpendicularly onto the surface you are working on either by direct vision or in the mirror.
- The oral cavity should be at mid-sternum height.
- Your forearms should be horizontal or no more than 25° up from horizontal, and elbows should be tucked in.
- Head should be tilted no more than 20° in any direction.
- Move your chair or the patient so you can maintain this position for 80% of your working time.
- Keep the other 20% for treating those patients who cannot lie in a supine position (e.g., pregnant women or bariatric patients).
- Keep your delivery unit at elbow height to avoid overstretching.

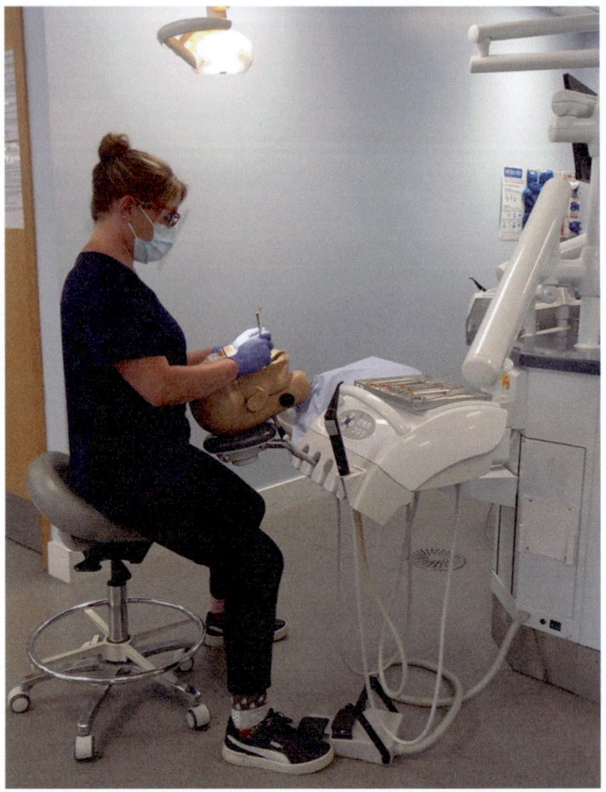

Fig. 49.2 Seated posture. (Courtesy of Peninsula Dental School staff and Carol Robinson)

Even with gold standard posture, staying in one position for too long—known as prolonged static postures (PSPs)—can result in muscle stiffness and disorders [10]. Make sure you move around every now and then to avoid PSPs!

49.2.3 Posture for the Dental Nurse

- Sit in an upright position.
- Should be sitting higher than the clinician so that the dental nurse's eyes are approximately 10 cm above the clinician's (Fig. 49.3).
- Stand up if you need to! [11]

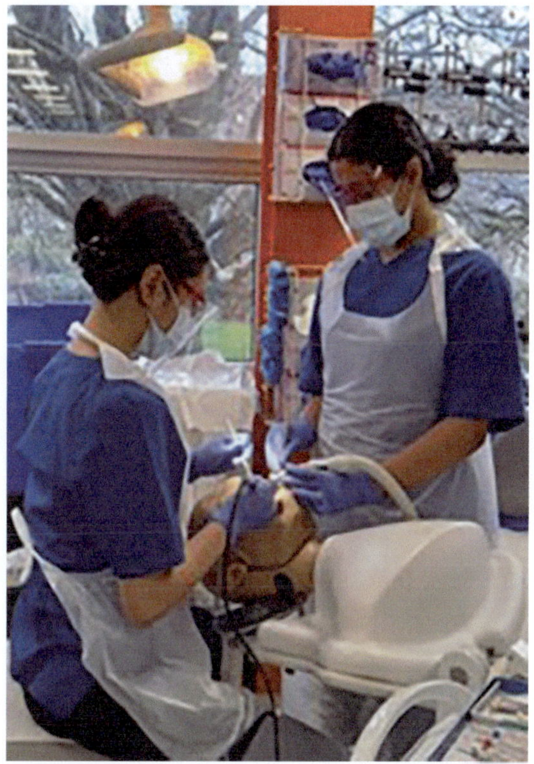

Fig. 49.3 Gold standard clinician and dental nurse posture. (Courtesy of students at Peninsula Dental School and Carol Robinson)

49.3 How to Sit Correctly at a Screen

You may need to adjust the height of either your desk, chair, table or screen to achieve the optimal seated position (Fig. 49.4).

- Sit with both feet flat on the floor, lower legs vertical and a 90° angle behind your knees [4, 6].
- Sit up straight with relaxed shoulders [2].
- Allow the back of your chair to support you [5].
- Shoulder joints above hip joints [2].
- Forearms flat on desk or table [3].
- The top of your screen should be level with your eyes [1].
- The screen should be about an arm's length away [7].

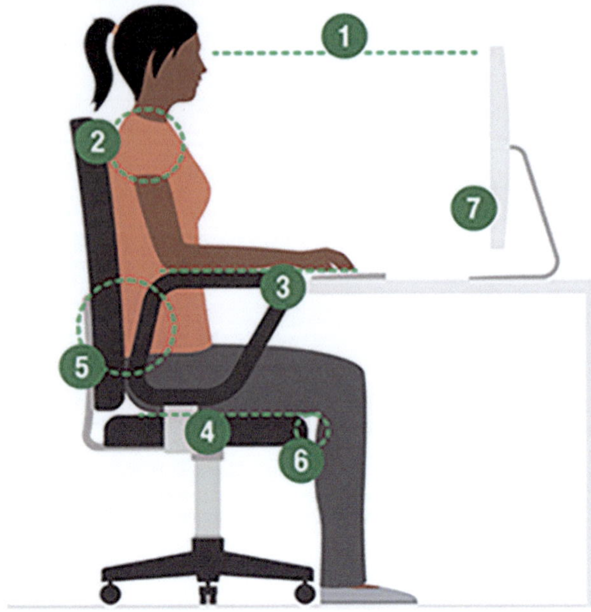

Fig. 49.4 How to sit at a screen. Contains public sector information published by the Health and Safety Executive and licensed under the https://www.nationalarchives.gov.uk/doc/open-government-licence/version/3/

49.4 Adjust the Patient

- The patient should lie supine; only then can you achieve good posture yourself.
- Ensure they have pulled themselves right back into the angle of the chair.
- Adjust the double articulating headrest correctly: Practise with a colleague to find how comfortable this is, even though it looks very odd.
- The headrest should support the head on the back of the skull on the mastoid bone.
- Use a wipeable cushion or folded towel if the gap between chair and headrest is long.
- Adjust the headrest so the patient's chin is up when treating upper teeth, down when treating lower teeth (Fig. 49.5).
- Ask the patient to move their head as required.

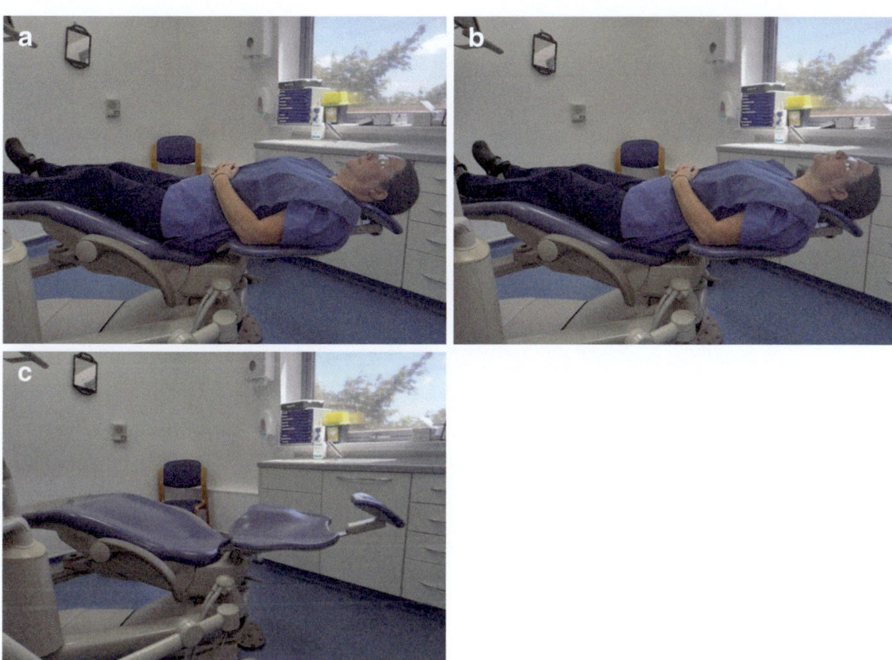

Fig. 49.5 (**a**) Chin down is good for working on lower teeth. (**b**) Chin up is preferred for upper teeth. (**c**) Note the position of the headrest. (Courtesy of Staff at Peninsula Dental School and Carol Robinson)

49.5 Proper Use of Lighting

- Your operating light should be positioned so the light runs parallel to your line of vision.
- Use your mirror to reflect the light into the cavity, no shadows (Fig. 49.6a)!
- If you use a light on your loupes, do not forget to use the operating light (Fig. 49.6b). Your dental nurse would like to see as well.

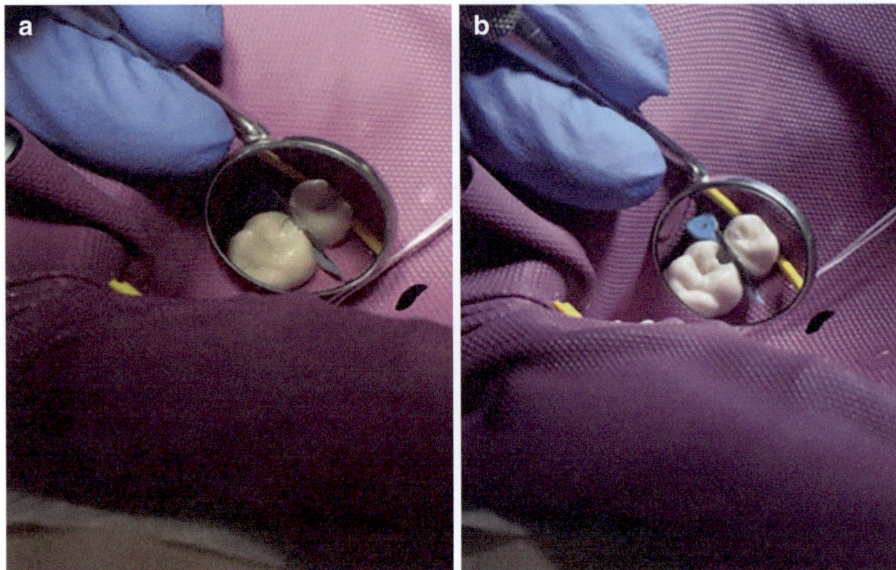

Fig. 49.6 (**a**) Improper use of lighting can cause shadows. (**b**) Adjusting the operating light to reflect the light back from the mirror into the cavity is a game changer. (Courtesy of Carol Robinson)

Fig. 49.7 Periodontal tray courtesy of Peninsula Dental School and Carol Robinson

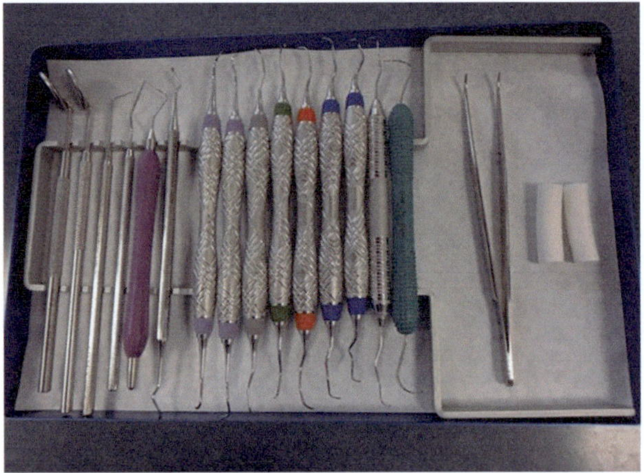

49.6 Use Sharp, Ergonomically Designed Instruments [12]

- Use light instruments that have a large diameter (Fig. 49.7).
- Instruments with a textured grip are easier to grasp, beneficial during scaling (PMPR) as the amount of force required is reduced.
- Hand fatigue can be minimised by using sharpened instruments.
- Instruments may be sharpened in practice with the right tool and technique or can be sent for professional sharpening.

49.7 Buy an Ergonomic Seat

Buying an ergonomic seat, especially one that is saddle shaped, is a great investment and can make achieving good posture so much easier. Once adjusted correctly, this will allow you to sit with a correctly aligned spine. Try out various makes until you find the one that suits you best. Tilting the seat 5–15° allows for a closer position to the patient with less lower back strain. If chairs cannot be tilted, then a wedge-shaped cushion can be used.

49.8 Use Magnification Loupes

You are executing precise movements in a dark, wet cave that keeps moving. Use of magnification loupes with a direct light source not only helps meet your visual demands but has demonstrated improved posture and reduced musculoskeletal pain [13, 14].

- Choose a pair of loupes that suit your daily needs and has an angle of declination of 40° and a light to go with it.
- General dentistry needs no more than 3.5× magnification. Save high magnification and costs for the specialists!
- Try refractive loupes; they ensure the neck stays upright.

See Figs. 49.8 and 49.9.

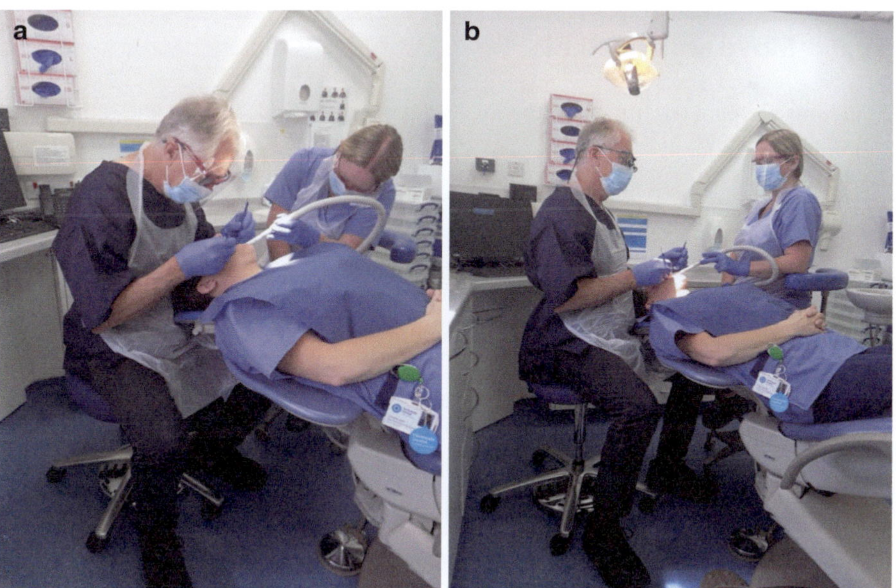

Fig. 49.8 (**a**) Poor posture from both clinician and dental nurse. (**b**) Improved by sitting correctly on saddle seat, wearing loupes and correcting position of operating light. (Courtesy of staff at Peninsula Dental School and Carol Robinson)

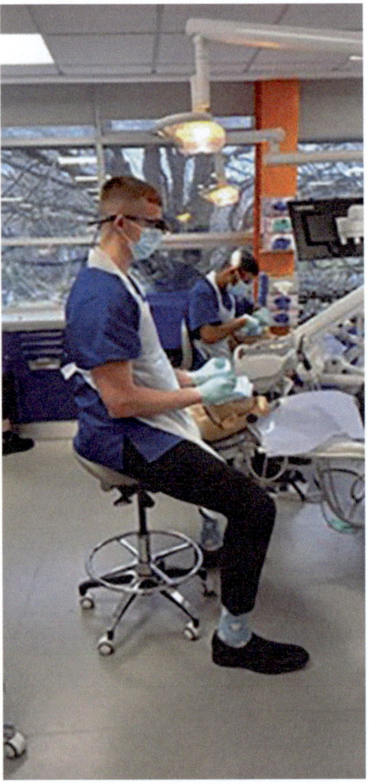

Fig. 49.9 Refractive loupes and a saddle seat allowing excellent seated posture for an extremely tall ex-basketball player. (Courtesy of student from Peninsula Dental School and Carol Robinson)

49.9 Move and Stretch!

Static muscle pain occurs when the load on the muscles is constant and unrelenting throughout an activity.

- Stand up and move about between patients.
- Walk or bike to work if you can or go for a short stroll at lunchtime.
- Stretch your neck, shoulders, lower back, hands and wrists regularly—especially between patients and at the end of the day.
- Take a few seconds during a long procedure to be mindful of posture and muscle strain.
- Ten minutes of daily stretching can make a world of difference, as will attending a Pilates or yoga class for a full body stretch.
- Make friends with your physiotherapist, osteopath, chiropractor or massage therapist.

There are several online materials available to correct posture, avoid fatigue and move better. Some of these include exercises to avoid wrist and hand strain [15] and videos of exercises and tips for better posture by physiotherapists [16].

49.10 Conclusion

The tips provided in this article are pragmatic and achievable by all, with the benefits being abundant. Using these tips may be the difference between an early ill-health retirement and a long fruitful career as a dental professional.

Photos Permissions obtained for this publication.

References

1. Kawtharani AA, Chemeisani A, Salman F, Younes AH, Msheik A. Neck and musculoskeletal pain among dentists: a review of the literature. Cureus. 2023;15(1):e33609. https://doi.org/10.7759/cureus.33609.
2. Lietz J, Kozak A, Nienhaus A. Prevalence and occupational risk factors of musculoskeletal diseases and pain among dental professionals in Western countries: a systematic literature review and meta-analysis. PLoS One. 2018;13(12):e0208628. https://doi.org/10.1371/journal.pone.0208628.
3. Chenna D, Pentapati KC, Kumar M, Madi M, Siddiq H. Prevalence of musculoskeletal disorders among dental healthcare providers: a systematic review and meta-analysis. F1000Res. 2022;11:1062. https://doi.org/10.12688/f1000research.124904.2.
4. Edrees A, Abu Rayyan I, Splieth CH, Alkilzy M, Barbe AG, Wicht MJ. Musculoskeletal disorders and risk indicators for pain chronification among German dentists: a cross-sectional questionnaire-based study. J Am Dent Assoc. 2024;155:536–45.
5. Brown J, Burke FJ, Macdonald EB, et al. Dental practitioners and ill health retirement: causes, outcomes and re-employment. Br Dent J. 2010;209(5):E7. https://doi.org/10.1038/sj.bdj.2010.813.
6. Al-Emara Z, Karaharju-Suvanto T, Furu P, Furu H. Musculoskeletal disorders and work ability among dentists and dental students in Finland. Work. 2024;78(1):73–81. https://doi.org/10.3233/WOR-23030.
7. FDI, World Dental Federation. Ergonomics and posture guidelines for oral health professionals. 2021. https://www.fdiworlddental.org/ergonomics-and-posture-guidelines-oral-health-professionals. Accessed May 2024.
8. Hokwerda O, de Ruijter R, Shaw S. Adopting a healthy sitting posture during patient treatment. 2009. https://www.rug.nl/research/ctm/kenniscentrum/ergonomie/pdfergonomie/1adoptingahealthysittingworkingpostureduringpatienttreatment.(jan2009).pdf. Accessed May 2024.
9. Breslin M, Cook S. No turning back: posture in dental practice. BDJ Team. 2015;2(10):15164. https://doi.org/10.1038/bdjteam.2015.164.
10. De Sio S, Traversini V, Rinaldo F, et al. Ergonomic risk and preventive measures of musculoskeletal disorders in the dentistry environment: an umbrella review. PeerJ. 2018;6:e4154. https://doi.org/10.7717/peerj.4154.
11. Paul E. Posture technique. Br Dent J. 2008;204:169–70.
12. HuFriedy Group. Ergonomics in the dental office—how to care for patients while also caring for yourself. 2020. https://hufriedygroup.eu/en/blog/ergonomics-dental-office-how-care-patients-while-also-caring-yourself. Accessed May 2024.
13. Plessas A, Bernardes DM. The role of ergonomic saddle seats and magnification loupes in the prevention of musculoskeletal disorders. A systematic review. Int J Dent Hyg. 2018;16:430–40.
14. Lietz J, Ulusoy N, Nienhaus A. Prevention of musculoskeletal diseases and pain among dental professionals through ergonomic interventions: a systematic literature review. Int J Environ Res Public Health. 2020;17(10):3482. https://doi.org/10.3390/ijerph17103482.

15. Ultradent Products Inc. Say goodbye to wrist and hand fatigue. 2018. https://blog.ultradent.com/5-easy-exercises-to-help-dental-professionals-prevent-hand-and-wrist-fatigue. Accessed Apr 2024.
16. Posturedontics: Dr Bethany Valachi. Solving work related pain in dentistry. https://posturedontics.com/product-category/online-course/. Accessed Apr 2024.

Preventative Dentistry in Primary Care 50

Ines Avery, Safiya Robinson, Yen Lin, and Ewen McColl

Learning Points
- Understand the importance of prevention and how this relates to core aspects of dental care provision.
- Recognise the various avenues for prevention and specifically fluoride delivery.
- Recall the need to tailor preventative regimes for each patient and that these may change when presenting factors either increase or decrease.

50.1 Introduction

Stabilisation of primary disease is a key pillar of successful treatment in the provision of dental care. As well as managing periodontal disease, managing caries is a crucial component of a successful treatment plan. Treatment plans are often divided into the following phases.

50.2 Phased Treatment

1. Emergency treatment.
2. Elimination of active disease to achieve oral stability.
3. Rehabilitation/reconstruction phase.
4. Maintenance/monitoring phase.

I. Avery · S. Robinson · Y. Lin
Dental Education, Peninsula Dental School (University of Plymouth), Plymouth, UK

E. McColl (✉)
Peninsula Dental School, Plymouth, UK
e-mail: ewen.mccoll@plymouth.ac.uk

E. McColl, A. Alani (eds.), *Practical Tips in Clinical Dentistry*, BDJ Clinician's Guides, https://doi.org/10.1007/978-3-031-90355-7_50

Whilst the focus is often on phases 1 and 3, achieving oral stability is the foundation of future success. Often in the rush to progress to phase 3, not enough time is spent on phase 2 given the time pressures in busy practices. However, if we do not relay the appropriate preventative messages to our patients, treatment carried out in phase 3 will inevitably fail. In this short article, we discuss some of our experiential tips for preventative care in primary care.

50.3 Optimising Fluoride Dose Depending on Caries Risk

Our recommendations regarding fluoride doses will differ depending on the patient's caries risk [1]. Establishing your patient's current fluoride exposure is important to tailor recommendations. Asking questions such as 'What toothpaste do you use?' can be helpful, as well as the number of times they brush a day, and whether they rinse their mouth or spit after toothbrushing. However, there has been a rise in 'social media dentistry' and unlicensed toothpastes that can lead patients to making uninformed decisions [2]. Therefore, it is essential for dentists to investigate the content of toothpastes if a patient reports using a brand you are not familiar with, to ensure that the patient is exposed to the appropriate fluoride content.

It is also important to remember that your patient might be exposed to other sources of fluoride. Therefore, one should consider this when assigning an appropriate caries risk and if any of these apply to your area of practice:

(a) **Fluoridated water and milk**—Fluoridation of water is rare in the United Kingdom; there are very few areas with naturally fluoridated water (some areas in County Durham, Staffordshire, Hampshire and Berkshire). It is only added to 10% of areas in England (Cumbria, Cheshire, Tyneside, Northumbria, Durham, Humberside, Lincolnshire, Nottinghamshire, Derbyshire, West Midlands and Bedfordshire) [3] and completely absent in Scotland, Wales and Northern Ireland [1]. Fluoridation of milk is also rare, but when used, it is given to early years and school children in areas of high caries incidence with no fluoridated water [1]. There is a limited number of studies done on its efficacy, and a Cochrane review concluded that it can lower caries risk; however, there was no mention of any adverse side effects, such as fluorosis [4].

(b) **High-fluoride toothpaste**—If a patient is deemed to be at an increased caries risk, one should consider increasing their fluoride availability until caries risk is able to be reduced by the patient [1]. This could be in the form of a prescription of high-fluoride toothpaste, fluoride varnish application or fluoridated mouthwashes. Regarding high-fluoride toothpastes, they should be considered for children with a high caries risk between the ages of 10 and 16 (2800 ppm) and over 16 as well as adults (5000 ppm) [1]. The evidence regarding its efficacy and benefits is limited, focusing mainly on radicular caries [1]. Their chronic use should also be avoided, and children as well as adults with additional needs may require supervision when using them [1].

(c) **Fluoride varnish**—Fluoride varnish at 22,600 ppm (2.26% NaF) is a medium that is mostly safe and well received by patients and should be regularly applied when a child attends a recall appointment [5]. Adverse reactions to colophony in patients with an allergy to plaster adhesives and severe asthma can occur; therefore, colophony-free varnishes should be used when possible [6]. It has been agreed that its use is accepted by Muslims, as its alcohol content is very low and is being used for medical purposes rather than for recreational purposes with an intoxication intent [1].

(d) **Fluoridated mouthwashes**—Mouthwashes can be used daily (230 ppm) or weekly (~900 ppm), with no current evidence on the efficacy of one versus the other [1]. It is important to stress to patients that mouthwashes should be used at a different time from toothbrushing to increase the effects of fluoride, as there is a large group of patients that believe mouthwash should be used after brushing [7, 8].

50.4 Tailoring Interdental Cleaning to Individual Patients

There are several different products in the market aimed at interdental cleaning, including dental floss, dental tape, interdental brushes, oral irrigators, etc. It can be difficult to decide which product to recommend. Evidence suggests that interdental brushes could be more effective than floss; however, there are several factors that need to be taken into account when making a bespoke interdental cleaning plan [9].

Assessing patients' embrasure types can help with the selection of interdental cleaning aids.

According to Liang et al. [10], there are three different types of embrasures (Table 50.1), and each type will benefit from different interdental cleaning aids. This should also be considered in combination with patient engagement, manual dexterity and patterns of plaque deposition. Table 50.2 illustrates a summary of the recommendations proposed by Liang et al. [10].

It is also worth reminding patients that they should start interdental cleaning by the age of 18; however, this can be started earlier if there is gingival inflammation present since attachment loss can be observed in early teenage years [9]. Interdental brush sizing is shown in Figs. 50.1 and 50.2.

Table 50.1 Embrasure types according to Liang et al. 2020 [10]

Embrasure type	Description
Type I	Closed interdental space filled with interdental papilla
Type II	Open interdental space with interdental papilla filling 51–75% of space
Type III	Open interdental space with interdental papilla filling up to 50% of space

Table 50.2 Interdental cleaning recommendations based on patient characteristics

Patient characteristics	Recommendations
Type 1 embrasure, motivated, good manual dexterity	• Dental floss
Type 1 embrasure, low motivation and/or low dexterity	• Small diameter interdental brushing, as long as there is space for passive insertion (Figs. 50.1 and 50.2) • Alternatively, rubber interdental bristle, flossette or irrigators • (If orthodontic appliance is present, irrigators are highly recommended)
Type II or III embrasures, regardless of motivation and dexterity	• Interdental brushes • Gum stimulators can reduce inflammation and bleeding • C-shape flossing technique or interdental brush with a lingual approach dependent on residual plaque accumulation

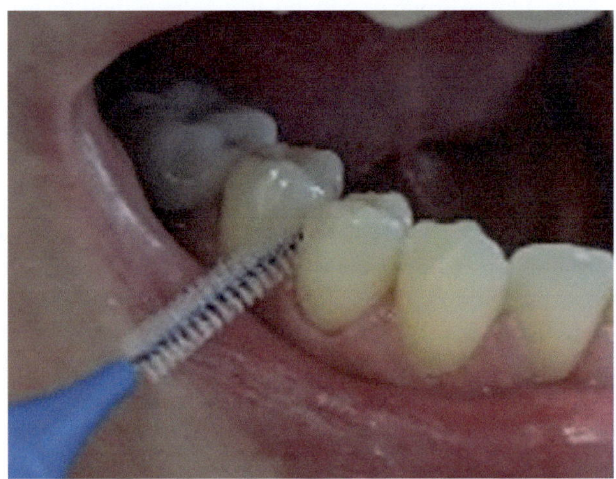

Fig. 50.1 Interdental brush sizing for type 1 embrasure. The brush is too large for the embrasure

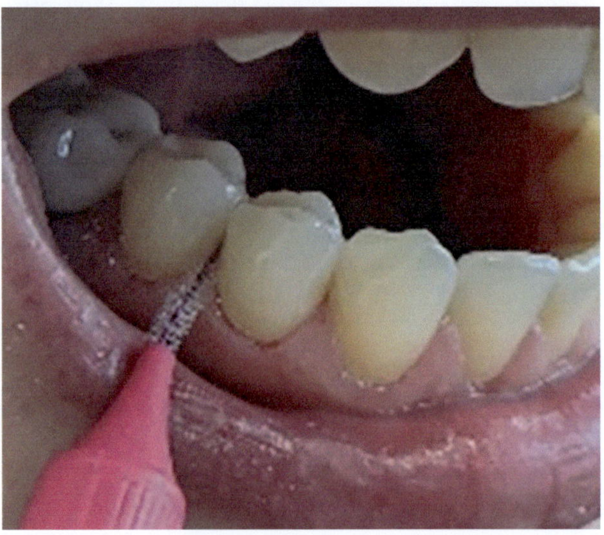

Fig. 50.2 An adequate interdental brush size for the embrasure

50.5 Toothbrushing Advice Based on Evidence

Giving toothbrushing advice is one of the main preventative measures that the majority of clinicians use [11]. There is strong evidence that brushing twice a day with fluoride toothpaste, before bed and at another time, is an effective biofilm removal technique that supports oral health [12]. Choosing a toothbrush that fits your patient is an important step in oral health instructions, so there are several factors to consider:

(a) **Powered versus manual toothbrush**—There is evidence that a powered toothbrush is more effective in biofilm removal and has both long- and short-term reduction in periodontal issues [9, 13]. There is, however, effective plaque removal with both types of toothbrushes, and no conclusive evidence regarding a superior mode of brushing, be it sonic or rotary [9]. It is important to tailor toothbrushing techniques to the toothbrush the patient is using, as using an electric toothbrush with a manual toothbrush technique can be more inefficient.
(b) **Bristles**—A toothbrush with a round head and medium bristles is appropriate for the majority of patients; however, recommendations should be done with the knowledge of the patient's toothpaste, as studies suggest that a medium to high abrasive paste can lead to higher dentine loss when used with medium and firm bristle toothbrushes [14].
(c) **Brushing time**—DBOH ('Delivering better oral health') recommends brushing for at least 2 min, which can be achieved with the aid of a timer, whether with an app on a smartphone, for example, BrushDJ or an egg timer [9]. There are, however, studies that suggest that this might not be sufficient to achieve sufficient plaque removal [15].
(d) **Brushing children's teeth**—Children's brushing should be supervised until the age of 7; however, further supervision might be required if brushing is proving to be ineffective with further support and encouragement [9]. Supervision will guarantee the correct amount of fluoride is dispensed, and it will ensure that the child does not eat or lick the toothpaste before it is used, avoiding fluoride overexposure [9].

50.6 Diet Advice and Sugar Intake

The intake of free sugars has reduced recently in children, but this has not been observed in adults [16]. Explaining to patients the definition of 'free sugars' can be very helpful in the management of their diet. Some patients will believe that sugars marketed as 'healthy', for example, honey, will not be damaging for their teeth. Raising awareness that any sugar that is added by a manufacturer, including natural sugars, such as those found in fruit juices and honey, constitutes a free sugar and can increase their caries risk. Increasing their vegetable, whole fruit and fibre intake will benefit not just their general but oral health as well [16]. Referring patients back to the Eatwell Guide will also help to reinforce their knowledge and fill in any gaps that the patient might not have grasped during their appointment [17].

A visual aid, such as the illustration of Stephan's curve [widely available online and often used at dental school], can be a good behavioural change tool, as it demonstrates the effect that sugar and acidic foods and beverages can have if not restricted to three sugar attacks daily [18].

Changing your patients' views on the types of food they purchase and encouraging them to check the product's label for sugar content as well as its position in the list of ingredients (Box 50.1) can be a good motivator for habit change [16].

Box 50.1 The Ingredients List of a Well-Known Hazelnut Spread Snack, Displaying Sugar at the Top

Wafer filled with hazelnut spread with cocoa.

Ingredients:

Hazelnut spread with cocoa 81.5% (sugar, palm oil, **hazelnuts** [13%]).
Skimmed **milk** powder (8.7%).
Fat-reduced cocoa (7.4%).
Emulsifier.
Lecithin (**soya**, vanillin).
Wheat flour.
Baker's yeast.
Powdered **barley's** malt extract.
Salt.
Skimmed **milk** powder.
Emulsifier.
Lecithin (**soya**).
Wheat proteins.
Whey proteins (**milk**).
Water.

When it comes to babies and young children, it should be highlighted that there are several benefits to breastfeeding, including a lower caries risk for babies that are breastfed for the first 12 months [19]. There is a potential for an increased caries risk for children that are breastfed for over 12 months; however, it becomes difficult to confirm the main aetiological factor due to ingestion of solids, which may include processed foods and sugars [19, 20].

Parents should be reminded that as soon as their children's teeth have erupted, they will need to be brushed. This should be done as close as possible to bedtime, even if there are night-time feeds or if the infant falls asleep at the breast/bottle. It is also helpful to remind parents that if a baby is bottle-fed, only milk, cooled boiled water or formula should be used, and anything with added sugars should not be used. Bottle use should also be discontinued after 12 months [16].

Another thing to be wary of is sugar in medications. Some liquid preparations contain sugars, so it is important to highlight this to the patient and potentially request a sugar-free preparation from their general practitioner (GP). If this is not possible, one should consider fitting medication times around meals [16].

50.7 Fissure Sealants

Resin-based fissure sealants are recommended for children that have an increased caries risk. This should be done on all erupting fissured teeth, especially molars [21]. There is less evidence regarding glass ionomer and resin-modified glass ionomer cements; however, they have a place if there is no opportunity or optimal clinical conditions to use a resin-based fissure sealant [22].

The provision of proximal resin-based sealants has proved to be more effective than glass ionomer [23]. This can be done when there is direct exposure and access to the proximal wall on children with an increased caries risk [21].

There can be little success after placement of fissure sealants, which is likely due to its highly sensitive technique [21]. Studies show that there is no difference in the outcome between sealed and non-sealed teeth; however, this is likely due to sealant failure [24]. The technique for correct sealant placement can be prone to error, which will affect not just the longevity of the sealants but also its function. Therefore, there should be a regular check of the integrity of sealants. One should assess them for wear, leakage and retention problems, ensuring that they are maintained properly and continue to prevent caries [21].

Here are a few tips that can minimise operator error:

- Ensuring good tooth surface cleaning, with pumice, air abrasion or hydrogen peroxide [25].
- Ensuring adequate moisture control. Exposure to salivary proteins will contaminate the enamel; hence, re-etching might be required [26]. Rubber dam should be used when possible [27].
- A four-handed approach has been associated with improved retention [26].
- Assessing the sealant for any voids, material deficiencies or air bubbles before curing will help to ensure retention [28].

50.8 Behaviour and Mindset Change

We know that many oral diseases can be prevented or managed by improving patients' healthy behaviours and suggesting the interventions we have already discussed. However, achieving behaviour change with our patients can be easier said than done. Indeed, change is influenced by a number of factors, including environmental and socioeconomic. Therefore, it is important to manage our own expectations around what that change looks like.

Behaviour change is a cycle, an ongoing process – not something that happens immediately or in a linear fashion [29].

This means that as clinicians, we need to accept that patients' behaviours will not change overnight and be willing to take the journey with the patient towards improving their oral health, remembering that information does not lead automatically to transformation and behaviour change. It also means that behaviour change is an ongoing process, not only for the patient but for us as practitioners too. We need to persevere as we encourage our patient to take the relevant steps, often repeatedly, as behaviour change can take many attempts.

Behaviour change can take up to 9 months and may be more effective when a patient is at a key point in life, as they may be more ready to change when stepping into a new chapter [29]. Milestones such as parenthood, entering retirement or finishing school are notably a good time to attempt behaviour change.

Our instructions will need to be tailored to the individual patient, taking into account whether or not they are ready to change. We can do this through discussion with the patient and deciding with them not only if they are ready to change but what changes they have the capacity to make. There are a number of behaviour change models that we can use to achieve this. The COM-B model states that a person must have the capability, opportunity and motivation to change their behaviour [30].

A part of this involves us as dental practitioners laying the groundwork for change by:

- Raising awareness of the issue and the fact that there are options to prevent/control disease through oral health improvement.
- Assessing the patient's capability, opportunity and motivation to change.
- Supporting patients who are ready to change by showing them what changes they can make and how. We can also set SMART goals, identify barriers to change and make suggestions to overcome these, plan for relapses in behaviour and provide encouragement and praise for any small shifts and changes.

Oral health interventions designed to influence a patient's behaviour can be delivered by various members of the dental team. Once we have decided who in our practice will be delivering these oral health interventions with the patient, we need to ensure that we build rapport and empathy with the patient and decide how we are going to deliver the intervention to them. This should be decided along with the assessment of the patient's readiness to change, to ensure that the method suits the patient and where they are in their journey of behaviour change. Face to face is the preferred method, by one or more team members, but this can be supplemented by printed or digital resources [31]. The duration of advice can range from brief to more in-depth interventions [31].

50.9 Recall Intervals and Caries Risk Assessment

Since caries risk assessment is used to predict the future likelihood of caries and its progression, it will help us to decide how often we need to recall our patients and take bitewing radiographs [32]. This will, in turn, reduce the prevalence of caries developing and progressing to the point of causing pain or infection.

Factors that can be taken into account for predicting caries risk include past experience of caries, oral hygiene, dietary habits, salivary changes and socio-economic factors [33]. A patient who presents with one or more of the above criteria is considered to be at an increased caries risk and, according to FGDP guidance, can be justified in having bitewing radiographs taken every 6 months and a recall interval from 6 months to 1 year [34, 35].

Even with the use of caries risk assessment tools, the determination of recall times for patients is down to clinical judgement in accordance with NICE guidelines (Table 50.3). In addition, the British Society of Paediatric Dentistry recommends that children have their first dental check-up by age 1 [36]. As clinicians, it is our responsibility to be familiar with NICE and FGDP (CGDent) guidance, decide which system for assessing caries risk works best within your practice and ensure that you justify both your recall time and your radiograph intervals in your clinical records [34, 35].

Table 50.3 Dental recalls adapted from NICE guidelines [35]

		Children and young people (under 18 years)	Adults (18 years or older)
Step 1	Consider patient's age; this sets range of recall interval	3–12 months	3–24 months
Step 2	Consider modifying factors (see NICE guidance) including medical, social and dental histories and clinical examination	3–12 months	3–24 months
Step 3	Integrate diagnostic and prognostic information with clinical judgement to recommend interval to next oral health review	3–12 months	3–24 months
Step 4	Discuss recommended interval with patient and record agreed interval or reason for disagreement	Discussion	Discussion
Step 5	At next oral health review, consider whether the interval was appropriate and adjust accordingly—depending on patient's ability to maintain oral health between recalls	Reassess	Reassess

50.10 Conclusions

There are many ways to help our patients prevent dental decay, even when we and our patients are pressed for time as is likely in a busy primary care practice. Fortunately, interventions that often do not take much time can be impactful if applied correctly. It is essential that we tailor our preventative advice to suit our patients' individual situations. In this short paper, we have highlighted some of the key factors in caries prevention that in combination with behaviour change and recall intervals will help to minimise the prevalence of caries.

References

1. Department of Health & Social Care, NHS England, NHS Improvement, Office for Health Improvement and Disparities. Delivering better oral health: an evidence-based toolkit for prevention. Chapter 9: Fluoride. 2021. https://www.gov.uk/government/publications/delivering-better-oral-health-an-evidence-based-toolkit-for-prevention/chapter-9-fluoride. Accessed Mar 2024.
2. Ooi HL, Kelleher MGD. Instagram dentistry. Prim Dent J. 2021;10:13–9.
3. British Fluoridation Society. Extent of water fluoridation. Updated 2020. https://bfsweb.org/extent/. Accessed Mar 2024.
4. Yeung CA, Chong LY, Glenny A-M. Fluoridated milk for preventing dental caries. Cochrane Database Syst Rev. 2015. https://doi.org/10.1002/14651858.CD003876.pub4.
5. Mascarenhas AK. Is fluoride varnish safe?: validating the safety of fluoride varnish. J Am Dent Assoc. 2021;152:364–8.
6. Brown PM, Fox K, Field EA, Randall C. UK Dental Medicines Advisory Service: questions asked by dentists—part 4: prescribing of high-strength fluoride toothpastes and use of fluoride varnishes in dental practice. Br Dent J. 2021;231:623–8.
7. Marinho VCC, Chong LY, Worthington HV, Walsh T. Fluoride mouthrinses for preventing dental caries in children and adolescents. Cochrane Database Syst Rev. 2016;7(7):CD002284. https://doi.org/10.1002/14651858.CD002284.pub2.
8. Satish S, Rudraswamy S, Hommerhalli JSP, Doggalli N, Sunitha S, Srinivas S. An exploratory insight into public's perception and preference of mouthwash during COVID-19 pandemic. Univ J Public Health. 2022;10:569–75.
9. Department of Health & Social Care, NHS England, NHS Improvement, Office for Health Improvement and Disparities. Delivering better oral health: an evidence-based toolkit for prevention. Chapter 8: Oral hygiene. 2021. https://www.gov.uk/government/publications/delivering-better-oral-health-an-evidence-based-toolkit-for-prevention/chapter-8-oral-hygiene. Accessed Mar 2024.
10. Liang P, Ye S, McComas M, Kwon T, Wang C-W. Evidence-based strategies for interdental cleaning: a practical decision tree and review of the literature. Quintessence Int. 2021;52:84–95.
11. Rashid M, Ellis A, Deery C. A practical guide to caries prevention in children. Dent Update. 2020;47:849–53.
12. Schnabl D, Wiesmüller V, Hönlinger V, Wimmer S, Bruckmoser E, Kapferer-Seebacher I. Cleansing efficacy of an auto-cleaning electronic toothbrushing device: a randomized-controlled crossover pilot study. Clin Oral Investig. 2021;25:247–53.
13. Elkerbout TA, Slot DE, Rosema NAM, Van der Weijden GA. How effective is a powered toothbrush as compared to a manual toothbrush? A systematic review and meta-analysis of single brushing exercises. Int J Dent Hyg. 2020;18:17–26.

14. Turssi CP, Binsaleh F, Lippert F, et al. Interplay between toothbrush stiffness and dentifrice abrasivity on the development of non-carious cervical lesions. Clin Oral Investig. 2019;23:3551–6.
15. Saghiri MA, Amanabi M, Vakhnovetsky J, Amini SB, Samadi E. Effects of brushing duration on the efficacy of dental plaque removal: an in vitro study. Int J Dent Hyg. 2023;21:618–23.
16. Department of Health & Social Care, NHS England, NHS Improvement, Office for Health Improvement and Disparities. Delivering better oral health: an evidence-based toolkit for prevention. Chapter 10: Healthier eating. 2021. https://www.gov.uk/government/publications/delivering-better-oral-health-an-evidence-based-toolkit-for-prevention/chapter-10-healthier-eating. Accessed Mar 2024.
17. Office for Health Improvement and Disparities. The Eatwell Guide. Updated January 2024. https://www.gov.uk/government/publications/the-eatwell-guide. Accessed Mar 2024.
18. Clarke L, Stevens C. Preventing dental caries in children: why improving children's oral health is everybody's business. Paediatr Child Health. 2019;29:536–42.
19. Cui L, Li X, Tian Y, et al. Breastfeeding and early childhood caries: a meta-analysis of observational studies. Asia Pac J Clin Nutr. 2017;26:867–80.
20. Maura Adelina H, Geanina B, Oana-Maria R, et al. Breastfeeding and dental caries in children—a review. Rom J Oral Rehabil. 2020;12:175–80.
21. Department of Health & Social Care, NHS England, NHS Improvement, Office for Health Improvement and Disparities. Delivering better oral health: an evidence-based toolkit for prevention. Chapter 4: Dental caries. 2021. https://www.gov.uk/government/publications/delivering-better-oral-health-an-evidence-based-toolkit-for-prevention/chapter-4-dental-caries. Accessed Mar 2024.
22. Mummery TA, Popat R. Glass ionomer cement as a preventative fissure sealant for first permanent molars in high caries risk patients waiting general anaesthetic—a case series. BDJ Open. 2022;8(1):25. https://doi.org/10.1038/s41405-022-00119-3.
23. Splieth C, Kanzow P, Wiegand A, Schmoeckel J, Jablonski-Momeni A. How to intervene in the caries process: proximal caries in adolescents and adults—a systematic review and meta-analysis. Clin Oral Investig. 2020;24:1623–36.
24. Chabadel O, Véronneau J, Montal S, Tramini P, Moulis E. Effectiveness of pit and fissure sealants on primary molars: a 2-yr split-mouth randomized clinical trial. Eur J Oral Sci. 2021;129(1):e12758. https://doi.org/10.1111/eos.12758.
25. Cvikl B, Moritz A, Bekes K. Pit and fissure sealants—a comprehensive review. Dent J (Basel). 2018;6(2):18. https://doi.org/10.3390/dj6020018.
26. Naaman R, El-Housseiny AA, Alamoudi N. The use of pit and fissure sealants—a literature review. Dent J (Basel). 2017;5(4):34. https://doi.org/10.3390/dj5040034.
27. Mattar RE, Sulimany AM, Binsaleh SS, Hamdan HM, Al-Majed IM. Evaluation of fissure sealant retention rates using isolite in comparison with rubber dam and cotton roll isolation techniques: a randomized clinical trial. Int J Paediatr Dent. 2023;33:12–9.
28. Wells MH. Pit and fissure sealants: scientific and clinical rationale. In: Nowak AJ, Christensen JR, Mabry TR, Townsend JA, Wells MH, editors. Pediatric dentistry. 6th ed. Philadelphia: Elsevier; 2019. p. 461–81.
29. Department of Health & Social Care, NHS England, NHS Improvement, Office for Health Improvement and Disparities. Delivering better oral health: an evidence-based toolkit for prevention. Chapter 3: Behaviour change. 2021. https://www.gov.uk/government/publications/delivering-better-oral-health-an-evidence-based-toolkit-for-prevention/chapter-3-behaviour-change. Accessed Mar 2024.
30. Michie S, van Stralen MM, West R. The behaviour change wheel: a new method for characterising and designing behaviour change interventions. Implement Sci. 2011;6:42. https://doi.org/10.1186/1748-5908-6-42.
31. Department of Health & Social Care, NHS England, NHS Improvement, Office for Health Improvement and Disparities. Delivering better oral health: an evidence-based toolkit for prevention. 2021. https://www.gov.uk/government/publications/delivering-better-oral-health-an-evidence-based-toolkit-for-prevention. Accessed Mar 2024.

32. Muraleedhar Seetha S, Thomas V, Sivaram R, Sreedharan S, Nayar BR. Caries Risk Assessment and Referral Tool (CRA-RT)—a novel risk scoring system for early childhood caries in community settings. Community Dent Oral Epidemiol. 2020;48:379–86.
33. Mejàre I, Axelsson S, Dahlén G, et al. Caries risk assessment. A systematic review. Acta Odontol Scand. 2014;72:81–91.
34. Horner K, Eaton KA. Selection criteria for dental radiography. FGDP(UK). 2018. https://cgdent.uk/selection-criteria-for-dental-radiography/. Accessed Mar 2024.
35. NICE. Dental recall: recall interval between routine dental examinations. 2004. https://www.nice.org.uk/guidance/cg19/resources/dental-recall-recall-interval-between-routine-dental-examinations-pdf-250576826821. Accessed Mar 2024.
36. British Society of Paediatric Dentistry. Dental check by one. https://www.bspd.co.uk/Patients/Dental-Check-by-One. Accessed Mar 2024.

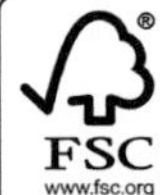

MIX
Papier aus verantwortungsvollen Quellen
Paper from responsible sources
FSC® C105338

If you have any concerns about our products,
you can contact us on
ProductSafety@springernature.com

In case Publisher is established outside the EU,
the EU authorized representative is:
Springer Nature Customer Service Center GmbH
Europaplatz 3, 69115 Heidelberg, Germany

Printed by Libri Plureos GmbH
in Hamburg, Germany